WITHDRAWN

Laura Katz Olson, PhD
Editor

The Graying of the World: Who Will Care for the Frail Elderly?

Pre-publication
REVIEWS,
COMMENTARIES,
EVALUATIONS . . .

"**T**he increase in the percentage of older persons in the United States population is now a rather well-known fact. Many Americans do not realize, however, that the increase in the percentage of the elderly is a worldwide phenomenon. Thus, there is much to be learned from an examination of public policy for the care of the aged in different countries.

LAURA OLSON'S *THE GRAYING OF THE WORLD: WHO WILL CARE FOR THE FRAIL ELDERLY?* REPRESENTS A UNIQUE AND VERY VALUABLE CONTRIBUTION TO THE LITERATURE. Although there have been some previous comparative studies of aging policy in various

countries in the literature, the Olson volume breaks new ground in its extensiveness and scope. Policies for care of the aging in eleven different countries on three different continents are presented and analyzed by experts who offer their own unique perspectives of the critical issues facing aging persons and policy makers in each country. The editor's introductory chapter is an excellent analysis of the major themes presented in the volume: social welfare policy, medical and social services, long-term care–both institutional and community based–and family caregiving.

This book will be a valuable resource for policy makers, gerontologists, and students."

David E. Biegel, PhD
*Henry L. Zucker Professor
of Social Work Practice,
Mandel School of Applied
Social Sciences,
Case Western Reserve University*

" *The Graying of the World* is well worth reading. Unlike many cross-national anthologies that deal with policies toward aging, it is far more than a collection of program descriptions. The editor, Laura Katz Olson, has established an effective team of scholars to help her probe the ideological, political, economic, and institutional dimensions of how different political systems–those of the United States, Sweden, Finland, Israel, Great Britain, Canada, France, Germany, Japan, China, and pre-war Yugoslavia–have dealt with the challenges of caring for increasing numbers of frail elderly persons. ANYONE INTERESTED IN LONG-TERM CARE POLICIES AND PROGRAMS WILL FIND THIS VOLUME TO BE A VALUABLE RESOURCE."

Robert H. Binstock, PhD
*Henry R. Luce Professor of Aging,
Health, and Society,
Case Western Reserve University*

The Haworth Press, Inc.

The Graying of the World
Who Will Care for the Frail Elderly?

THE HAWORTH PRESS
Aging and Gerontology

New, Recent, and Forthcoming Titles:

Long Term Care Administration: The Management of Institutional and Non-Institutional Components of the Continuum of Care by Ben Abramovice

Psychiatry in the Nursing Home: Assessment, Evaluation, and Intervention by D. Peter Birkett

Women and Aging: Celebrating Ourselves by Ruth Raymond Thone

Victims of Dementia: Services, Support, and Care by Wm. Michael Clemmer

Dietetic Service Operation Handbook: Practical Applications in Geriatric Care by Karen S. Thatcher Kolasa

A Guide to Psychological Practice in Geriatric Long-Term Care by Peter A. Lichtenberg

The Graying of the World: Who Will Care for the Frail Elderly? edited by Laura Katz Olson

The Graying of the World
Who Will Care for the Frail Elderly?

Laura Katz Olson, PhD
Editor

The Haworth Press
New York • London • Norwood (Australia)

The Haworth Press, Inc., 10 Alice Street, Binghamton, NY 13904-1580

Library of Congress Cataloging-in-Publication Data

The Graying of the world : who will care for the frail elderly? / Laura Katz Olson, editor.
     p.   cm.
    Includes bibliographical references and index.
    ISBN 1-56024-364-3 (acid-free paper).
    1. Frail elderly–Care–Government policy. 2. Old age assistance. 3. Frail elderly–Long–term care. 4. Privatization. I. Olson, Laura Katz, 1945- .
HV1451.G725   1993
362.6′1–dc20

                                                92-1661
                                               CIP

For my grandmothers,
Lily Samnik Katz
and
Annie Goldsmith Zager

CONTENTS

ABOUT THE EDITOR

Laura Katz Olson, PhD, Professor of Government at Lehigh University in Bethlehem, Pennsylvania, specializes in aging and public policy. She is the author of *The Political Economy of Aging: The State, Private Power, and Social Welfare* and co-editor of *Aging and Public Policy: The Politics of Growing Old in America.* She has published widely in the field of aging on topics such as private pension funds, the Social Security System, problems of older women, and long-term care. She has also been active in community organizations on behalf of the elderly. Dr. Olson has worked as a policy analyst for the Social Security Administration and has been a Gerontological Fellow and Fulbright Scholar.

Contributors

Michel Frossard is a professor of Economics, professor of Health Economics and Planning, and director of the Centre Pluridisciplinaire de Gèrontologie in Grenoble, France. He also is a consultant to local authorities in planning for the elderly. Professor Frossard has published widely on economic issues related to older people in France. His main research areas are health, preretirement, cost comparisons between home care and residential facilities, and planning.

Anne-Marie Guillemard is a professor at University Panthèon Sorbonne and a Research Fellow at the Center for the Study of Social Movements, in Paris. She received her doctorate in Sociology at the Sorbonne in 1971. Dr. Guillemard is the author of several books on aging, including *Old Age and the Welfare State, Le dèclin du social,* and *Time for Retirement.* She also has written numerous book chapters and articles on social policy and aging in France and from an international perspective.

David Guttmann is the Dean of the School of Social Work at the University of Haifa in Israel. He received his MSW at the University of Maryland, and his doctorate at the Catholic School University of America in Washington, D.C., where he served as Assistant Dean for Academic Affairs and Director of the Center for the Study of Aging. Dr. Guttmann is the author of *European American Elderly, Jewish Elderly in the English Speaking Countries,* and coeditor of *European American Elderly: A Guide for Practice.* In addition, he has written many chapters on aging, and has conducted workshops and seminars on the topic in South America, South Africa, and Hungary. Guttmann's main research interests include delivery of services to the elderly, aging and ethnicity, social work education, and logotherapeutic intervention.

Riitta-Liisa Heikkinen is a researcher in the Department of Health Sciences and the Gerontology Research Center at the University of

Jyväskylä, Finland. She received her doctorate in the Faculty of Educational Sciences from Tampere University, Finland in 1988 and docent in Nursing Science from Tampere University (Faculty of Medicine) in 1990. Dr. Heikkinen has been involved in numerous research projects in the field of gerontology, including a comparative study on health care of the elderly in eleven nations, and a study of functional capacity and health among individuals seventy-five years old in the Nordic countries. Heikkinen also has published numerous articles and book chapters on medical and social issues pertaining to the elderly.

Marianne Heinemann-Knoch is director and founder of a nonprofit organization, the Institute of Gerontology, in Munich, Germany. She received her doctorate in economics and social sciences at the University of Augsburg, Germany in 1976. Dr. Heinemann-Knoch has engaged in research and taught at the universities of Stuttgart, Munich, and Augsburg. Her research and written work are in the areas of social policies for the aged, care of the frail elderly, and the problems faced by caregivers.

Ariela Lowenstein is the coordinator of the Center for Research and Study of Aging at the University of Haifa in Israel. She also is chairperson of the Israeli Gerontological Society and serves on the executive board of the Social Sciences Section of the European Society of Gerontology. She received her doctorate at the Hebrew University of Jerusalem, Israel. Dr. Lowenstein has authored and coauthored numerous monographs, book chapters, and articles dealing with social aspects of aging, the family and caregiving, widowhood, rehabilitation, and the development and evaluation of services for the elderly. She is active in service developments for the elderly in Israel, cooperating with the Brookdale Institute and the Association for Planning and Development of Services for the Elderly.

Sheila Marjorie Neysmith is an associate professor in Social Work at the University of Toronto in Canada. She received her doctorate in Social Welfare from Columbia University in 1976. She has been awarded several research grants to study the frail elderly, and the roles of the community and family in their care. Dr. Neysmith is the author of numerous book chapters and journal articles focusing on aging in Canada and elsewhere. The most recent include: "Canadian

Social Services and Social Work Practice in the Field of Aging" (1988); "Closing the Gap between Health Policy and the Service Needs of Tomorrow's Elderly" (1989); and "Developing Dependency Among Third World Elderly: A Need for New Directions in the Nineties" (1990). She is currently working on a book entitled *Social Policies for an Aging Population.*

Harry Kaneharu Nishio is a professor in the Department of Sociology at the University of Toronto in Canada. He received his doctorate in sociology from the University of California, Berkeley, in 1966. He is coauthor of *Quantitative Japanese Economic History.* Dr. Nishio also is the author of several articles and book chapters, including several in Japanese, on aging and Japan. He is currently doing research at KIBI International University in Okayama, Japan.

Laura Katz Olson is a professor in the Department of Government at Lehigh University in Bethlehem, Pennsylvania. She received her doctorate at the University of Colorado, Boulder, in 1974. She is author of *The Political Economy of Aging: The State, Private Power, and Social Welfare* and coeditor of *Aging and Public Policy: The Politics of Growing Old in America.* She has been a Fulbright Scholar, Gerontological Fellow, and a NASPAA Fellow at the Social Security Administration in Baltimore. Dr. Olson has published widely in the field of aging and has been active in community organizations on behalf of the elderly.

Philip G. Olson is director of the Center on Rural Elderly at the University of Missouri in Kansas City, Missouri. He received his doctorate in Sociology from Purdue University in 1959, and engaged in postdoctoral studies in Sociology at the University of Chicago from 1978 to 1979. In addition to receiving a number of research and training grants to aging, Dr. Olson has authored many journal articles and book chapters, including several in Chinese, on the situation of the elderly in the People's Republic of China. His research interest focuses on the rural elderly population. Dr. Olson currently is coediting a book entitled *Social Support for the Elderly in the Third World.* He has also worked with the Chinese to develop professional sociology at universities in the People's Republic of China.

James H. Seroka is head of the Division of Humanities and Social Science and professor of Political Science at Penn State University at Erie, the Behrend College. He received his doctorate in political science at Michigan State University in 1976. He is coauthor of *Political Organizations in Socialist Yugoslavia,* editor of *Rural Public Administration,* and coeditor of *Developed Socialism in the Soviet Bloc* and *Contemporary Political Systems: Classifications and Typologies.* Dr. Seroka also has written nearly fifty journal articles and book chapters on East European politics, and comparative policy making and public management.

Gerdt Sundström is a senior researcher at the Institute of Gerontology in Jönköping, Sweden. He holds a doctorate in social work from the University of Stockholm, where he previously worked as a university lecturer. Dr. Sundström has published extensively in the field of gerontology. He also has lectured in Sweden and abroad on old age care, family sociology, and related fields.

Mats Thorslund is senior researcher and associate professor with the Swedish Medical Research Council's Health Services Research and a consultant on care of the elderly to the Ministry of Social Affairs. Based in Uppsala, Sweden, his work for the last ten years has aimed at understanding the effects of policy changes on the elderly care system, on families, and on elderly persons themselves. He also is a former chair of the Swedish Association of Medical Sociology. Dr. Thorslund is the author of numerous articles dealing with home-based care for the elderly in Sweden.

Alan Walker is a professor of Social Policy and chairperson of the Department of Sociological Studies at the University of Sheffield in Great Britain. He has been researching and writing in the field of social gerontology for nearly twenty years. He is most closely associated with the development of the social construction and political economy of aging perspectives. He has authored or coauthored nine books in the fields of social gerontology and social policy, including *Social Planning* (1984), *Aging and Social Policy* (1986), and *The Caring Relationship: Elderly People and Their Families* (1989). He has published numerous journal articles and contributions to edited volumes on the subject of aging.

Lorna Warren is a Research Fellow in the Department of Sociological Studies at the University of Sheffield in Great Britain. Dr. Warren is working with Alan Walker on a major research project evaluating the Neighbourhood Support Units initiative in Sheffield and their role in the care of older people living at home. She has recently contributed to *New Perspectives in the Sociology of Health* (1990) and has also published on the subject of doing fieldwork *(Feminist Praxis,* No. 31).

Chapter 1

Introduction

Laura Katz Olson

This book was conceived several years ago following yet another of my diatribes on the scandalous conditions within American nursing homes. I had been arguing for years, both in my written work and lectures, that the American political economy is inherently incapable of providing for the real needs of the elderly, especially those who are frail. Moreover, after several decades of forcing most families to choose between self-care and deplorable, profiteering institutional facilities, U.S. public policy now has begun to compel even greater family responsibility. Such care-giving demands are, of course, placed on women who are already struggling to perform multiple roles both in the labor force and at home. At the same time, the U.S. is experiencing a rapid growth of frail older people, rendering the nation's ability to solve intractable long-term care questions even more problematic.

The proliferation of older people is not unique to American society. Such demographic changes are occurring throughout the world, especially within industrialized nations. In fact, compared to the U.S., many countries currently have or expect to experience in the next several decades an even greater percentage of their population aged seventy-five and over. In addition, based on longevity, the U.S. ranks only seventeenth among the thirty-three most industrialized states.

Not only is population aging universal, but it also is unprecedented historically. Our generation is the first ever to confront such large numbers of very old people in the population. Prolonged life spans into the extreme age groups generate large numbers of frail individuals, many of whom experience debilitating illnesses, and/or periods of invalidism. However, the degree of incapacitation, vulnerability, and powerlessness rendered by the chronic conditions of old age is largely dependent on the social context in which the elderly function. Therefore, the extent of dependency is inseparably linked to such factors as economic, psychological, social, and political structures and supports.

Rather than critique American policy anew, I decided to investigate how nations with dissimilar political economies are attending to the rising needs of their frail and disabled elderly. Surprisingly, there have been few such intercountry comparisons.

Among the multiple goals of this text was to find innovative strategies and model programs for elder care. For example, I sought to reveal which social arrangements, and the policies they engender, best allow chronically impaired older people to age with dignity. I also attempted to assess which nations, if any, are providing quality programs and services for the dependent elderly and their caregivers without shortchanging other needy groups or bankrupting their overall economy. What I found through the essays in this volume is that every country, regardless of its political economy, is struggling with varying political, social, economic, and psychological issues associated with caring for growing frail populations.

SOCIAL WELFARE POLICY

Not surprisingly, one of the primary differences among the nations is where the locus of responsibility for care resides. Thus, although in the 1990s all of the countries in this volume have become seriously concerned with the rising costs of supportive services for the elderly, they diverge on the question of who should (or will) bear the costs. They also vary on the issue of who, if anyone, will profit from service provision.

I argue in Chapter 2 that the American cultural emphasis on individualism and self-reliance, which lies on one end of the spectrum, fosters privately provided support, whether by the family or paid caregivers. Public spending to heal social ills, including elder care, tends to be severely constrained. Moreover, state-supported programs often become stigmatized due to such factors as restrictive income eligibility tests.

Concomitantly, the privatization of human services brings the profit motive to the forefront. Thus, access to services in the U.S. is often based on the ability to pay, resulting in large imbalances between need and the availabiltiy of service. Where the public sector funds proprietary care, accountability and the quality of services may be negatively affected as well. This is exemplified by the American nursing home industry, a multi-billion dollar, privately administered business with escalating public costs.

Societies with more collectivist approaches assume that frailty among the aged is a social problem engendering social solutions. For example, Sundström and Thorslund (Chapter 3), Heikkinen (Chapter 4), Guttmann and Lowenstein (Chapter 5), and Frossard and Guillemard (Chapter 8) note that in Sweden, Finland, Israel, and France, respectively, the public sector is responsible for its dependent older population. The individual and/or the family is not expected to shoulder the entire burden of care. In addition, although medical and social welfare services are available to all sectors of society in these countries, the elderly tend to be one of the more important target groups.

Health care and social services in Sweden, Finland, Israel, and France are presumed to be "rights." The dominant view is that the aged are entitled to receive all types of care; such aid is not a privilege for those who can afford to pay for it. Public services receive widespread support among citizens and political leaders. Consequently, social programs tend to comprise quality services that are provided with dignity.

In Britain and Canada, despite collectivist social security norms and an entitlement approach to health care, the state plays a relatively minor role in the direct provision of long-term care. For these services, the national governments rely on a residualist social welfare model. The family is the preferred caregiver; programs are developed only to fill gaps when kin are not available.

Walker and Warren (Chapter 6) indicate that until recently the public sector in Britain dominated for-profit and nonprofit organizations in the delivery of formal services. Since 1979, and the emergence of the Thatcher and Major governments, the for-profit sector has grown at the expense of publicly supported care. According to these authors, the promotion of greater privatization has ensued and further engenders challenges to basic values underlying the British welfare state.

Canada's approach to social welfare and the frail elderly parallels that of Britain, though Neysmith (Chapter 7) reminds us that Canada does not provide the mix of protective housing options that are available in Britain or the Scandinavian countries. The Canadian system fosters a mixed market approach, with the public and non-profit sectors providing a minimum level of services. Neysmith is concerned, however, since the for-profit sector has been playing an increasingly larger role in long-term care over the last decade.

Similarly, Heinemann-Knoch (Chapter 9) maintains that the German social welfare system utilizes the "subsidiary principle": the public sector intervenes only when individuals and their families are incapable of providing for themselves. Although the entire German population is now covered under health insurance, there is no similar provision for long-term care. In fact, the voluntary sector is primarily responsible for the organization and delivery of formal services, with the economically needy subsidized by the state.

Nishio (Chapter 10) proposes that Japanese-style welfarism eschews both self-reliance and individual dependence on privately contracted services. Although the nation acknowledges social obligations to older people, based on Japanese communal values, it places primary responsibility for their care on the family institution. Recent efforts to initiate publicly supported assistance entail a unique blend between the state and the private economic sector.

According to Olson (Chapter 11), frail older people in the People's Republic of China are a low priority in the allocation of public resources, despite the nation's communist-dominated political economy, strong communal ethos, and the alleged importance of the elderly in the development of society. State social welfare policies for the chronically ill aged tend to reinforce the role of the family, even in rural communes.

Seroka (Chapter 12) argues that the welfare statism model that existed in former Yugoslavia, in which the public sector assumes responsibility for economic and social needs, severely restricted the role of the individual, family, market, and other nongovernmental institutions in providing for the elderly. At the same time, while pensions and medical care were considered to be "rights," supportive services were not viewed similarly. Local interests, which solicited funds from work units in each republic, hold primary responsibility for social welfare programs. Since there was no lobbying for special populations such as the elderly, and the latter's needs were a low priority, there were few programs for frail older people. Moreover, due to severe national economic problems, by the end of the 1980s the social welfare system collapsed.

MEDICAL TREATMENT, SUPPORTIVE SERVICES, AND THE SOCIAL CONTEXT OF CARE

Objectives for long-term care services vary considerably among nations. They range from rehabilitation and the maintenance of a quality life, including independent living, to merely "warehousing" physically and mentally deteriorating populations. Aid can also focus on the caregiver, the care recipient, or both. Where the entire family is of primary concern, respite services and day care are more common. Successful long-term care also entails a continuum of interrelated health and social services as well as a supportive environment. Rehabilitation or the ability to cope with disabling physical and/or mental conditions often depends on social conditions and support systems.

Social welfare policy in Finland, Sweden, and more recently in Israel appear to reflect the importance of these interconnections more than in other nations. For example, in the Scandinavian countries, pensions, housing allowances, and upgraded housing conditions are viewed as essential components of elder care. In addition, both medical and social services are highly subsidized by the state and utilized by a significant percentage of frail older people. On the other hand, even in these nations health and support benefits are funded and administered separately.

Programs for the elderly in Finland apparently have had a medical focus, especially within old age homes. Heikkinen writes that the country intends to emphasize an intensifying cooperation and coordination between health care and social services at the national and local levels in its future development of old age policy. Coordination of social welfare and health care on behalf of the frail elderly has been a problem in Israel as well. Guttmann and Lowenstein maintain that one of the goals of the recently enacted Long-Term Care Insurance Law is to integrate medical and social services.

Despite the relatively comprehensive social welfare and health programs in France, jurisdictional separation of health and community services has curtailed the effectiveness of the nation's old age policies. Frossard and Guillemard argue that, among other problems, such dualism has contributed to the fragmentation of elder care, the diversion of community-based resources to the more able-bodied aged, and a medical focus, especially within institutions, for problems that include both social and health factors. They point out, however, that current reforms seek to enhance the coordination of the various types of programs, including housing.

According to Nishio, Japan also is attempting to develop additional and improved linkages between medical treatment in hospitals and clinics and supportive services, including preventive health measures, for its elderly population.

Many nations, including the United States, Canada, Britain, Germany, and the People's Republic of China, focus primarily on medical treatment for those individuals experiencing a diminishing capacity for self-care. Moreover, the evidence suggests that there is a relatively rigid separation in some countries between social services and health care. Heinemann-Knoch points out that this separation of health care and caregiving in Germany, for example, has generated greater dependency among frail older people than their conditions would warrant.

Public funding for the elderly in the United States is mostly provided for the medical aspects of long-term care needs, and even these are both narrowly defined and severely constricted. While Canada has extensive health services, Neysmith warns that the nation is subsidizing and supporting a medical model of social welfare. She contends that the state must redirect policy away from its exclusive focus on medical treatment if the needs of frail older people and their families are to be met.

In Britain, as shown by Walker and Warren, the costly National Health Service is state run and state funded; the more modest social services are a local responsibility financed through a mix of national and local sources.

Olson determines that greater priority is placed on medical care than on social services in the People's Republic of China, as well. In urban areas, though workers are provided with health insurance, long-term care services are not covered at all. In rural areas, where health facilities have been designed to supplement family care, few state-supported social services are available.

Seroka concludes that both medical and social services were inadequate in formr Yugoslavia, especially within rural areas; supportive services for the frail, preventive health programs, home care, and even hospitals and doctors were scarce in some areas.

REGIONAL AND LOCAL SERVICE IMBALANCES

In many nations there are strong regional variations and imbalances both in the need for elder care and available services. In assessing the network of social service stations throughout Germany, Heinemann-Knoch discovers considerable differences in types of assistance, personnel requirements, and funding levels. Frossard and Guillemard also point to major differences among the French departments in who receives service, the amount of aid available, and how such costs are distributed. Significantly, Neysmith finds that, in Canada, those provinces which provide the least community services have the highest incidence of institutionalization.

Walker and Warren mention the wide divergence among local authorities in levels of service provision in Britain, as well. Such differences are especially prevalent between rural and urban areas. In Japan, there is a high proportion of rural older people without adequate support, but Nishio warns that the cities will soon confront similar problems. Similarly, calling attention to an "urban bias" in China, Olson demonstrates that few state programs or policies are directed at the rural elderly. He implies that there is a similar bias under state socialism in Eastern Europe.

Indeed, Seroka confirms that there were serious inequities in services and protection for the elderly among the six republics and two provinces in former Yugoslavia. Not only do rural localities have a greater percentage of older people to support, but they also tend to be the most economically depressed. Since the early 1980s and accelerating during the 1990s, such problems have become even more pronounced as a result of economic and political crises.

Sundström also finds evidence of large regional variations in the provision of services in Sweden. In contrast to other nations, however, he determines that rural and poor areas actually receive more aid than less needy parts of the country. He hypothesizes that this is because of such factors as Sweden's homogeneity, redistributive policies, and national consensus on old age care.

INSTITUTIONAL CARE

Many of the countries in this volume have similar percentages of their frail population residing in institutional facilities. However, as noted in 1976 by Robert and Rosalie Kane in *Long Term Care in Six Countries: Implications for the United States,* no other nation has nursing homes similar to those in the U.S.; neglect or abuse does not appear to be a significant issue elsewhere. There have been efforts to improve institutional conditions in the U.S. through new rules and guidelines. However, given the current private market context of the nation's nursing home enterprise, most of these have been neither enforceable nor effective.

Although they vary both in type and quality of care, nearly all of the institutional facilities in other nations provide more normal, homelike environments than in the U.S. Where nursing home placement is inevitable, many nations are attempting to develop residences with even more humane environments.

In Finland, over 90 percent of old people's homes are communal-owned, with the remainder run under the jurisdiction of nonprofit organizations. Heikkinen mentions that the state is attempting to simultaneously place a ceiling on the number of full-time institutionalized elderly (the rate has remained relatively stable at 5 percent since the 1960s), provide for more part-time and short-term treatment opportunities, upgrade its facilities, provide greater freedom to its residents, integrate better with surrounding communities, and deliver more rehabilitative services. She points out that the nation imposes high standards for training personnel, though salary levels are comparatively low.

In Sweden, where nearly all institutional facilities also are publicly owned and operated, similar efforts are underway. According to Sundström and Thorslund, these include attempts to make them more homelike, encourage rehabilitation, and provide for part-time residency and respite care. Despite limitations placed on the building of new facilities, 5 to 6 percent of the elderly are institutionalized and nearly a third, mostly those in advanced ages and with weak family ties, eventually reside in an old-age home.

Although Israel has a relatively low rate of institutionalization, the large influx of immigrants over the last several decades has generated long waiting lists, and consequently a steady expansion in the number of available places. During the 1980s, the number of old-age homes grew by 30 percent, with increased involvement by the proprietary sector. However, the majority of institutions are either nonprofit (voluntary) or state facilities; only about a third are profit-making institutions. Moreover, funding for nursing home care is now often covered by insurance.

Despite relatively large public costs, institutional facilities have played a small role in the British long-term care system. Since 1979, however, Social Security subsidies to the private sector have fostered the rapid growth of private nursing and residential homes and a decline in the once predominant public-sector local authority homes. Walker and Warren claim that there is mounting evidence that such changes have engendered growing abuse, misuse of drugs, fraud, lack of proper hygiene, fire hazards and other problems similar to those experienced in the American nursing home industry. There is also increasing premature and/or unnecessary institutionalization.

Current funding patterns in Canada favor institutional care, especially for those frail elderly without family to care for them. Neysmith indicates that the nation has a relatively large percentage of its population residing in these facilities which, depending on the province, are labelled alternatively nursing homes, homes for the aged, chronic care facilities, and even "meeting places." Approximately 7.5 percent of those individuals aged 65 and over, and nearly 36 percent of those aged eighty-five and over, are institutionalized. Neysmith also mentions that although some provinces such as Ontario rely heavily on proprietary services, given the nation's commitment to a public health care model such privatized facilities are an increasingly contentious issue politically.

Prior to 1961, institutions in Germany were mostly substandard and available primarily to economically needy individuals who did not have any family to care for them. Heinemann-Knoch contends that, although the number of nursing homes and residential homes has expanded and their quality has improved since that time, there are long and growing waiting lists, and poor conditions persist. The resident population is increasingly older and more frail, with the facilities serving mostly a custodial function. Moreover, because of high costs relative to pension income, about two-thirds of the inhabitants are dependent on relatives or social assistance.

In France, although public policy has not traditionally favored nursing homes, hospital-type long-term care facilities were set up during the 1970s in order to remove older people from acute-care hospitals. The Health Funds provide a fixed sum for each resident; the remaining costs are paid by the patient, the family, or welfare. According to Frossard and Guillemard, these facilities are overly large, poorly designed, and generally do not offer a quality life. Although recently some older people have been placed in small-scale facilities with collective services, there are few such innovations.

Japan currently has one of the lowest percentages of institutionalized older people; less than 2 percent of the population aged 65 and over lives in homes for the aged. However, Nishio discloses that the country has been forced to expand the number of beds in special nursing homes and Senior Health Centers in order to accommodate the rapidly growing need for institutional care, especially among those experiencing mental disorders.

Few of the aged in the People's Republic of China and former Yugoslavia are institutionalized, as well. According to Olson, in China such facilities are available mainly to the childless and ambulatory population. Although a massive campaign to build old age homes at the end of the 1950s failed, there is renewed interest in their construction since the early 1980s. Seroka notes that nursing homes in former Yugoslavia were limited to major urban areas, where there were long waiting lists. In some republics the only available institutional care was within an overcrowded hospital system.

The steady increase in the number and percentage of mentally impaired older people tends to be a world-wide issue. The percentages of the older population with some form of dementia currently range from about 5 to 7 percent; in most industrialized nations nearly a quarter of those individuals aged 75 and over are impaired. Yet the response to the needs of people with dementia and their caregivers ranges enormously among nations.

For example, in Britain, despite a rise in the need for care, mental hospitals have been closed since the late 1970s, thrusting mentally disabled individuals into the community, where services have declined. In Finland, on the other hand, each of the nation's twenty-one hospital districts has its own separate mental hospital. The communes also are experimenting with alternative means for treating such patients in the community.

HOME AND COMMUNITY-BASED SERVICES

Countries differ considerably, especially in the last two decades, in their commitment to in-home and community services for the frail elderly. In the U.S., recent efforts to maintain older people at home have been motivated primarily by financial considerations, and have been accompanied by fewer public sector dollars. In many other nations, monetary inducements similarly have motivated a strong interest in noninstitutional forms of care. However, in some countries there is also a growing determination to avoid premature or unnecessary institutionalization; institutional care increasingly is viewed as the alternative rather than the primary means for care.

Both Swedish and Finnish health and social welfare services originally had been geared toward institutional care. Sundström and Thorslund and Heikkinen advise that the priority placed on community and home services in their respective nations over the last several decades is due to both economic and humanitarian factors. Significantly, frail older people in need of services are eligible for them regardless of whether or not they have relatives capable of caring for them. Approximately one-fifth of the aged in Sweden and

Finland receive some home assistance for which they pay only a fraction of the cost.

Sundström and Thorslund notes that in Sweden, agencies responsible for the elderly tend to agree that the majority of old age homes should be closed and replaced by more assistance in the home environment. Service apartments have partially replaced institutional facilities. In addition, communes in Finland are now required to supply older people with service homes which include a wide range of supportive services, meals, and the like.

In the 1960s, Israel shifted from a focus on institutional care to community-based services, as well; during the last decade these services, including day care, grew rapidly as did public and private sheltered housing and collective homes for independent older people. The basic goals of long-term care in Israel have been to foster independent living among the elderly and aid their caregivers while, at the same time, building sufficient old age homes for those in need. Currently, older people who meet certain eligibility requirements are entitled, without regard to income, to receive state-supported benefits either at home or in community facilities.

Similarly, since the early 1970s, French national policy has been directed toward home care of the frail elderly, both to meet the needs of older people who want to live independently and to control societal costs. As part of this Home-Maintenance Policy, new services and collective facilities were instituted throughout the nation. However, Frossard and Guillemard conclude that although such efforts have increased steadily over the last two decades, they have not been adequately targeted to those people most in need.

While community care also has been favored by successive postwar governments in Britain, in actuality these services have been subordinate to institutional interests, particularly in funding levels. Walker and Warren argue that the policies of the Thatcher era finally succeeded in promoting community care; however, the primary goals have been to control costs rather than to improve the quality of care.

Similar themes imbue Canadian long-term care policy. According to Neysmith, during the 1980s institutionalization lost favor to home care in public rhetoric. However, although community-based projects now have been established in all Canadian provinces, in actuality they have received low funding priority, and are evaluated primarily by their cost effectiveness and efficiency in delivering services. Moreover, recent efforts by political leaders to control social welfare costs overall suggest that there will be limited program growth to meet increasing needs over the next several decades.

In Germany, social service units, which developed during the 1970s, deliver in-home services for all needy individuals, regardless of age. Such assistance ranges from nursing care to neighborhood activities, and is funded through a combination of state and local subsidies, health insurance, social assistance, voluntary agencies, and client fees. However, Heinemann-Knoch concludes that, despite their extensive network and growth in actual services, these programs are not able to meet the needs of growing numbers of frail older people, especially those who are poor.

FAMILY CAREGIVERS: INCREASING BURDENS ON WOMEN

Although the barrier between the formal (public) and informal (individual/family) sectors of society is the most clearly defined and rigid in the U.S., it is slowly becoming more demarcated in some of the social welfare states: elder care is increasingly relegated to the discrete domestic domain. In fact, support for community care and greater demands placed on women may be inextricably linked.

Somewhat surprisingly, this volume indicates that many nations, encumbered by rising social welfare costs, are placing increasing obligations on family members, primarily women, for caregiving tasks. One of the most stark similarities among the nations is the gender-based concomitants of growing frail populations: each nation, though to a varying extent, has relied on and increasingly expects women to provide such services to their kin. Moreover, not only have more females added care of the superannuated to their productive and reproductive roles, but, in addition, these efforts tend to be both invisible and undervalued. However, as implied earlier, the actual concepts of dependency and caring tend to be perceived disparately in different societies.

Independent living, especially among the chronically ill, is high-

est in Sweden where decent public pensions, raised housing standards, and increases in home and community-based services have
increasingly allowed the elderly to cope on their own. Nevertheless,
we find that interdependence among the generations and the growth
of independent living can occur simultaneously. According to Sundström and Thorslund, family ties have strengthened in Sweden; in
many respects, the immediate family plays a more–not less–important role in the life of the aged than in the past. Moreover, adult
children often rely on their parents for aid in a number of ways,
including economic support and babysitting.

Despite the growth of supportive services, the family still plays
the dominant role in the actual care of chronically ill spouses and
parents; formal care is used more extensively and intensely by those
who lack available kin. Significantly, such "caring" in Sweden and
Finland, whether by kin, homemakers, or institutions, remains in
the women's domain.

Independent living also is extremely common in France where
over 90 percent of the 65 and over population reside in their own
home. In addition, 75 percent of dependent older people live in the
community; in many cases this is due to professional help alone.
However, despite the importance of the latter, most elder care is
provided by family members.

Likewise, in the U.S., Britain, Canada, and Germany, large and
increasing percentages of older people, mostly women, live alone.
Despite recent policies encouraging traditional family roles and
nonstate forms of care, most of the care in these countries already is
provided by wives and adult daughters; the limits to what women
can do appear to have been reached. In all of these nations, caregivers risk their own health as well as their emotional and financial
stability.

Although Israel has experienced some decline in multigenerational households, it has a lower proportion of older people who are
living alone than other industrialized nations. Guttmann and Lowenstein claim that such factors as the Jewish tradition of "honoring
one's parents," and a low divorce rate may partially account for this
phenomenon. On the other hand, the Jewish tradition of mutual aid
and collective responsibility has encouraged a vast network of state-
supported and voluntary sector services. Yet, the family still plays

the major role in caregiving. In fact, Israeli law directs that the availability of kin should be taken into account when assessing an older person's eligibility for services.

In Japan, over 60 percent of older people aged 65 and over, and nearly 80 percent of those aged 80 and over, live with their adult children; fewer than 10 percent live alone. Nishio points out that "dependency" by older people on the family is culturally sanctioned; familism, based on the Confucian concept of filial piety, promotes mutual support, cooperation, and obligation among the generations.

Similarly, Olson notes that in the People's Republic of China the tradition of reverence toward elders, along with the concept of family reciprocity, ensures elder care for the vast majority of older people. Aging parents receiving support contribute to the household through such tasks as child care, gardening, cooking, and the like. However, the evidence suggests that increasing numbers of elders are either living alone or would prefer to do so.

Even in Japan and China, where Confucianism mandates male filial responsibility for aging parents, it is the daughters-in-law who provide the actual care. Nishio finds that the increase in frail older people has placed growing obligations on daughters-in-law; most must quit, take a leave of absence, or change their jobs when they assume caregiving responsibilities. According to Olson, the paucity of social services and the decline in health services for the elderly in rural areas since the 1980s have placed greater responsibility on daughters-in-law in China as well. Although community and in-home services have increased rapidly in urban areas since the early 1980s, they are provided primarily to childless older people.

In former Yugoslavia, the extended family tradition had withered considerably; growing numbers of older people lived alone with very limited family support. Seroka writes that younger cohorts tended to leave agricultural areas and villages for urban centers, abandoning their elders. He contends that the acute housing crisis further limited the possibility of adult children caring for their frail parents. The reality is that most of the elderly relied on each other for support and assistance.

AN OVERVIEW OF CHAPTERS

In Chapter 2, I analyze long-term care policy in the United States. As suggested earlier, since the issues associated with old age and frailty are viewed as private problems, individuals and their families must provide for their own needs. Eligibility for publicly subsidized support, which mostly funds institutional care, is based on personal insolvency. This combination of a reliance on individual resources and a welfare approach to caregiving has generated a two-class system of elder care.

At the same time, the public sector is subsidizing an overly costly, profit-making nursing home industry that has failed dramatically to meet the basic health and safety requirements of frail older people; even less emphasis is placed on providing quality care. Faced with growing numbers of frail older people in need and spiral costs, political leaders are seeking alternatives to institutional care. However, their primary concern is to control expenditures rather than to offer effective, quality services. Moreover, the emphasis on in-home services has been accompanied by a systematic reduction in public resources for social welfare needs overall.

Increasing privatization, an emphasis on community care, and fewer public resources all signify increased expectations and burdens on women, particularly spouses and adult daughters. Yet, contemporary females in the U.S. are increasingly incapable of meeting these additional demands without sacrificing their own social, economic, and psychological well-being. In addition, employees in the long-term care industries, who primarily are women, tend to be overworked, underpaid, untrained, and lack opportunities for advancement. Among other problems, this has lead to poor quality care, personnel shortages, and high rates of turnover and absenteeism.

I conclude that the public sector in the U.S. has not provided the appropriate environment or supportive services for those suffering from chronic ailments, thus preventing many older people from meeting their maximum human potential. Further, public policy must more adequately address the social, economic, and health needs of the entire society, especially since the well-being of all generations is interlocked.

Sundström and Thorslund evaluate Swedish old age care in Chapter 3. They note that few other nations have such a high life expectancy (80.1 years for women and 74.1 years for men) or as great a percentage of older people in the population (18 percent). At the same time, Sweden provides probably one of the most extensive and costly social welfare systems, especially for the aged. Few of the frail elderly are isolated or face unmet needs for care; most are satisfied with the quality of the services, as well.

Decent pension systems, housing allowances, medical care, and heavily subsidized services foster reciprocity among the generations rather than dependency in old age. Sundström and Thorslund show that, while spouses and adult children provide substantial aid to their elders, the latter are increasingly more significant to their family.

The authors note that, despite support among all generations for elder care programs, political and economic trends indicate that the public provision of care will not expand to meet growing service needs in the future. They argue that the current focus on the oldest and frailest elderly without kin will increasingly burden relatives, especially women. Consequently, they call for greater effort to encourage and support families in their caring roles. Sundström and Thorslund also warn that one response to less public aid is the growth of privatization, which will be accompanied by growing inequities between the "haves" and the "have nots," as well as contribute to growing personnel shortages in the public sector.

Heikkinen examines the Finnish system of long-term care in Chapter 4. She notes that the nation has had a relatively high rate of institutionalization but now is attempting to promote more community living, even for the frail and mentally impaired population.

In Finland, services are publicly supported and delivered, with older people paying only a small percentage of the actual cost. They are also provided to those in need regardless of their family situation. Heikkinen notes that the communes are experimenting with improved service provision, including those aimed at rehabilitation and prevention. At the same time, income security is assured to most older Finnish people through the national pension scheme.

According to Heikkinen, national studies indicate that steady growth in social and health care services, and its associated costs, are both justifiable and feasible. However, the author argues that such assumptions may be overly optimistic: population aging, along with deteriorating economic conditions in the country, may prevent the continuation of expansive old-age policies. She also points out that there will be a shortage of labor in the service sector as women continue to move into higher paying occupations. She proposes that if the state intends to maintain the current high level and quality of institutional and community services it must increase wages, allow more flexible hours, and encourage the entry of male workers.

In Chapter 5, Guttmann and Lowenstein evaluate elder care in Israel. They point out that Israel is unique in a number of ways. For example, the constant influx of elderly immigrants, including those aged seventy-five and over, generates both unpredictable demographic changes and ever-increasing needs for new and innovative services. In fact, the majority of elderly are not native born and comprise about 100 different ethnic and cultural subgroups.

Guttmann and Lowenstein argue that Israel's 1986 Long-term Care Act, which is one of the most complex pieces of legislation enacted in the nation, is unprecedented among the social security legislation of the industrialized world. It not only has legalized older people's "right" to state-supported care, but also has fostered an extensive and creative network of social and health services throughout the country. Public, voluntary, and, more recently, proprietary agencies are all involved in these programs, services, and facilities.

Nevertheless, Guttmann and Lowenstein remind us that gaps remain between the need for and the provision of services. In addition, the authors warn that the recent trend toward privatization of hospitals, nursing homes, sheltered housing, and home care will enlarge the gap between the "haves" and the "have nots" among the aged.

In Chapter 6, Walker and Warren critique the British system of long-term care. They point to the growing percentage of older people, particularly at advanced ages, and the commensurate increase in need for care within this group. Yet, since 1979, the state has pursued a policy of residualism. In pressing for cost reductions in social welfare, British political leaders have fostered a reduced public sector role, increased marketization of services, a decline in mental health facilities, and a massive increase in private institutional care.

The authors assert that along with the ideology of "familism," these social policies are dramatically increasing family burdens, especially for wives and adult daughters. They also argue that state funding priorities, rather than suitability, are the driving force in the types of care available, especially for the mentally impaired.

Despite the language embodied in the newly enacted Community Care Act of 1990 suggesting greater responsiveness to frail older people and their families, Walker and Warren allege that the overriding concerns continue to be cost containment and enhanced marketization of services; the evidence suggests that, in reality, the needs of caregivers will not be taken into account.

Walker and Warren provide evidence that there are a number of innovative and successful small scale local initiatives focusing on such issues as rehabilitation and support for caregivers. However, these tend to be only short-term demonstration projects that have not fundamentally altered the provision of care in Britain.

Neysmith critiques the Canadian approach to long-term care in Chapter 7, and alleges that the current cost crisis milieu is socially constructed. She maintains that the nation has the necessary human and material resources to plan for its elderly. The high and growing expenditures of public dollars on health care are not caused by demographic pressures but rather by the state's emphasis on traditional, costly medical services. Canada must redirect real health dollars to community-based care services if the country is to keep pace with the needs of an aging population.

Neysmith presumes that the frail elderly ought to have a basic right to long-term care. She also points out that the Canadian familial model of care burdens wives and daughters disproportionately and argues for more programs aimed at supporting and supplementing the family. Moreover, she warns against the continued growth of for-profit services, noting that such privatization exacerbates the inequitable distribution of elder care.

Neysmith concludes that universal access to publicly supported and delivered services is a necessary beginning for long-term care policy. However, in order to ensure equitable and quality services to the frail elderly and their families, Canada must reduce the economic and gender inequalities inherent in society.

France is the focus of Chapter 8. Frossard and Guillemard note that due to lower fertility rates and longer life expectancies, France has experienced population aging earlier and more extensively than nearly any other nation. At the same time, with the exception of Scandinavia, the country has one of the more comprehensive social welfare systems in Europe, including services, benefits, and pensions for older people.

Frossard and Guillemard argue that it is not a rational system: elder care consists of a disparate collection of programs that do not adequately serve the needs of the frail elderly and their families. They find, for example, that because housing and home care policies are not integrated, a continuum of long-term care options is not available to the older population. However, current reforms are attempting to ameliorate such problems.

The authors also indicate that, despite a commitment to community care of the aged, departmental policymakers have not been able to devise and implement gerontological plans successfully. Such individuals tend to have inadequate training in planning, economic analyses, and organizational theory. They also lack a full understanding of the role of politics in decision making.

Frossard and Guillemard warn that there is a growing number of aged who live alone and risk becoming dependent on care services. Consequently, critical issues confront French policymakers, including how services and costs for the frail elderly can be equitably distributed in the coming decades.

In Chapter 9, Heinemann-Knoch suggests that social security legislation in Germany is primarily concerned with labor force participation and, as such, provides only for medical treatment, worker disability and old age pensions. The risks of frailty and impairment during old age, which are mostly excluded from coverage, remain within the private domain of the individual, her family, and voluntary organizations. Elder care developed from and continues to be part of a tradition of Christian charity and welfare for the poor.

Heinemann-Knoch maintains that unnecessary dependency in old age is fostered by various aspects of German social policy. For example, the health care system funds only potentially treatable illnesses and excludes chronic diseases and geriatric rehabilitation. She argues that the costs of health care are rapidly growing, without commensurate improvements in the type or quality of medical services. Moreover, frail older women tend to live in substandard housing; sheltered housing with domiciliary services, in particular, is lacking.

The author concludes that long-term care in Germany is sorely inadequate. Both community and institutional care are not available to a large percentage of frail older people, especially those who have low incomes; personnel problems are prevalent, including low wages, staff shortages, and inadequate training; day care and short-term care are both expensive and in short supply; and the availability of potential family caregivers among women is steadily decreasing. Problems related to elder care, as well as numerous other social and economic questions, have been exacerbated by a unified Germany.

In Chapter 10, Nishio argues that Japan is unique among the industrialized countries in that multigenerational households are both prevalent and preferred by family members, including adult children. Consequently, Japan has much fewer publicly supported services, such as home helpers, as compared with other social welfare states. He does note that even in Japan there has been a decline in extended family households.

Nishio contends that demographic trends will make it particularly difficult for Japan to adjust to population aging. With fewer than 7 percent of the population aged sixty-five and over prior to 1970, the nation currently has one of the fastest growing aging societies. The rapid increase in the number of people in need of assistance with daily activities has precipitated costly demands on the public sector by the elderly and their caretakers, with which the state has not been able to keep pace. Nishio comments that since Japan will have the oldest age structure in the world by 2020, with over 11 percent of the population aged 75 and over, these problems will worsen considerably unless Japan adequately prepares for them.

In Chapter 11, Olson examines the changing situation of the frail elderly in the People's Republic of China. He writes that during the era of Mao Zedong (beginning in 1949) there was an attempt to purge the system of traditional values, including veneration of the old, since these ideas were viewed as antithetical to the new social, economic, and political goals of the Communist Party.

Since 1976 (the post-Mao China era), The People's Republic has embarked on full-scale modernization efforts, including a serious reduction in population growth, economic revisions, and party reform. Olson signifies that these developments have had a considerable impact on the older population, especially those who are frail. For example, homes for the aged were built during the 1980s to symbolize community support for the childless, and reassure younger families subject to the one-child policy.

Olson implies that the People's Republic of China is confronting a situation different from that in more industrialized nations. He maintains that China is faced with the dilemma of growing proportions of frail elderly while also attempting both to develop economically and to meet the basic needs of all generations, including the massive peasant population.

As a result, national leaders are minimizing the role of the state in elder care as well as limiting the growth of costly medical treatment programs. The emphasis is on local or community initiatives rather than on centralized programs. However, the family has primary responsibility for most of the actual care of its frail kin, even in the urban areas where the state now plays a major role in providing economic support for the retired population.

Seroka evaluates the social welfare system of socialist Yugoslavia in Chapter 12. He writes that beginning in 1974 the former nation adopted a unique approach to social policy making–self-management. Local interests within the republics and provinces were responsible for providing services, competing among themselves for funds from the multitude of work units.

The author denotes that there was no comprehensive policy for the elderly at either the national or communal levels. Older Yugoslavians, particularly those who were frail, had been at a competitive disadvantage within the system. A substantial percentage, especially in rural areas, was deprived of essential health and social services; many lacked decent pensions and adequate housing as well. Even in urban localities the gap between need and service delivery was wide. The latter programs ranged from nonexistent to decent, depending on the region; however, they never approached the level of accessibility or quality available in Western Europe.

Moreover, socialist Yugoslavia experienced growing income inequalities, marked deterioration in its gross domestic product and living standards, high unemployment, and the aging of its population. As these problems increased in the 1980s, and resources for social programs diminished, the state could not deliver on its cradle-to-grave promises; social welfare statism virtually collapsed even before the dissolution of the nation itself. However, the author concludes that the U.S. market approach to social welfare would be unacceptable in the context of Eastern Europe politics and society. After the ethnic and other political struggles are resolved, the most feasible alternative for the new nations emerging from socialist Yugoslavia will be to adopt the cooperative social welfare pluralism found in western Europe.

Finally, it should be noted that many of the nations included in this study have experienced or are continuing to experience momentous social, economic, and/or political upheaval during the formation of the book. Israel sustained Scud missile attacks by Iraq; the People's Republic of China confronted massive student demonstrations; socialist Yugoslavia has been dissolved and succeeded by five separate and antagonistic entities; Germany is enduring the historical unification of FRG and GDR, along with the multitude of problems it is generating; Britain changed its Prime Minister for the first time in eleven years, though it failed to alter its policy course; and in 1991, Carl Bildt, Sweden's first conservative prime minister in sixty years, proposed dramatic policy shifts including tax cuts and privatization of some welfare services.

Chapter 2

Public Policy and Privatization: Long-Term Care in the United States

Laura Katz Olson

Similar to other industrialized nations, the United States has experienced an enormous growth in its older population. Rising from 3.1 million people age 65 and over in 1900, and representing only 4 percent of the population, this age group accounted for thirty-two million people by 1990, or over 12 percent of the total. It is projected that by the year 2030 the number of elderly will double to approximately 65 million; at that time nearly one-fifth of the population will be sixty-five years of age or older (Stone and Fletcher 1988).

The extreme age group constitutes the fastest growing sector, a trend that began as early as the 1940s and has accelerated since the 1960s. Currently there are 2.8 million people age 85 and over, or 1 percent of the population. In ten years this number is expected to reach 4.9 million, and by the year 2030 to extend to 8.6 million or more people, or 3 percent of the total population (Stone and Fletcher 1988).

Population aging has been fostered by an admixture of increasing longevity, declining fertility, and immigration. The decline of the younger population during the 1960s contributed considerably to the abrupt and largely unanticipated demographic changes. Birth rates fell steadily from 3.68 children per female in the late 1950s to 1.8 children per female by the late 1970s. This sharp decrease in fertility, however, leveled off in the 1980s and 1990s (Preston 1984).

During the first half of the twentieth century, there were limited gains in life expectancy, and these occurred mostly at the younger ages. Any progress was primarily due to better nutrition and public sanitation, the discovery of antibiotics, greater control over acute infectious diseases, and the reduction in the incidence of infant mortality (Kayser-Jones 1981, 4). Beginning in 1940 mortality declined significantly, and since 1970 improvements in longevity have occurred somewhat among the middle-aged and older populations; a reduction in cardiovascular diseases, the leading cause of death in the U.S., has fostered moderate advances in life expectancy among seniors. Currently, the average life expectancy at birth is 71.3 for men, and 78.3 for women.

Chronic diseases and the disabilities they induce are prevalent among older people, especially those in the extreme age groups. Although most older people are healthier today than in past decades, a trend that is expected to continue, there will be more frail and debilitated elderly overall as the number of very old people grows.

The incidence and severity of arthritis, multiple types of heart conditions (cardiovascular and cerebrovascular diseases), high blood pressure (hypertension), diabetes, osteoporosis, and rheumatism, the most frequent chronic conditions among the elderly, tend to increase with age. Moreover, success in the prevention, treatment, or cure of chronic disabilities has been significantly less than that of acute and infectious illnesses. For the most part, the diseases afflicting the aged can, at best, be controlled or stabilized rather than cured.

Mental disorders in particular, including Alzheimer's disease, have become more prevalent with increasing old age. According to Brickner and his associates (1987, 86), about 1 percent of people over the age of sixty-five develop senile dementia every year. By the late 1980s, slightly over 1 million older people were afflicted with severe dementia and another 3 million suffered from milder symptoms of the disorder.

Since the primary illnesses of the very old are chronic rather than acute diseases, more sustained and progressively intensified care is required. Older age groups therefore increasingly represent a greater number of functionally impaired individuals with needs for various types and levels of long-term care. In fact, the incidence of dependency in the performance of basic activities of daily living, such as eating, bathing, toileting, dressing, and getting out of bed, doubles with each successive age group until age 75; after that, the prevalence of dependency triples (Branch and Meyers 1988).

It is important to note that most elderly are not seriously impaired and cope satisfactorily with their physical limitations or disabilities on their own. About one-third of all noninstitutionalized people age 85 and over in the U.S. currently are independent, while another one-third need only limited assistance in performing their daily activities. On the other hand, one-third of the total require substantial aid from others (Longino 1988).

According to the Pepper Commission (1990, 108), there are 7 million older people requiring help with basic tasks, a number that is expected to increase to 13.8 million by 2030. In addition, under current conditions and policies, the 1.5 million elderly needing nursing home care will increase to 5.3 million.

Increased life expectancy, even among seniors, has been greater for women than for men. As a result, the frail elderly population is increasingly feminized. Moreover, due primarily to widowhood and, to a lesser extent, divorce, women are more likely than men to reside in an institution or to live alone in the community. Approximately 26 percent of the men and 46 percent of the women age 85 and over who are not institutionalized live alone. Among those age 85 and over, 50 percent of the men are married compared to only 8 percent of the women (Rosenwaike 1985). Divorce has increased steadily, particularly at older ages; one-sixth of all divorces are in the over 45 age group (Lesnoff-Caravaglia 1984).

Most frail older people, including those with serious disabilities, live in their own home or with a family member, rather than in an institution. Only 5 percent of all older people and one-fifth of the disabled elderly reside in a nursing home at any one point in time. The incidence of institutionalization, however, increases with age: 17 percent of men and 28 percent of women age 85 and over live in a nursing home (Rosenwaike 1985, 95). In addition, approximately 36 to 45 percent of all older people will spend some time in such an institution, and 20 percent will die there (Pepper Commission 1990, 92).

According to the 1982 Long-term Care Survey conducted by the

Department of Health and Human Services, only one-fifth of older people who are functionally disabled reside in nursing homes (Brody 1990). Health status and functional capacity are not good indicators of impending institutionalization: for every person age 65 and over in a nursing home, there are approximately two individuals in the community with similar impairments (Johnson and Grant 1985, 37).

APPROACHES TO LONG-TERM CARE

The U.S. has not developed a comprehensive national policy for long-term care. Nor is there an assumption that frail older people are entitled to receive publicly supported aid. On the contrary, the issues and problems of old age are viewed as private problems requiring private solutions. The American ethos of individualism and self-reliance, and the policies based on these, presuppose that individuals and their families should and will provide for their own social, financial, and service needs. As the Kanes's note, nowhere else in the world are the expectations for care so firmly placed on the backs of the elderly and their families (Kane and Kane 1976, 187).

In addition to family assistance, the preferred methods of self-support for the chronically impaired include the encouragement of personal savings, private pensions plans, and more recently such programs as private long-term care insurance and Home Equity Conversions. Policy makers argue that by expanding their capacity to pay, the aged will be able to purchase the services they need in the private sector. However, as one major study has concluded, at best only a small minority of older people will ever be capable of meeting their long-term care needs through their own efforts alone. The vast majority of the elderly will require some form of supplementary help (Rivlin and Wiener 1988).

Publicly subsidized support tends to be available only to those without personal economic resources and family caregivers. The government is viewed as the provider of last resort, generally requiring a means test in order to qualify; eligibility for long-term care is based on personal insolvency. Thus, publicly supported nursing home care, and the even more constricted funding for home-based services, are provided predominantly to elderly people who do not have a family network, and who have been poor their whole lives or are newly impoverished.

Nearly all public funding for long-term care is provided under the Medicaid program, which is designed and administered by the states under general federal guidelines. The national government contributes between 50 and 80 percent of the costs. The original impetus for the legislation, which was enacted in 1965, was to allow limited access to health care by the very poor, particularly single mothers on welfare. It was never intended to provide significant amounts of long-term care to the elderly. Yet, by 1990, the elderly represented nearly 20 percent of the 26 million Medicaid recipients and about 40 percent of the program's total expenditures of $70 billion (Pepper Commission 1990, 30). It has been estimated that under current policy Medicaid expenditures will increase three-fold, with nursing home fees representing nearly 50 percent of all costs over the next three decades (Rivlin and Wiener 1988, 155).

In order to qualify for coverage under Medicaid, the elderly must meet restrictive income and asset eligibility standards, which for most people means exhausting all of their resources. (In 1988, an older person could retain only $1,900 in assets.) Moreover, it is often difficult for low income people to obtain a nursing home bed. A large percentage of institutionalized older people funded through Medicaid are "conversion" cases who enter as private-paying clients; after nursing home costs impoverish them, they can qualify for Medicaid. Growing numbers of nursing homes will not accept Medicaid-funded applicants (Huttman 1985, 220).

Spouses of institutionalized older people may also be forced to deplete most of their resources. Financial hardship is particularly acute when the institutionalized individual had been the sole provider. The dependent can retain only exempt assets, including a house, car, and personal belongings, and a specified monthly income, which varies from state to state.

Medicare, the 1965 health care legislation for the elderly, provides even fewer resources for long-term care. Scarcely 4 percent, or $3.4 billion out of a total $78.9 billion in Medicare funding in 1988, was expended on long-term care. Only the frail elderly aged 65 and over who require skilled care are even eligible for personal services. Since Medicare does not cover custodial services alone, whether at home or in an institution, most functionally impaired older people are not served under the program.

Neither Medicaid nor Medicare provides a significant amount of funding for home care services. Out of a total $25.9 billion spent on long-term care in 1988 under these programs, only $5.9 billion was devoted to home care; Medicaid and Medicare contributed $3.3 billion, and $2.6 billion, respectively (Pepper Commission 1990, 93).

Moreover, the combination of a reliance on individual resources and a welfare approach to public support, as noted by Rivlin and Wiener (1988), has fostered a two-class system of elder care. Formal in-home services, in particular, are concentrated among the economically privileged. Since there is a difference between real needs existing in the community (demand) and the ability to pay for appropriate services (market demand), a large percentage of older people with limited income are not able to obtain home-based services at all. The Brookings Institution has estimated that long-term care costs will probably escalate faster than the cost of living; the elderly will be even less able to afford home-based services in the future (Rivlin and Wiener 1988).

The type and quality of care available and received in the U.S. thus is dependent mostly on costs, who pays them, profitability, and other factors unrelated to the actual service needs of the frail elderly. Patterns of care, for example, are largely influenced by government funding sources favoring institutionalization. Throughout U.S. history, the approach to most social problems, including poverty, has been some form of institutional treatment. Accordingly, institutional care has been the predominant mode of public support for the poor, disabled aged without family. Over the last several decades, the concept of long-term care has become synonymous with nursing homes (Koff 1982).

Further, rather than providing services directly, the public sector in the U.S. serves to subsidize private firms. Human services and long-term care in particular have been increasingly privatized. Not only do the real needs of the elderly and their families go unmet, but this has led to an overly costly system. Over 80 percent of all nursing homes are for-profit institutions. By the early 1980s, for-profit institutions emerged in the previously nonprofit home-care field, as well; the proprietary share steadily grew to 30 percent by 1990 (Scharlach and Boyd 1989).

NURSING HOMES

During the early years, there was only a small percentage of frail older people in need of care. Those lacking both financial resources and kin were placed in almshouses and, in later years, in state mental institutions. It was not until the passage of the Social Security Act in 1935, with its prohibition on funding for public facilities, that the nursing home emerged in the U.S. (This federal prohibition against payments to persons in public facilities was rescinded in 1950.) These institutions, which initially were small, private boarding homes, spread during the 1950s and even more dramatically after 1965 as a result of Medicare and Medicaid. In an attempt to shift costs to the federal government, states increasingly moved older, mentally disabled patients from state-funded mental hospitals to nursing homes or other private facilities now funded under Medicaid. (Hashimi 1988, 127). According to one source, there was neither screening on who was to be discharged nor psychiatric services available in these new facilities (Moss and Halamandaris 1977, 107). At the same time, the Hill-Burton hospital construction program, the Small Business Administration, and the Federal Housing Administration mortgage insurance program provided capital to entrepreneurs for the building or enlargement of nursing institutions.

As nursing homes became an increasingly lucrative financial investment, generating high profits, the smaller facilities gradually disappeared. Big business entered the field during the late 1960s, and according to Moss and Halamandaris (1977), nursing homes developed into "the hottest item on the stock exchange." By 1989, there were over 16,000 nursing homes, mostly for-profit facilities, providing for 1.5 million elderly.

Market speculation, and more recently mergers and acquisitions by large corporations, have dramatically consolidated nursing home ownership and control. By the 1980s, chains captured two-fifths of the market. Margolis (1990, 157) estimates that by the year 2000, big business will control nearly 60 percent of the total. Over half of the $5 billion in profits accrued by the top fifty nursing homes in 1985 went to two major companies: Beverly Enterprises and Hillhaven Corporation. In his study of the subject, Margolis (1990, 158) concludes:

> What the chains usually do with their profits is of no use either to the residents or the general public. Instead of upgrading services, they increase dividends to stockholders, instead of building new facilities, they swallow up existing ones, thereby adding not a single bed to the nation's inadequate pool.

Large nursing home establishments have begun diversifying into other ventures such as pharmaceutical supplies, home-health care, and homemaker services (Harrington and Swan 1985). Conglomerates unrelated to long-term care, including Avon Products and Marriott Corporation, have entered the market as well (Margolis 1990, 157).

Profit maximization, the priority value for the private sector, has served as the guiding principle in the provision of nursing home care. This has produced a costly, publicly supported, "private" system that fails to meet the needs of millions of chronically ill older people. Approximately one-half of all nursing home revenues accrue from government funding, mostly from Medicaid; the latter accounted for about 63 percent of all beds (Margolis 1990, 163).

As Barney (1974) remarks, nursing homes are in the business domain, and organized according to business principles. She acutely observes:

> . . . it would be fair to say that in many instances it has succeeded in meeting its marketplace standards, the same standards which give us our great supermarkets, for example.

These institutions have failed, however, to produce an adequate human environment.

Services are organized to meet the needs of administrators and stockholders rather than those of residents or their families. As the Kanes contend, faith in the marketplace as a means of assuring quality and reducing cost may be misdirected in the case of long-term care (Kane and Kane 1985, 265). The pursuit of profits over human needs has negatively affected the quality, accessibility, and affordability of care.

The relentless search for profits by nursing home owners has prompted providers to compete for the most lucrative markets and leave others uncovered. The for-profit institutions and, increasingly, the non-profit organizations are unwilling to serve both the poor and the more difficult (and thus more expensive) cases; yet these older people tend to have the greatest needs.

The number of for-profit institutions in most other nations is negligible (Kane and Kane 1976, 175). As a result, no other country has developed the American equivalent of the nursing home; it is truly a unique institution. As indicated sardonically by Johnson and Grant (1985, 3), these facilities "have been described as 'houses of death,' 'human junkyards,' 'warehouses for the dying,' and 'travesties on the word home.'"

The vast majority of homes fail to provide for the basic health and safety needs of the occupants. Most are substandard facilities that do not comply with even minimum federal and state standards of care; many violations are serious and life-threatening, including lack of clean food, proper administration of drugs, and decent personal hygiene. Due to a scarcity of physicians, a significant percentage of patients do not receive needed lab tests or adequate medical attention. Many suffer from poor nutrition, insufficient nursing care, and generally squalid conditions.

Even less emphasis is placed on their fully human needs. On the contrary, most nursing home residents experience a decline in their social, psychological, and physical functioning after placement. According to Johnson and Grant (1985), in the U.S. these facilities tend to dehumanize residents through denial of privacy; deindividuation and disculturation (loss of sense of self and continuity in the social environment); rigid controls on personal autonomy; and segregation from the outside world.

In nearly all nursing homes, the personal lives of residents are strictly organized; most are denied their basic civil rights. One Congressional study disclosed that 70 percent of institutionalized people have no privacy, are prohibited from making simple personal choices such as when to get up or go to sleep, and are not allowed to maintain personal possessions. They also are not protected against theft or, in many cases, emotional or physical abuse (HSCA 1985). Residents frequently are required to wear name bands which are permanently placed on their wrists.

In their cross-national studies, the Kanes found that there is a higher quality of care outside the U.S., including institutions that foster comfort and dignity for the chronically ill (1976). Similarly, in a comparative study of U.S. and British institutions, Kayser-Jones (1981) found that only in the U.S. are the residents treated as if they had no value whatsoever, with devastating and debilitating consequences.

The American nursing home tends to be organized around the medical model, which fosters a hospital-like environment. The major focus is on custodial care; meaningful social activities, psychological care, or rehabilitative services generally are not provided. Patients are cast in a sick role where withdrawal from social activities predominate; they are kept both disabled and dependent. For example, despite the fact that a significant portion of nursing home residents suffer from mental disorders, and many others evidence a high incidence of psychiatric symptoms, few facilities offer any psychological evaluation or treatment. The latter can include reality orientation, milieu therapy, remotivation therapy, and behavior modification.

Johnson and Grant (1985, 81-83) maintain that a significant percentage of older patients assumed to be suffering from an organic brain disorder may, instead, be afflicted with a reversible acute illness. They point out that psychiatric evaluations could differentiate those clients with conditions susceptible to effective treatment.

While most chronic disorders afflicting the elderly cannot be entirely eliminated, rehabilitative services can help to reduce or alleviate disabilities, or to provide retraining so that the individual can function at his or her maximum level of capacity within the limits of the disability. Mendelson (1974, 11) alleges that even when rehabilitative equipment is purchased by a facility in order to qualify for Medicare reimbursement, such machines often are not even used.

In a substantial number of cases, patients are chemically controlled through psychotropic drugs. One study revealed that up to 75 percent of all residents have such prescriptions (Hashimi 1988).

Through the use of thorazine and Mellaril, patients are kept quiet; many are reduced to an empty shell. Arluke and Peterson (1981) propose that

> by managing behavior in this manner the cause of the problem is attributed to the older person, it is the individual that we seek to change. By focusing on the symptoms and defining them as senile psychosis, we ignore the possibility that their behavior is not an illness but an adaptation to a social situation . . . (this) . . . lends itself to the individualization of social problems.

Physical restraints also are routinely utilized to control patients, resulting in decreased muscle tone, and eventually permanent immobility. Such immobilized individuals are more susceptible to incontinence, bedsores, apathy, and depression.

In 1987, as part of the Omnibus Reconciliation Act (OBRA), Congress passed a major nursing home reform package; one major provision severely limits the use of both chemical and physical restraints. In particular, the law mandates that these can be used only in emergencies, on the order of a physician, or, in the case of physical restraints, with the permission of the resident or her guardian. OBRA also attempts to improve staff training, resident's rights, admission procedures, nursing services, and the overall safety and quality of institutional care.

However, it is unlikely that these guidelines will improve conditions considerably; previous regulations have not assured serious institutional changes. Moreover, as of 1991, the regulations have not even been implemented.

IN-HOME AND COMMUNITY-BASED SERVICES

Publicly supported institutional care under Medicaid had begun as a limited government responsibility to a relatively small older population; by the 1980s, demand had increased far beyond what was anticipated when the program was enacted. At the same time, nursing home charges increased dramatically, as did the public sector's share of these costs. Growing numbers of older people began to rely on Medicaid for nursing home fees, especially among middle-income households, many of whom impoverished themselves after only a year or less of care. Consequently, concern over expenditures for institutionalization began to intensify among policymakers. State governments in particular became anxious about the escalating fiscal crisis in their Medicaid programs. In fact, the latter had become the single largest item in many state budgets.

In an effort to curtail the spiraling costs of institutional services, national and state political leaders began to search for alternative, less costly ways of providing for publicly supported long-term care. Accordingly, these policymakers turned their attention to in-home services. Limited federal funding became available primarily for home-care demonstrations projects under several programs, including amendments to the Social Security Act (title XX), Medicaid (Section 2176 Waivers), and the older Americans Act (OAA).

In 1980, Congress also instituted the National Long Term Care Channeling Demonstration Program. Funding became available from the Administration on Aging (AoA) and the Health Care Financing Administration (HCFA) to establish a system of long-term care in ten local sites utilizing a case management approach. This national channeling experiment focused exclusively on those elderly who not only were at risk for institutionalization but also who could be expected to live independently in the community with some assistance. These projects focused primarily on efficient service management (Eustis, Greenberg, and Patten 1984, 107).

The overriding goal of these programs was to demonstrate whether the cost of providing in-home or community services would be less than that of nursing home care. Given this perspective, policymakers primarily have been interested in cost-based questions rather than in the quality or effectiveness of services.

At the forefront of concern is apprehension by political leaders that publicly supported home care would replace or undermine family input rather than delay or prevent institutionalization. If formal services substitute for family and friends, decisionmakers argue that latent demands would emerge. As a result, even if per capita costs were lower, public outlays overall would be significantly higher. Potential claimants for services include dependent frail people living in the community through their own choice. They also encompass those frail elderly who have encountered a shortage of nursing home beds.

An antithetical position advanced by other observers is that greater publicly supported home care would ensure more rather than less family support. According to some gerontologists, by easing the burden on the caregiver and thus decreasing tensions within the family, formal services prevent or at least delay institutionalization. One study found, for example, that although families play the primary role in maintaining the chronically ill older person at home, both children and spouses require outside help in order to sustain such care over time (Johnson and Catalano 1983).

Similarly, Hooyman and Lustbader (1986, 6) note that the absence of supportive services leads to a greater chance for institutionalization of the ill relative. Since chronic diseases tend to be progressive, and custodial responsibilities intensify over time, a significant percentage of caregivers eventually experience debilitating mental or physical impairments. As Huttman (1985, 91-92) denotes:

> Today's family often lacks . . . the structural, organizational, and economic resources to care for the elderly ill over a long period of time. The stress of care increases along with the stages of the parent's illness. Over time, many adult children caring for their ill parents develop attitudes ranging from irritation to exasperation to desparation . . . Prolonged illness increases tension for family members, especially when support from outside sources diminishes.

Other gerontological research shows that formal services are generally effective in delaying or preventing institutionalization only when supplemented by informal supports (Dunlap 1980). Yet, as suggested earlier, the limited available publicly supported in-home care in the U.S. focuses primarily on the frail elderly without family aid.

Indeed, several studies have found that formal services complement rather than substitute for family care. Caro demonstrates that even when public sector services are abundantly available, the family still assumes most of the responsibility (Caro 1986). However, such care may be enhanced to include greater emotional and psychological support.

Home care services have not significantly replaced nursing homes in the U.S. primarily because it has not been proven that the former save costs; the evidence is mixed on whether savings actually occur (Benjamin 1985). Some studies of demonstration projects have concluded that while families are not replaced entirely, total long-term care costs may, in fact, increase (Stephens and Christianson 1986; Caro 1986; Pepper Commission 1990; and Edelman and Hughs 1990).

Cost limitations have been assured through stringent policy guidelines. Nearly all of the limited efforts to expand or coordinate non-institutional types of care over the last two decades have focused primarily on the Medicaid-eligible frail elderly. Further, expenditures and number of people served under the largest program, Section 2176 Waivers, could not exceed what they otherwise would have been for nursing home care. In 1986, only 79,000 aged or disabled people were served (Pepper Commission 1990, 97-99).

For the most part, new in-home services have been funded by channeling existing resources from established programs. There also has been a failure to institutionalize successful in-home service pilot programs. In many localities where money has been available for demonstration projects, continuous funding is tenuous. The New York State Nursing Home Without Walls, which began in 1978, ended in the early 1980s. The national channeling experiment was terminated in 1985, after only five years. A significant number of other projects have been similarly dismantled.

Most state efforts are focused on coordination among existing home-care programs. Further, according to the Pepper Commission (1990, 97), five states, with only one-third of the older population in the U.S., account for approximately two-thirds of all in-home and community-based expenditures.

Community-based assistance such as respite services, especially daycare, has been particularly underfunded. Adult day care did not even exist in the U.S. prior to 1970. Financed mostly under title XX of the Social Security Act, but also through the Older Americans Act and Medicaid, pilot programs emerged during the 1970s in the ongoing effort to combat high institutional costs.

Day care, however, has not proven to be cost effective. As a result, there has been only limited growth in the number of facilities. Lack of continuous funding for demonstration projects has added significantly to the paucity of these programs. In addition to limited supply and stringent eligibility rules, day care facilities tend not to serve the more seriously impaired people (Huttman 1985). In addition, the price of day care in the private sector, when available, is prohibitive. Consequently, this community-based service remains inaccessible to the vast majority of older people.

For the most part, the U.S. has extremely fragmented and limited publicly supported in-home or community-based services. At the same time, home-care in the private sector has altered dramatically. Over the last decade, the U.S. has witnessed the growth of profit-making homemaker and home health agencies in this previously nonprofit field. Concomitantly, nonprofit agencies have been increasing charges, including copayments, eliminating free care for those with limited income, and reducing or eliminating less "profitable" programs and services. Thus, the paucity of public sector services will be felt even more acutely in the next several decades by those who can not afford to purchase them.

FAMILY CAREGIVING IN THE U.S.

Since the early 1970s, the U.S. has experienced declining rates of productivity growth, rising budget deficits, high unemployment, a reduced competitive economy worldwide, and a host of other economic and social problems. In response, policymakers in the 1980s and beyond began addressing social problems by focusing almost exclusively on greater efficiency and controlling or cutting costs.

At the same time, the aging of the U.S. population overall, and the emergence of growing numbers of frail elderly in particular, have been viewed increasingly as contributing substantially to the fiscal crisis. According to most public officials, the demands of the elderly are consuming a disproportionate share of the national budget. As Daniels (1988) suggests:

> There is a growing perception that the old and the young are locked in fierce competition for a critical but scarce resource, public funds for human services.

Pressure to contain growing government costs over the last two decades has led to a retrenchment in Medicaid and other programs serving the elderly, including more stringent eligibility requirements and caps on reimbursement rates for nursing homes. Since many institutions have been unwilling to accept current government fee levels, greater numbers of indigent, disabled older people must be cared for by their families, in the community. Similarly, the institution of Diagnostically-Related Groups (DRGs) under Medicare has limited the length of hospital stays, forcing sicker and quicker hospital discharges. This cost-containment measure has contributed to a growing shortage of nursing home beds as well.

At the same time, fiscal austerity has fostered policymakers' interests in less costly alternatives to institutionalization. However, this has been accompanied by a systematic reduction in public resources for supportive social services and other forms of community aid.

Consequently, privatization, community care, "restoring traditional values," and the growing numbers of frail elderly all mean increasing expectations of and burdens on the family. As Retsinas (1986, 171) writes:

> Policy-makers have accordingly reified 'the community' into the salvation of these wheelchair-bound nursing home denizens . . . Not only will community-based care be inherently better, but it will also be cheaper, or so policy-makers hope. Where such policies are widely accepted, families can be encouraged, prompted, even forced to keep Mom with them.

Yet, studies clearly show that families already provide about 80 percent of all long-term care in the U.S. The vast majority of frail, older people who live outside of institutions depend exclusively on their family; others, who may pay professionals for some aid, tend to rely on family and, to a lesser extent, friends for at least some portion of their care (Stone, Cafferata, and Sangl 1987, 1).

Most of the burden of informal care, however, is provided by one family member who is usually female; responsibilities of caring for a chronically ill relative tend not to be shared. Women represent over 70 percent of all caregivers, including adult daughters (30 percent), wives (23 percent), and other female relatives, many of whom are daughters-in-law and sisters (20 percent). Husbands provide 13 percent of total care, followed by sons (9 percent), and other male relatives (7 percent) (Brody 1990, 35).

Elderly males generally are cared for by their spouses, while older women rely on their adult children. Daughters tend to provide personal care, health care, and household chores; sons are more likely to assist with household repairs and financial management. Sons also generally receive more support from their spouses than do daughters (Abel 1987, 16). Moreover, one study suggests that married children provide fewer hours of care than do divorced, widowed, and never-married children (Stoller 1983).

Family members in general, and women in particular, are not only the major caregivers in the U.S., but studies show that the vast majority prefer to provide such care rather than to institutionalize their relatives. Both older people and their families strongly resist nursing home placement, viewing it only as a last resort after all other alternatives have been tried. According to one observer,

> adult children report the placement of a parent into a nursing home as one of the most unhappy events of their lives. Studies conducted among adult children of nursing home residents demonstrate that 29 percent to 45 percent tried to avoid placement by moving the dependent adult into their homes for care. (Buckwalter and Hall 1987)

In fact, as pointed out by several researchers, older people are institutionalized primarily when their caretaker becomes exhausted, ill, or dies (Morycz 1985; Hooyman and Lustbader 1986, 90).

Even former caregivers of institutionalized dementia patients often view institutionalization as a personal failure, despite the overwhelmingly difficult task of caring for such patients at home (Buckwalter and Hall 1987). In addition, when institutionalization is necessary or unavoidable, families continue to devote considerable time, effort, and emotional energy to their incapacitated kin.

Most caregivers are unprepared for both the role itself and the intensity of the task. In a recent study, Abel (1989) found that very few of the females caring for their parents anticipated doing so; the vast majority were shocked by the type of disease that struck, and were surprised at the suddenness and depth of need.

According to a national profile of caregivers, 80 percent assist their relatives seven days a week, averaging four hours a day (Stone, Cafferata, and Sangl 1987). It has been estimated that those aiding the very frail elderly average two hours daily on personal and medical care, with an additional four hours devoted to household tasks and companionship (Stephens and Christianson 1986, 50). Certain types of disabilities requiring continuous nursing care and advanced mental disorders require even more intensive effort. As Fahey (1984) indicates:

> Because of the extensive burden of care (for Alzheimer's disease), the caregiver is commonly described as the disease's "second victim."

Moreover, the burden heightens over time as patients become increasingly disabled.

Sustained caregiving fosters enormous stress on individuals and their families. According to one study, about half of all caregivers suffer moderate to severe psychological stress, from 15 to 33 percent are affected physically, and nearly 20 percent face financial problems. A high percentage of caregivers also experience increased tension with other family members, including spouses, children, siblings, and care recipients themselves. Where the caregiver and parent share a household, strain tends to be even greater. About 36 percent of the extremely disabled elderly reside in the home of an adult child (Brody 1990).

Many caregivers, particularly women, also sacrifice both their current employment and economic future, including decent pensions. Approximately 44 percent of caregiving daughters now work and, for many, their income is essential for supporting themselves and their family (Brody 1990, 214). A significant percentage of working caregivers are forced to quit their jobs either temporarily or permanently. Many of those who remain in the labor force have to reduce the number of working hours, seek less demanding employment, adjust work schedules, endure periodic interruptions, and/or forego career advancement.

Stoller (1983) argues that working women spend similar amounts of time as do their nonworking counterparts on caregiving tasks, indicating that the former sacrifice other facets of their lives, particularly "personal" time. In fact, several studies show that the greatest sacrifices are in socializing with friends, leisure activities, and vacations (Cantor 1983; Burnley 1987).

The question, of course, is whether American women can continue to provide nearly all of the long-term care in the future. Paradoxically, the family is expected to provide even more caregiving in the 1990s and beyond, when it is least able to do so. There are unique features of contemporary society that contribute to the infeasibility of greater amounts of elder care by adult children, especially daughters, or even spouses.

With the growth in the oldest age group and its prolonged periods of impairment, an increasing percentage of the population is forced to confront the issue of care for a frail relative. Currently, over 80 percent of people in their 40s have at least one surviving parent (Hooyman and Lustbader 1986, 3-4). According to Rivlin and Wiener (1988, 180), the chance of individuals age 60 and over having a parent alive is expected to increase from 7 to nearly 30 percent over the next three decades. Given current assumptions of filial obligation, caregiving will become an integral part of the adult life-cycle.

There also are more people that each individual or family will potentially be required to care for, including two sets of parents and even grandparents. The four-generation family now is common; approximately 50 percent of older people with adult children have great-grandchildren (Hooyman and Lustbader 1986, 3). Moreover, with longer life spans and more sophisticated medical technology, adult children are called upon to provide more intensive care for longer periods of time than in the past.

Lower fertility rates and childbearing at later ages have meant a decrease in family size, with fewer children available to share caregiving responsibilities. Caregiving children as well as spouses are increasingly in advanced age themselves. According to one source, the average age of wives delivering long-term care is sixty-five; nearly one-third are over the age of seventy-four. The majority of caregiving daughters are over the age of fifty (Sommers and Shields 1987, 21). Moreover, one study determined that fully one-third of people caring for the frail elderly experience health problems of their own, including disabling conditions (Stephens and Christianson 1986, 27).

While the "problem" of elder care has been relegated to the ever-increasing domain of women's work, contemporary females have even less time for caregiving than in the past. Women tend to face multiple and competing demands, including those of child care (often as single parents), paid employment, and other household and family needs.

Growing numbers of women participate in the labor force, especially middle-aged wives who traditionally have provided most of the caregiving duties. While in 1950 only 38 percent of all women between the ages of 45 and 54 worked, by 1990 this percentage grew to over 60 percent and is expected to rise steadily. Labeled the "sandwich generation," or "women in the middle," many of these women are caught between caring for both dependent children and frail older relatives. For others, caregiving is thrust upon them just as their youngest child is leaving the home (Brody 1981).

The emergence of alternative family configurations, resulting from remarriage, has obscured caretaking obligations. The fragility of these "blended" families, due to a high divorce rate among the remarried, further complicates the situation (Brody 1990, 17). As Retsinas (1986, 18) points out:

> The lines of "family," . . . have blurred in the last decade. Divorce, remarriage, stepchildren, half-children–relationships are, both legally and emotionally, less emphatically delineated . . . . When an 80-year old man is incapacitated from a stroke, is his wife of ten years the primary caregiver? If she herself is frail, do her children assume the responsibility for their stepfather, even though they may barely know him? Are the children from his first marriage responsible for him . . . . As individual geneological diagrams have grown more complicated, so too the demarcation of families has grown more difficult.

Moreover, whether due to widowhood or, increasingly, divorce, a significant percentage of daughters are likely to face the financial, emotional, and physical responsibilities of caregiving alone. High divorce rates at older ages over the last several decades portend less spousal care as well.

In addition, there is a tendency for Americans to equate *caring about* and *caring for*. This has been internalized, particularly by women, and built into the social structure and social policies. Yet, affection and warmth for one's parent does not necessarily translate into caregiving; a daughter can care deeply about her chronically ill mother without actually providing the physical care herself (Dalley 1988; Brody 1990).

Older people themselves value personal independence and autonomy. Most individuals, including those with functional impairments, strive to maintain their own residence for as long as possible. At the same time, they endeavor not to burden their adult children. Older people move in with their children, primarily daughters, only when it is no longer possible to live alone (Brody 1990). As Rosenmayr and Kockeis have remarked (1963), the elderly tend to prefer "intimacy at a distance."

In fact, affection and closeness actually can dissipate under the real strains of caregiving (Jarrett 1985). Some researchers have found that the stress of excessive caregiver burden can contribute to elder abuse (Rathbone-McCuan 1984; Caro 1986; Steinmetz 1988). It has been estimated that nearly 4 percent of the older population in the U.S. are victims of emotional, physical, or financial abuse (PA Attorney General 1988).

Abel (1987, 38) contends that the use of formal services can actually enhance the relationship between caregivers and care recipients as well as contribute to the latter's dignity. According to Finley, Roberts, and Banahan (1988):

> Perhaps the warmth and affectionate relationship desired between adult children and their parents are achieved only when the children are freed from day-to-day survival responsibilities such as economic support or activities of daily living. Freedom from the bonds of obligation and guilt associated with failure to meet such obligations . . . might release and encourage family members to develop the type of family bonds valued in an institution considered based on emotional association.

Some researchers have found that institutionalization of a sick parent or spouse may strengthen family ties by reducing stress (Koff 1982, 17).

Given changing social conditions and the high emotional, physical, and financial costs of caregiving, increasing pressure on adult children and spouses to personally take care of their frail relative's every need would be socially irresponsible (Brody 1981). There must be limits to the caregiving burden on adult children and spouses, as well as the option not to provide care. In the U.S., caregivers usually do not have a choice as to whether to assume full responsibility for their chronically ill relatives; due to the high and escalating costs of in-home and institutional services, as well as their limited availability, accessability, and/or poor quality, women often are forced to provide the care themselves.

WORKERS IN THE SERVICE SECTOR

In long-term care, employees contribute substantially to the well-being of the frail elderly. The personnel are most important to the quality of care supplied by home care agencies or nursing homes; the relationship between the practitioner and client is crucial.

Although the quality of care in institutions is dependent to a large extent on the personnel, nursing homes and home-health agencies tend to be the employers of last resort. Employees tend to be over-worked, underpaid, and lack opportunities for advancement. Moreover, employers tend to rely on unlicensed and untrained people. In fact, there is no other health field in the U.S. that has such a high percentage of unskilled workers, comprising about 75 percent of the total (Johnson and Grant 1985, 123). Women, blacks, and ethnic minorities represent the overwhelming percentage of workers in the long-term care industry. Nearly 90 percent of nurses aides, orderlies, and attendants in nursing homes are female.

Wages are extremely low. Nursing aides, for example, averaged less than four dollars per hour in 1986 (Margolis 1990, 162). The Service Employees International Union recently found that many of the 110,000 workers employed in the $2 billion Beverly Enterprises actually qualified for food stamps and Medicaid. Although aides, orderlies, and attendants are projected to be among the fastest growing job categories over the next several decades, it has been projected that wages will remain below the poverty line (SEIU 1989). Employees in long-term care generally are denied health care benefits and pension plans as well.

Consequently, there is a shortage of personnel both in homemaker organizations and nursing homes. These industries also experience a high rate of turnover, absenteeism, and vacancies. In nursing homes, the annual turnover rate often reaches 75 percent.

Workers in nursing homes and home care agencies tend to confront a contradiction between their concern for the frail elderly and the realities of their own working conditions. Dalley (1988, 136) claims that such individuals have the following choices: make the best of a bad job; experience mental or physical illness themselves; or adhere to the job description, ignoring the real needs of their patients. Employees who are exploited and dehumanized themselves, while working under inhumane conditions, will have great difficulty in treating their patients in a caring, dignified manner.

ALTERNATIVE HOUSING OPTIONS AND INCOME CLASS

Housing and the Frail Elderly Poor

Labeled alternately Board and Care Homes, Personal Care, Adult Care, Family Care, Adult Congregate Living Facilities, or Domiciliary Care, depending on the state, these residential options provide room and board, and in some cases personal services, for the frail elderly (Hilker 1987). Most of the residents are female, poor, and often disabled and/or mentally ill, with no place else to go (U.S. Congress 1989).

Board and Care Homes have grown rapidly over the last several decades in response to the deinstitutionalization of the mentally ill, enactment of the Supplementary Security Income Program (SSI), and the growing shortage of in-home services and nursing home beds for the poor. Some states have increasingly encouraged the use of these facilities in lieu of nursing homes in order to save costs. Financial support for these "private" facilities depends primarily on SSI, which provides a minimum level of income for the elderly poor. Over 72 percent of the residents rely on SSI alone. By the late 1980s, federal and state government outlays for SSI-supported Board and Care Homes amounted to over $7 billion (U.S. Congress 1989, 39).

Although states are required to set minimum standards for these dwellings, few states enforce them. In most localities, these residences are substandard, unregulated, and unlicensed. Many of the homes offer squalid conditions, and their residents are often subjected to various forms of abuse, including sexual violence, theft, control of residents through drugs, and inadequate nutrition. According to a recent government report (1989, 39):

> Warehousing, exploitation and abuse in the board and care industry is far from an isolated and localized problem involving a few mentally impaired elderly. Rather, fraud and abuse in board and care homes is a nationwide scandal of epic proportions.

Despite these problems, it has been projected that the number of Board and Care Homes, and the percentage of frail older people residing in them, will continue to rise steadily.

Subsidized low-income housing for the elderly, including congregate housing, provides additional shelter options for those with few economic resources. However, the number of units is limited, and most facilities have long waiting lists. Moreover, the very frail or functionally incapacitated applicant is not eligible for these accomodations. Although administrators have attempted to institute some support services for current residents as they age, most of the seriously impaired residents are forced to move, usually to nursing homes (Lawton, Moss, and Grimes 1985).

Housing and the Economically Well-Off Frail Elderly

Not all older people are poor and the market has responded to those with ample income. Continuing Care Retirement Communities (CCRCs), or Life-Care Community Housing, for example, have become increasingly available for those with sufficient income to pay the substantial entry and monthly fees. In some cases, residents are required to contribute all of their assets. Generally included in these contracts are housing, supportive services, and, in most cases, health and nursing care.

In 1987, there were 680 lifecare communities, with an average of 245 residents each (Huttman 1985). Although most of these "guarantee" a continuum of care, including nursing home services, in reality many charge additional fees for the latter. In addition, a large number of these developments have gone bankrupt, leaving their elderly residents without any financial resources (Rivlin and Wiener 1988, 17-23).

Other types of retirement communities have been increasing as well, although most of these do not provide for the frail, dependent resident. These housing options include: Retirement New Towns which offer health care, support services, and leisure activities; Retirement Villages which provide only recreational activities, although limited health services are sometimes available; Retirement Subdivisions which tend to supply housing only; and Retirement Residences which have some leisure activities, congregate meals, and sometimes laundry and transportation services (Pastalan 1983).

One comprehensive study of retirement communities found that by the late 1970s there were about 2,400 of these developments, housing over 1 million residents (Pastalan 1983). In 1989, Mariott Corporation announced its intention to invest over $1 billion to build 150 new senior citizen communities by 1994; they are expected to house about 25,000 people at a per capita monthly cost of $1,000 to $2,000.

Most retirement communities have encountered increasingly aging populations, which foster growing costs. High interest rates, inflation, and other problems have further added to their fiscal problems. Consequently, retirement communities have become more expensive for older people to move into, as well as for those already dwelling there to maintain. In some cases, escalating maintenance, service, and user fees have forced residents to find alternative housing; this is especially devastating, for the frail elderly.

CONCLUSION

While aging is a universal phenomenon, the way we age is linked to the social context. Chronic diseases do not necessarily entail dependency; their debilitating effects can only be understood and ameliorated within the context of the interrelatedness of social, environmental, and economic conditions. The public sector in the U.S. has not provided the appropriate environment for those suffering from chronic ailments, thus preventing many older people from reaching their maximum human potential. A significant percentage of the very old experience inadequate income, including poverty conditions, low-quality housing, and insufficient health care.

Most of the frail elderly also lack access to publicly supported in-home and community services, and quality institutional care. Among other benefits, decent formal services would serve to compensate for losses resulting from chronic disabilities; they can do this while protecting the dignity and self-respect of the recipient. Consequently, a significant number of the partially disabled elderly, who with appropriate supportive services would be able to maintain their lifestyle and independence, are unable to do so. Daniels (1988, 8) points out that

> people with only mild disabilities, who could maintain normal patterns of living if they had modest help, cannot find or finance the home care and social support services they need. Ultimately, millions of elderly are forced into premature and inappropriate levels of dependency on their families or institutions.

It is one of the ironies of U.S. public policy that, in promoting individualism and self-reliance, the structural arrangements tend to foster dependency.

For many older people, the emphasis on individualism also means social isolation. Streib, Folts, and Hilker (1984, 245-246), in their study of shared living for the elderly, contend that in many instances such arrangements are preferable to bringing support services into the individual's home. They argue further that an overemphasis on independence at older ages may be counterproductive.

In addition, rather than rendering only caretaking functions, nursing homes could potentially provide socially created settings that would enable residents to capitalize on their capabilities and opportunities, however limited. In contrast, institutional care is viewed in this country as a means of merely maintaining an older person at his or her basic functioning level.

Policymakers should invest resources in new forms of group care that maximize the potential of the chronically ill. For example, a homelike setting, along with mechanisms encouraging participation in decisions affecting their lives, would allow nursing home residents to better fulfill their human potential. Just as importantly, as pointed out by Kayser-Jones (1981), care must be provided in such a way as to show the residents that "we value them as human beings." A profit-making environment is unsuitable for the development of such facilities. The frail elderly can not age with dignity unless they receive public support as a right. This would allow older people to have maximum choice in their living arrangements. A sense of control over one's life is essential for maintaining personal integrity, and should be supported by public policy to the fullest extent possible. Impoverished nursing home residents have no resources with which to exert any control over their lives or even their care.

The vast majority of older people and their families attempt to avoid institutionalization at all costs. Numerous Congressional studies and reports, gerontological research, and newspaper exposés all have exhaustively enumerated the dire situation of nursing home residents in the U.S. At best, policymakers over the last two decades have promulgated a thicket of regulations, most of which have been inadequately enforced and largely ignored.

Over 90 percent of public funds for long-term care in the U.S. still accrues to nursing homes; institutional placement remains the only viable alternative for a significant percentage of elderly people and their families. While institutional care may be necessary and even beneficial in some cases, it must be seen as an alternative to community supports, not as a primary means of care (Landsberger 1985, 219).

Additionally, U.S. policy generally addresses distinct and separate stages in the life cycle, often with an emphasis on the end stages. Yet, the situation of a chronically ill individual tends to represent an accumulation of a lifetime's experience. In the absence of a comprehensive and affordable health care system for younger generations, the vast majority of Americans enter middle and old age vulnerable. At the same time, the paucity of affordable, quality supportive services for the frail elderly has engendered greater expectations of and burdens on the family. Sustained caregiving responsibilities often entail high emotional, personal, physical, and financial costs for women of all ages.

Public policy must recognize the social, economic, and health needs of the entire society. By focusing attention on the elderly alone, policymakers encourage intergenerational conflict; the reality is that the well-being of the different generations is interlocked.

REFERENCES

Abel, Emily K. 1987. *Love is Not Enough: Family Care of the Frail Elderly.* Washington, DC: American Public Health Association.

Abel, Emily K. 1989. "The Ambiguities of Social Support: Adult Daughters Caring for Frail Elderly Parents." *Journal of Aging Studies,* Fall, 1(3): 211-230.

Arluke, Arnold, and Peterson, John. 1981. "Accidental Medicalization of Old Age and Its Social Control Implications." In *Dimensions: Aging, Culture, and Health.* Edited by Christine L. Frey. New York: Bergin Press, 271-284.

Barney, Jane L. 1974. "Community Presence as a Key to Quality of Life in Nursing Homes." *American Journal of Public Health,* March, 3(64): 265-268.

Benjamin, A. E., Jr. 1985. "Community-Based Long Term Care." In *Long Term Care of the Elderly: Public Policy Issues.* Edited by Charlene Harrington, Robert J. Newcomer, and Carroll L. Esters. Beverly Hills, CA: Sage, 197-211.

Branch, Laurence G., and Meyers, Allan R. 1988. "Long Term Care in the U.S." In *North American Elders: United States and Canadian Perspectives.* Edited by Eloise Rathbone-McCuan and Betty Havens. Westport, CT: Greenwood Press, 89-110.

Brickner, Philip W.; Lechich, Anthony J.; Lipsman, Roberta; and Scharer, Linda. 1987. *Long-Term Health Care: Providing a Spectrum of Services to the Aged.* New York: Basic Books.

Brody, Elaine M. 1981. "Women in the Middle' and Family Help to Older People." *The Gerontologist,* 5(21): 471-480.

Brody, Elaine. 1990. *Women in the Middle: Their Parent-Care Years.* New York: Springer Publishing Co.

Buckwalter, Kathleen, and Hall, Geri. 1987. "Families of the Institutionalized Older Adult." In *Aging, Health, and Family: Long-Term Care.* Edited by Timothy H. Brubaker. Newbury Park, CA: Sage, 176-196.

Burnley, Cynthia. 1987. "Caregiving: The Impact on Emotional Support for Never-Married Women." *Journal of Aging Studies,* 3(1): 253-264.

Cantor, Marjorie H. 1983. "Strain Among Caregivers: A Study of Experience in the United States." *The Gerontologist,* 23: 597-603.

Caro, Francis G. 1986. "Relieving Informal Caregiver Burden Through Organized Services." In *Elder Abuse: Conflict in the Family.* Edited by Karl A. Pillemer and Rosalie S. Wolf. Dover, MA: Auburn House Publishing Co., 283-296.

Dalley, Gillian. 1988. *Ideologies of Caring: Rethinking Community and Collectivism.* London: MacMillan Education LTD.

Daniels, Norman. 1988. *Am I My Parent's Keeper?* New York: Oxford University Press.

Dunlap, Burton D. 1980. "Expanded Home-Based Care for the Impaired Elderly: Solution or Pipe Dream." *American Journal of Public Health,* 70: 514-519.

Edelman, Perry, and Hughs, Susan. 1990. "The Impact of Community Care on Provision of Informal Care to Homebound Elderly Persons." *The Journal of Gerontology,* March, 2(45): 570-588.

Eustis, Nancy; Greenberg, Jay; and Patten, Sharon. 1984. *Long-Term Care for Older Persons: A Policy Perspective.* Monterey, CA: Brooks/Cole.

Fahey, Monsignor Charles J. 1984. "National Perspectives on Issues of Long-Term Care." In *Coordinated Service Delivery Systems for the Elderly: New Approaches for Care and Referral in New York State.* Edited by Ruth Bennett, and Susana Frisch. Binghamton, NY: Haworth Press, 5-13.

Finley, Nancy; Roberts, M. Diane; and Banahan, Benjamin. 1988. "Motivators and Inhibitors of Attitudes of Filial Obligation Toward Aging Parents." *The Gerontologist,* 1(28): 73-78.

Harrington, Charlene, and Swan, James. 1985. "Institutional Long Term Care Services." In *Long Term Care of the Elderly: Public Policy Issues.* Edited by Charlene Harrison, Robert Newcomer, and Carroll Estes. Beverly Hills, CA: Sage, 153-176.

Hashimi, Joan. 1988. "U.S. Elders with Chronic Mental Disorder." In *North American Elders: United States and Canadian Perspectives.* Edited by Eloise Rathbone-McCuan and Betty Havens. Westport, CT: Greenwood Press, 123-139.

Hilker, Mary. 1987. "Families and Supportive Residential Settings as Long-Term Care Options." In *Aging, Health, and Family: Long-Term Care.* Edited by Timothy H. Brubaker. Newbury Parl, CA: Sage, 234-246.

Hooyman, Nancy R., and Lustbader, Wendy. 1986. *Taking Care: Supporting Older People and Their Families.* New York: The Free Press.

Huttman, Elizabeth D. 1985. *Social Services for the Elderly.* New York: The Free Press.

Jarrett, William H. 1985. "Caregiving Within Kinship Systems: Is Affection Really Necessary?" *The Gerontologist,* 25(1): 5-10.

Johnson, Colleen L., and Catalano, Donald J. 1983. "A Longitudinal Study of Family Supports to Impaired Elderly." *The Gerontologist,* 23: 612-628.

Johnson, Colleen, and Grant, Leslie. 1985. *The Nursing Home in American Society.* Baltimore: John Hopkins Press.

Kane, Robert L., and Kane, Rosalie. 1976. *Long-Term Care in Six Countries: Implications for the United States.* Washington, DC: U.S. Department of Health, Education, and Welfare.

Kane, Robert L., and Kane, Rosalie. 1985. *A Will and a Way: What the United States Can Learn from Canada About Caring for the Elderly.* New York: Columbia University Press.

Kayser-Jones, Jeanie Schmit. 1981. *Old, Alone, and Neglected: Care of the Aged in Scotland and the United States.* Berkeley, CA: University of California Press.

Koff, Theodore H. 1982. *Long-Term Care: An Approach to Serving the Frail Elderly.* Boston: Little, Brown, and Co.

Landsberger, Betty H. 1985. *Long-Term Care of the Elderly: A Comparative View of Layers of Care.* New York: St. Martin's Press.

Lawton, M. Powell; Moss, Miriam; and Grimes, Miriam. 1985. "The Changing Service Needs of Older Tenants in Planned Housing." *The Gerontologist,* 25: 258-264.

Lesnoff-Caravaglia, Gari. 1984. "Double Stigmation: Female and Old." In *The World of the Older Woman: Conflicts and Resolutions.* Edited by Gari Lesnoff-Caravaglia. New York: Human Sciences Press, 11-20.

Longino, Charles F. 1988. "Who Are the Oldest Americans?" *The Gerontologist,* 28(4): 515-523.

Margolis, Richard J. 1990. *Risking Old Age in America.* Boulder, Colorado: Westview Press.

Mendelson, M. A. 1974. *Tender Loving Greed: How the Incredibly Lucrative Nursing Home Industry Is Exploiting America's Old People and Defrauding Us All.* New York: Alfred A. Knopf.

Morycz, R. K. 1985. "Caregiving Strain and the Desire to Institutionalize Family Members with Alzheimer's Disease." *Research on Aging,* 7: 329-361.

Moss, Frank, and Halamandaris, Val J. 1977. *Too Old, Too Sick, Too Bad: Nursing Homes in America.* Germantown, MD: Aspen Systems Corp.

Pastalan, Leon. 1983. *Retirement Communities: An American Original.* New York: Hawthorn Books.

Pennsylvania Attorney General's Family Violence Task Force. 1988. *Violence Against Elders.* A Report to LeRoy S. Zimmerman, Attorney General, September, Harrisburg, Pennsylvania: Office of the Attorney General.

Pepper Commission, U.S. Bipartisan Commission on Comprehensive Health Care. 1990. *A Call for Action: Final Report,* September, Washington, DC: U.S. Government Printing Office.

Preston, Samuel H. 1984. "Children and the Elderly: Divergent Paths for America's Dependents." *Demography,* 4(21): 435-457.

Rathbone-McCuan, Eloise. 1984. "The Abused Older Woman: A Discussion of Abuses and Rape." In *The World of the Older Woman: Conflicts and Resolutions.* Edited by Gari Lesnoff-Caravaglia. New York: Human Sciences Press, 49-69.

Retsinas, Joan. 1986. *It's OK, Mom: The Nursing Home from a Sociological Perspective.* New York: Tiresias Press.

Rivlin, Alice M., and Wiener, Joshua. 1988. *Caring for the Disabled Elderly: Who Will Pay?* Washington, DC: Brookings Institution.

Rosenmayr, R., and Kockeis, L. 1963. "Propositions for a Sociological Theory of Aging and the Family." *International Social Review Journal,* 15: 410-426.

Rosenwaike, Ira. 1985. *The Extreme Aged in America: A Portrait of An Expanding Population.* Westport, CT: Greenwood Press.

Scharlach, Andrew E., and Boyd, Sandra. 1989. "Caregiving and Employment: Results of an Employee Study." *The Gerontologist,* 29(3): 382-387.

Service Employees International Union (SEIU). 1989. *Solutions for the New Work Force.* Cabin John, MD: Seven Locks Press.

Sommers, Tish, and Shields, Laurie. 1987. *Women Take Care: The Consequences of Caregiving in Today's Society.* Gainesville, Florida: Triad Publications.

Steinmetz, Suzanne K. 1988. *Duty Bound: Elder Abuse and Family Care.* Newbury Park, CA: Sage.

Stephens, S. A., and Christianson, T. B. 1986. *Informal Care of the Elderly.* Lexington, Mass.: Lexington Books.

Stoller, Eleanor P. 1983. "Parental Caregiving by Adult Children." *Journal of Marriage and the Family,* November, 851-858.

Stone, Leroy O., and Fletcher, Susan. 1988. "Demographic Variations in North America." In *North American Elders: United States and Canadian Perspectives.* Edited by Eloise Rathbone-McCuan and Betty Havens. Westport, CT: Greenwood Press, 9-36.

Stone, Robyn; Cafferata, Gail; and Sangl, Judith. 1987. *Caregivers of the Elderly: A National Profile.* Washington, DC: Dept. of Health and Human Services, U.S. Public Health Service.

Streib, Gordon F.; Folts, Edward W.; and Hilker, Mary Anne. 1984. *Old Homes—New Families: Shared Living for the Elderly.* New York: Columbia University Press.

U.S. House, Select Committee on Aging (HSCA). 1985. *The Rights of America's Institutionalized Aged: Lost in Confinement.* Hearings before the Subcommittee on Health and Long-Term Care, 99th Cong., 1st Sess., September 18, Washington, DC: Government Printing Office.

U.S. Senate, Special Committee on Aging, and U.S. House, Select Committee on Aging. 1989. *Board and Care: A Failure in Public Policy.* Joint Hearings before the Subcommittee on Health and Long-Term Care and the Subcommittee on Housing and Consumer Interest, 100th Cong., 1st Sess., March 9, Washington, DC: Government Printing Office.

ADDITIONAL READING

Amoss, Pamela T., and Harrell, Stevan, eds. 1981. *Other Ways of Growing Old: Anthropological Perspectives.* Stanford, CA: Stanford University Press.

Baggett, Sharon A. 1989. *Residential Care for the Elderly: Critical Issues in Public Policy.* Westport, CT: Greenwood Press.

Bennett, Ruth; Frisch, Susanna eds. 1984. *Coordinated Service Delivery Systems for the Elderly: New Approaches for Care and Referral in New York State.* New York: Haworth Press.

Bowker, Lee H. 1982. *Humanizing Institutions for the Aged.* Lexington, MA: Lexington Books.

Brocklehurst, J.C. 1975. *Geriatric Care in Advanced Societies.* Lancaster, England: Blackburn Times Press.

Brody, Elaine M. 1985. "Parent Care as a Normative Family Stress." *The Gerontologist,* 25(1): 19-29.

Brody, Elaine M. 1984. "What Should Adult Children do for their Elderly Parents?: Opinions and Preferences of Three Generations of Women." *Journal of Gerontology,* November, 39(6): 736-747.

Brown, Lynn E. 1986. "Taking in Each Other's Laundry–The Service Economy." *New England Economic Review,* July/August, 25-34.

Brubaker, Ellie. 1986. "Caring for a Dependent Spouse: Three Case Studies. *American Behavioral Scientist,* 29: 485-496.

Brubaker, Timothy, ed. 1987. *Aging, Health, and Family: Long-Term Care.* Newbury Park, CA: Sage.

Butler, Robert N., ed. 1985. *Productive Aging: Enhancing Vitality in Later Life.* New York: Springer Publishing Co.

Butler, Robert N. 1971. *Why Survive?: Being Old in America.* New York: Harper and Row.

Butler, Robert; Oberlink, Mia R.; and Schechter, Mal eds. 1990. *The Promise of Productive Aging: From Biology to Social Policy.* New York: Springer Publishing Co.

Chappell, Neena L. 1985. "Social Support and the Receipt of Home Care Services." *The Gerontologist,* 25: 47-54.

Corbin, Juliet M., and Strauss, Anselm. 1988. *Unending Work and Care: Managing Chronic Illness at Home.* San Francisco: Jossey Bass.

Coward, Raymond T., and Lee, Gary R., eds. 1985. *The Elderly in Rural Society.* New York: Springer Publishing Co.

Fry, Christine L., ed. 1980. *Aging in Culture and Society: Comparative Viewpoints and Strategies.* New York: Bergin Press.

Fry, Christine L., ed. 1981. *Dimensions: Aging, Culture, and Health.* New York: Bergin Press.

Garvin, Richard M., and Burger, Robert E. 1968. *Where They Go To Die: The Tragedy of America's Aged.* New York: Delacorte Press.

Glasscote, Raymond M., and Beigel, Allan. 1976. *Old Folks At Home: A Field Study of Nursing and Board-and-Care Homes.* Washington, DC: The Joint Information Service.

Goffman, E. 1961. *Asylums.* Garden City, New York: Doubleday Press.

Gottesman, Leonard E. 1988. "Nursing Home Performance as Related to Resident Traits, Ownership, Size, and Source of Payment." *American Journal of Public Health,* 64: 269-276.

Gubrium, Jaber F. 1988. "Family Responsibility and Caregiving in the Qualitative Analysis of the Alzheimer's Disease Experience." *Journal of Marriage and the Family,* February, 50: 197-207.

Gubrium, Jaber F. 1975. *Living and Dying at Murray Manor.* New York: St. Martin's Press.

Gwyther, Lisa P., and George, Linda K. 1986. Symposium. "Caregivers for Dementia Patients: Complete Determinants of Well-Being and Burden. Introduction." *The Gerontologist,* 26: 245-247.

Harrington, Charlene; Newcomer, Robert J.; and Estes, Carroll L., eds. 1985. *Long Term Care of the Elderly: Public Policy Issues.* Beverly Hills, CA: Sage.

Johnson, Colleen, and Catalano, Donald J. 1983. "A Longitudinal Study of Family Supports for Impaired Elderly." *The Gerontologist,* 23: 612-618.

Kamerman, Sheila B., and Kahn, Alfred J., eds. 1989. *Privatization and the Welfare State.* Princeton, NJ: Princeton University Press.

Kane, Nancy M. 1989. "The Home Care Crisis of the Nineties." *The Gerontologist,* 29(1): 24-31.

Kane, Rosalie A. 1989. "Editorial: Toward Competent, Caring Paid Caregivers." *The Gerontologist,* 29(3): 292.

Kaye, Lenard W. 1985. "Home Care for the Aged: A Fragile Partnership." *Social Work,* 30: 312-317.

Kemper, Peter. 1990. "Case Management Agency Systems of Administering Long-Term Care: Evidence from the Channeling Demonstration." *The Gerontologist,* 30(6): 817-824.

Kosberg, Jordon I. 1973. "Differences in Propietary Institutions Caring for Affluent and Nonaffluent Elderly." *The Gerontologist,* 13: 299-304.

Lang, A., and Brody, Elaine. 1983. "Characteristics of Middle-Aged Daughters and Help to Their Elderly Mothers." *Journal of Marriage and the Family,* 45: 193-202.

Lewis, Michael, and Miller, Joann L. 1984. *Research in Social Problems.* Greenwich, CT: Jai Press.

Linsk, Nathan; Keigher, Sharon M.; and Osterbusch, Suzanne E. 1988. "States' Policies Regarding Paid Family Caregiving." *The Gerontologist,* 28(2): 204-212.

Lyles, Yvonne M. 1986. "Impact of Medicare Diagnosis-Related Groups (DRGs) on Nursing Homes in the Portland, Oregon Metropolitan Area." *Journal of the American Geriatrics Society,* 34(8): 573-578.

Mitchell, Janet B. 1982. "Physician Visits to Nursing Homes." *The Gerontologist,* 22: 45-48.

Mor, Vincent; Sherwood, Sylvia; and Gutkin, Claire. 1986. "A National Study of Residential Care for the Aged." *The Gerontologist,* 26(4): 405-417.

Neuhaus, Ruby H., and Neuhaus, Robert H. 1982. *Successful Aging.* New York: Wiley and Sons.

OMB Watch. 1990. *Long-Term Care Policy: Where Are We Going?* April. Boston: University of Mass., Gerontology Institute.

Pillemer, Karl A., and Wolf, Rosalie S., eds. 1986. *Elder Abuse: Conflict in the Family.* Dover, MA: Auburn House Publishing Co.

Pinkston, Elsie, and Linsk, Nathan. 1984. *Care of the Elderly: A Family Approach.* New York: Pergamon Press.

Rathbone-McCuan, Eloise. 1982. *Isolated Elders: Health and Social Intervention.* Rockville, MO: Aspen Systems.

Rathbone-McCuan, Eloise, and Havens, Betty, eds. 1988. *North American Elders: United States and Canadian Perspectives.* Westport, CT: Greenwood Press.

Reif, Laura, and Trager, Brahna, eds. 1985. *International Perspectives on Long-Term Care*. Binghamton, NY: Haworth Press.

Rosenwaike, Ira, and Dolinsky, Arthur. 1987. "The Changing Demographic Determinants of the Growth of the Extreme Aged." *The Gerontologist*, 27: 275-280.

Saur, William J., and Coward, Raymond T., eds. 1985. *Social Support Networks and the Care of the Elderly: Theory, Research and Practice*. New York: Springer Publishing Co.

Scott, Jean Pearson, and Roberto, Karen A. 1985. "Use of Informal and Formal Support Networks by Rural Elderly Poor." *The Gerontologist*, 25: 624-630.

Seelbach, Wayne C., and Sauer, William J. 1977. "Filial Responsibility Expectations and Morale Among Aged Parents." *The Gerontologist*, 17: 492-499.

Shanas, Ethel. 1979. "The Family as a Social Support System in Old Age." *The Gerontologist*, 2(19): 169-174.

Sheild, Renee Rose. 1988. *Uneasy Endings: Daily Life in an American Nursing Home*. Ithaca, New York: Cornell University Press.

Sorkin, Alan L. 1986. *Health Care and the Changing Environment*. Lexington, MA: Lexington Press.

Tarman, Vera Ingrid. 1990. *Privatization and Health Care: The Case of Ontario Nursing Homes*. Toronto, Canada: Garamond Press.

Tobin, Sheldon S., and Lieberman, Morton A. 1976. *Last Home for the Aged*. San Francisco: Jossey-Bass Publishing Co.

U.S. House. 1987. *Prescription Drugs and the Elderly: The High Cost of Growing Old,* Hearings Before the Special Committee on Aging, 1st sess., July 20, Washington, DC: Government Printing Office.

U.S. Senate. 1990. *Aging in America: Trends and Projections,* An Information Paper to the Special Committee on Aging, February, Washington, DC: Government Printing Office.

U.S. Senate. 1986. *Nursing Home Care: The Unfinished Agenda,* An Information Paper prepared by the Staff for the Special Committee on Aging, May, Washington, DC: Government Printing Office.

Williams, G. H. 1983. "The Movement for Independent Living: An Evaluation and Critique." *Social Science and Medicine*, 15(17): 1002-1010.

Zarit, Steven H.; Todd, Pamela A.; and Zarit, Judith M. 1986. "Subjective Burden of Husbands and Wives as Caregivers: A Longitudinal Study." *The Gerontologist*, 26: 260-266.

Chapter 3

Caring for the Frail Elderly in Sweden

Gerdt Sundström
Mats Thorslund

INTRODUCTION

In terms of population, Sweden is a small country. Of its 8.5 million people, about 1.5 million or 17.8 percent are aged 65 or older; 4 percent of the population are aged 80 or older. Few other countries have such a large proportion of elderly in the population, and Sweden's average life expectancy is among the highest in the world–80.1 years for women, and 74.1 years for men.

The numbers of the very oldest in the population are continuing to rise, as they have done for some time. Those individuals aged 80 and over have increased by 31 percent since 1980. Over the next decade, the number of elderly people aged 85 to 89 years is expected to increase by over 40 percent, and those aged 90 and over by more than 75 percent.

Age is the single factor which demonstrates the strongest link with consumption of social, health, and medical services. In all probability, therefore, the increase in numbers of the very old will be accompanied by growing frailty and thus greater burdens on programs and services for the elderly.

SWEDISH OLD-AGE POLICY

Sweden has been able to provide comparatively good funding for a well-managed social welfare policy, not least in the field of old-age care. But of equally great interest are the explicit goals under which the old-age care system has operated. The most important of these are specified in the Social Services Act which went into effect in 1982. This is a framework legislation which emphasizes the right of the individual to receive municipal services at all stages of life. All those who need help for their day-to-day existence have the right to claim assistance if their needs cannot be met in any other way. The key concepts under the act are self-determination and normalization; the individual should be able to choose among various types of aid and services, while the system makes it easier for the elderly to continue living in their normal environment.

One characteristic feature of Swedish social welfare policy, distinguishing it from that of many other countries, is its general nature. A comparatively small proportion of public sector social programs are means-tested. Many forms of support are available to everyone in a given category, regardless of income. Everyone who has reached age 65 thus receives an old age pension, and everyone with children receives child allowances.

In 1983, a new Health and Medical Services Act came into effect. According to this act, health care and medical services are available to all members of society, thus ensuring a high standard of general health and care for all on equal terms. The elderly receive the necessary medical care within the publicly operated medical care apparatus and as part of the same social insurance system as younger people. Nearly all medical care is operated by public authorities, and a large proportion of doctors work in the public sector.

One important aim of Swedish old age care is to make it easier for the elderly to live independently. Comparatively generous pensions, along with housing allowances, allow retired older people to manage without other economic support from the state or their families. Although the average income of pensioners is below that of younger groups, most retirees have decent incomes and few live below the poverty level. Moreover, the great majority of elderly people in Sweden have good housing, even when there are shortages.

On average, the Swedish public sector taxes about half of a person's income. Of all public expenditures, about 33 percent goes toward social insurance and social welfare programs. This percentage now remains steady, but it climbed very rapidly during the

1970s. Of these social expenditures, in turn, more than 40 percent goes toward various types of old-age care.

The largest item is pensions, followed by housing allowances for pensioners. Old-age homes and nursing homes also are expensive, costing about four times as much as Home Help. The ratio between institutional and noninstitutional care has not changed significantly during the past 20 years.

The great majority of the Swedish population strongly supports taxation for old-age care, medical care, and related programs. When people are asked to choose between expenditures that mainly bene-fit the younger generations and those that primarily benefit the elderly, people aged 30 and upward tend to choose the latter.

THE FRAIL ELDERLY IN SWEDEN

One is hard pressed to find an unambiguous, overall indicator of frailty, as most people are affected by the standards of the environ-ment (especially by housing factors), by sex stereotypes, or by other factors that vary by culture and standards of living. For example, the inability to cook for oneself as stated by survey respondents is not well suited as a measure of frailty for international comparisons of old-age care (Habib and Sundström 1990). Some individuals have never cooked for themselves, including certain men and those people having high socioeconomic status, depending on the particu-lar country.

One indicator that has a long standing in gerontology, and that has been used in many studies, is outdoor mobility (unaided by another person). The first major international study to employ this (Shanas et al. 1968) found that between 8 percent and 14 percent of the elderly in Denmark, Britain, and the United States were frail in this sense ("housebound," including the bedfast). However, that study was confined to noninstitutionalized persons.

Using this definition, a major Swedish study in 1954 found that about 20 percent of older people, including the institutionalized, were frail. In 1977, a Stockholm study calculated that the propor-tion of frail elderly was approximately 14 percent (Fried 1979). It is possible that frailty, thus measured, has declined somewhat with new cohorts of old people having improved health and living conditions. Importantly, frail elders in Sweden have become more likely to live on their own, more so than in other countries. The changes between 1954 and 1975, the latest available major national study of frailty and living arrangements in Sweden, are depicted in Table 1.

Table 1 shows that most of the frail elderly live in their own home. Among frail elders living at home and without a spouse–a vulnerable group–a third lived together with offspring right after the war; twenty years later only a tenth did so. The most significant feature among the frail elderly is the large proportion that lives

TABLE 1. Swedish elderly* incapable of outdoor mobility,** by living arrangement (1954 and 1975).

	1954	1975
Living with their children		
Married	8%	2%
Not Married	16	5
Not living with their children		
Married	24	19
Not Married	32	44
Institutionalized	19	30
Total	100%	100%

* In 1954, age 67 and over. Represents 20 percent of the elderly population; In 1975, age 65 and over. Represents 12 percent of the elderly population.
** Totally incapable or capable only with personal support

Source: Habib and Sundström 1990.

alone, and the growth of that group. This has been made possible by raised housing standards, and by the enormous increase in home-making services (Home Help) of the welfare state. Yet, it is note-worthy that family support is most significant despite the expansion of public services.

More recent data for the total population on various aspects of frailty are given in Table 2. These data are presently available only by age groups, not by living arrangements or other factors. Obviously, a majority of the elderly are able to manage through advanced ages without the help of another person. Yet, somewhere after 80, many have problems, particularly with instrumental activities (shopping, cooking, cleaning, laundry.) But most do manage

TABLE 2. Percent of Swedish elderly* who manage daily activities on their own, by age. 1988.

ACTIVITY	65-74	75-84	85+	Total 65+
Shopping	89.8%	72.2%	40.7%	80.3%
Cooking	95.6	84.0	61.8	89.3
Cleaning	87.5	62.0	23.5	74.3
Laundry	89.3	65.9	30.4	77.1
Getting out of or into bed	99.1	97.3	93.1	98.0
Dress/undress	98.5	96.2	91.9	97.2
Toilet	99.7	98.2	95.1	98.8
Bath/shower	96.6	89.7	70.7	92.5
(N)	(824)	(622)	(283)	(1,729)

* Elderly living in their own home

Source: Statistics Sweden, (Ingrid Sjöberg), unpublished data from Undersöknin-gen av Levnadsförhållanden (ULF), 1988.

their personal care by themselves. As we will see later, they also tend to obtain any help they may need.

We may also illustrate frailty with data from a closely studied locality, Tierp (Table 3). Most of the elderly in Tierp manage indoors without problems. Many also manage outdoors, though there is a difference among the age groups. In some ways the oldest old remaining at home is a functional elite; yet some of these individuals are incapable of functioning outside the home. When they have to go outdoors they are usually helped by their children or, less commonly, by the Home Help service. In the age group 75-84, the spouse was the most important aid in outdoor activities; adult children or Home Help was much less significant (Habib and Sundström 1990; Johansson et al. 1991).

One important aspect of frailty and care is the gender dimension: most needy elders are women who are vulnerable in a number of ways. This has been explored elsewhere (Sundström 1991), but should be kept in mind. It implies, among other things, that they often have low incomes and generally live alone.

It also should be noted that cross-sectional data, such as we have been utilizing here, often provide a distorted view of what is "typical," what may be expected for any single individual, or what may be his or her real "risks". For example, dementia affects on average 5 percent of the elderly (over age 65). However, the long run risk of affliction is about 15 to 20 percent, or possibly even higher (Sundström et al. 1991).

In addition, although 5 to 6 percent of the Swedish elderly are in institutions at any one time, the long-term chance of ending up there is approximately from 25 to 30 percent (Samuelsson and Sundström 1988). We also know that, on average, about 15 percent of the elderly use Home Help, but that usage is significantly higher among certain sectors of the older population, or during specific periods of their lives.

Recent research in a small rural municipality provides evidence for understanding real institutional risks, Home Help usage, and family care. The investigator drew up a list of everyone age 55 and over who had died, and analyzed their health and care situations during the year prior to their death. Only 3 persons out of a total of 65 had died unexpectedly without any prior deterioration in their health. Fifteen percent had died in their homes, while 85 percent had died in an institution of some kind (nearly half in an acute-care ward, and the rest in an old-age home or nursing home). A quarter had been institutionalized their entire last year of life. The most common situation, however, was movement back and forth between the person's home and different institutions.

For those who had been cared for at home, families had been the significant caregivers, often supplemented by Home Help and Home Health Care. Among those who had been in their home for at least some time during their last year, 80 percent had used Home Help.

TABLE 3. Proportions with mobility problems in Tierp, 1986, by age*

Mobility Capacity	75 to 84	85 and over
Indoors		
On one's own	98.8%	98.1%
With help	0.6	0.4
Not at all	0.6	1.5
Outdoors		
On one's own	88.2	70.0
With help	9.3	13.9
Not at all	1.2	13.5
No answer	—	2.7
N	(161)	(269)

*Elderly living in their own home.

Source: The Tierp Data Base, (Thorslund 1991a), Institute for Social Medicine, University of Uppsala.

Yet, it was very unusual for Home Help to carry the total responsibility for service and care (Rinell Hermansson 1990).

VULNERABILITY–
RISING NUMBERS OF THE ELDERLY LIVE ALONE

It is not only frailty in itself that deserves attention, but also the immediate social environment of the elderly. The availability of help from a person nearby, especially a family member, is crucial in a number of ways. Although in previous works we have used coresidence of the elderly with their children as an indicator of elder care, we are now less sure about such measures. Coresidence, in fact, may indicate parental care of an offspring; the home of parents– even aging ones in the welfare state–may be a refuge for adult children who are unmarried and/or handicapped in some way (Sundström 1987). In our view, solitary living may be a better measure to employ, and usually is also somewhat easier to procure from statistical sources than data on joint residence with an offspring. Of course, living together may still provide emotional and other security to both parties.

In the Nordic countries, Denmark and Sweden have very high percentages of people age 70 and over living alone (53 percent and 46 percent, respectively), while the levels are considerably lower in Finland and Norway. In all of these countries the percentages have been rising. For example, during 1954 only 27 percent of noninstitutionalized older people age 67 and over lived alone in Sweden (Habib and Sundström 1990).

The figures are even higher for the oldest sectors of the population as well as for women. It is also noteworthy that living alone is a phenomenon that varies greatly inside each country, as shown in a recent study. Thus, in Stockholm seven out of ten women age 80 and over live alone, many of whom never married and are childless (Sundström and Berg 1990). In response to this data, it has been suggested by some policymakers that Swedish state subsidies to municipal old age care be weighted by the proportion of the aged that lives alone (Govt. Bill 1990/91:14).

In most countries the percentages are lower, ranging from 10 percent in Japan, 28 percent in Israel, and 15 to 20 percent in other

Mediterranean countries to the higher proportions in the Nordic nations discussed above. In Table 4 we provide additional comparative data, based on age and sex, for the percentages of elderly people living alone in seven countries, including Great Britain, Ireland, Finland, France, The Netherlands, Poland, and Sweden.

Obviously, this secular trend toward more solitary households will add heavily to "external" care needs among the future elderly in many countries. The relationship of these changes in household structure–often desired by both generations–to emergent needs for social services often has been overlooked. For example, Japan has 12 million older people compared to only 1.5 million elderly in Sweden, yet there are only a few hundred thousand more such individuals living alone in the former nation. These differences must be considered when patterns of care and provision of public support are analyzed.

HOME HELP SERVICES

For those needy elderly living alone in Sweden, Home Help is the primary formal support system. In fact, nearly 90 percent of the Home Help clients live by themselves. Significantly, the number of Home Help recipients grew rapidly in the 1960s and 1970s and more than tripled between 1964 and 1980. Lately, the tendency has been to give more home help to fewer clients, with emphasis on the oldest (aged 80 and over) and presumably the neediest. Currently, about 15 percent of the elderly population age 65 and over receives regular Home Help (Thorslund 1991b).

The municipal social service agencies are responsible for supplying Home Help services, which include shopping, cleaning, cooking, washing, and personal hygiene, to those elderly persons living at home who cannot cope on their own. The Home Help services as well as the health care and medical services provided by the county councils are heavily subsidized; the recipient pays only a fraction of the actual cost (usually 5 to 10 percent). As a precondition for receipt of such care and service, the older person must demonstrate a need.

The decision-making process in the care of the elderly in Sweden is highly decentralized. Quite often a single social worker (who may lack both professional qualifications and experience in assessing old people's needs) has to decide whether an elderly person requires Home Help and what the suitable number of hours should be (Thorslund and Johansson 1987). Practically all assessments appear to be subjective. Standardized scales are seldom used, and rarely are attempts made to define "need."

Despite these problems, the general consensus is that the home helpers do an excellent job and are apparently of vital importance to certain categories of elderly people. The availability of home helpers has allowed such individuals to manage autonomously in a dignified manner in their own homes, despite their advancing physical frailty.

In deciding the amount of Home Help a person needs, the social worker has to take a variety of factors into account, including age,

TABLE 4. Elderly people living alone, in seven countries, by age and sex (in percentages)

Age	Males							Females						
	a	b	c	d	e	f	g	a	b	c	d	e	f	g
65-69	12	13	13	11	9	8	21	32	18	37	31	30	26	41
70-74	19	15	17	14	12	12		42	24	46	39	40	30	
75-79	25	15	24	18	21	10	33	53	23	51	48	40	28	66
80-84	33			23							53			
85+				29				60			51			

Key to Column Heading: a. Great Britain, 1983; b. Ireland, 1979; c. Finland, 1980; d. France, 1982; e. Netherlands, 1981; f. Poland, 1978; g. Sweden, 1988-1989

Note: Swedish data include institutionalized elders (counted as living alone).

Source: a-f from Wall 1988.
g by courtesy of Statistics Sweden (Ingrid Sjöberg), based on Undersökningen Levnadsförhållanden (ULF) 1988-1989.

gender, marital status, living circumstances, ability to perform certain personal care and household tasks, physical and mental state, and the possibility of receiving help from relatives, friends, and neighbors. As can be expected, both official statistics and several studies show that the propensity to use Home Help is strongly correlated with these factors. In fact, many of these variables themselves are highly interrelated. For example, two studies estimated through multivariate analysis the net effects of different predictors on the use of Home Help at the individual level. They found that the two most important correlates of Home Help use were Instrumental Activities of Daily Living Limitations and living alone (Sundström 1983, Thorslund, Norström, and Wernberg 1991).

In a separate analysis by gender, the studies disclosed that disability weighs somewhat more for women, while living alone was a more important factor for men. Home Help thus appears to be a "health" service for women, and a "social" service for men (Sundström 1983; Thorslund, Norström, and Wernberg 1991). Living alone relates significantly to Home Help usage when utilizing aggregate macrodata as well: the rate of single households for the elderly is strongly correlated with Home Help coverage ratios among Swedish municipalities (Sundström and Berg 1990).

Interestingly, the evidence indicates that social class does not influence the provision and/or use of homemaking services in Sweden. To be sure, elderly members of the working class use the services more often and get more hours per recipient, but this is due to their greater frailty (they also die earlier), not to their social class. When comparing elderly of the same health, we find that the differences between classes vanish. (The same has been shown in Danish, Norwegian, and British studies–see Sundström 1992 and Hunt 1970.)

Regional variations are large in Sweden. On average, over 40 percent of the oldest age group (80+) received homemaking services at least once during 1989. However, one municipality provided as many as 72 percent of this age group with services; another municipality supplied as little as 19 percent of the total (SCB 1990). While the proportion of the elderly that lives alone is a significant predictor of Home Help service coverage, the percentage of older people in the municipality is strongly related to the total amount of old-age care.

Regional and economic factors explain part of the variation as well. Contrary to what one may expect, the rural and poor municipalities provide more services than do other areas. This is possible due to the tax redistribution system operating among municipalities in Sweden. Moreover, service differences are not based on the political composition of municipalities, indicating a consensus on old-age care in Sweden; the country's relative homogeneity probably plays a role as well (Berg and Sundström 1989).

OTHER COMMUNITY-BASED SERVICES

Aside from the home helper service, nearly all municipalities offer a number of other types of noninstitutional old-age care services that are either not subject to a needs assessment or less so than the home helper service. Some are provided in elderly people's homes, some in district day centers.

One of the most extensively used public amenities for pensioners is the on-call municipal transport service. Most often, it involves travel in an ordinary taxi at greatly reduced prices. The system is state subsidized, exists in all municipalities, and is used by a substantial percentage of the elderly. Interview studies show that 11 percent of those aged 60 to 84 and 23 percent of those aged 80 to 84 had recently made use of the transport service. Older people with limited mobility or with vision problems obviously use the transport service more often: the figures were 37 percent and 49 percent, respectively.

Another municipal service, chiropody, is used by more than 10 percent of the elderly. The cost is somewhat below the open market level for the same service. Food service, which is used by about 3 percent of the elderly, is available at district day centers and sometimes in school cafeterias at subsidized prices. Very few (1 percent) take advantage of meals-on-wheels; it is more common for a Home Helper to do the cooking in the elderly person's own home, which is considered a better alternative. Hairdressing is another service used by very few (two percent). Considering the climate in Sweden, it should perhaps be noted that many municipalities provide subsidized snowclearing services for pensioners.

District day centers are an important part of the public sector's old-age care programs. Eight out of ten municipalities have such centers, and they are open to all pensioners. Most of them are located in service buildings, while some have an independent location. There are no statistics on the percentage of elderly people who use the 1,000 or so day centers, but an educated guess would be one pensioner out of twenty.

The most important activity at the centers appears to be simply maintaining social contacts, aside from the hobby programs available. Many day centers also have public baths, hairdressing, chiropody, gymnastics, cafeterias, excursion programs, and the like. However, healthy pensioners appear to be taking over the centers at the expense of those who are frail.

SERVICE APARTMENTS

Housing, along with economic resources, are major factors in the ability of the elderly to live independently. Most of the elderly in Sweden live in "ordinary" dwellings. However, 2 percent of pensioners live in service apartments owned and managed by the municipality.

These sheltered accomodations are in buildings containing 20 to 100 housing units, most of which were built during the 1970s and 1980s. The availability of service apartments, allocation policies, and thus the age and fitness range of the occupants, vary among the municipalities. Overall, tenants tend to be pensioners who have ordinary rent contracts with the local authority; they pay market rents and are eligible for municipal housing allowances.

The apartments consist of from one to three rooms plus a kitchen and bathroom. Subsidized municipal Home Help is obtainable by residents (after means testing) in the same way as it is available to those living in ordinary homes. These services are provided by staff members who perform the same function as the municipal Home Helper.

DO THE FRAIL ELDERLY IN SWEDEN GET THE HELP THEY NEED?

There are stereotypes, especially among professionals in the social services and in the health care sector, that many needy elderly are left unaided or get very unsatisfactory care. Although there may be some neglected frail elderly, such situations are not widespread nor are they increasing.

Recent studies indicate that over the last several decades fewer of the aged are isolated or face unmet needs for care (Sundström 1983; Jonsson and Lundberg 1984). A number of local and national studies have found that very few of the aged have unsatisfied needs for help and support. Nationwide surveys disclose that only 4 percent of the married (or otherwise coresident aged) and 7 percent of those who live alone need help but do not get it (43 percent and 31 percent, respectively, manage without any help at all) (Sjöberg 1985).

Despite the large variations in public services (and single households) among geographic areas, research shows that there are only small local differences in unmet needs. Moreover, a dearth of services in some areas has not meant that elderly persons live in neglect and misery. To some degree this may be explained by mechanisms of adaptation. The more important reason, however, is that even in the welfare state the family is still the most important provider of care and therefore is likely to act as a "buffer," compensating for services not publicly provided (Sundström 1986; Hokenstad and Johansson 1990).

A major question that arises when discussing unmet needs is whether we know exactly who should be receiving care. Similarly, we must address the issue of whether services are actually provided to those most in need. Table 5 gives a panorama of the supply of public care and services to the elderly in the municipality of Jönköping.

Jönköping is at the national Swedish average in its provision of both institutional and noninstitutional types of care for the elderly. For those noninstitutionalized elderly who use Home Help, one study in Jönköping found that nearly all get the help they need, both according to their own definition and by assessments done by the Home Help supervisor and the field worker. Further, most of the clients express subjective satisfaction with the services they receive (Sundström and Cronholm 1988).

Another study of older people aged 84 to 90 in the same municipality also disclosed that there are very few unmet needs for help

(OCTO-project, unpublished). About a third of the total receive no public support: they either do not require any help at all or get what they need solely from their family.

Additional research has addressed the issue of health visits, utilizing data from the municipality of Tierp. Swedish legislation on health care and the social services states that it is the task of the authority responsible for a particular service to ensure that the needs of the entire local population are satisfied. Yet, very few systematic health visits or other outreach activities to probe potential needs actually occur. Consequently, it is not entirely clear whether all those in need are being served. Are there hidden needs in the elderly population? If such needs come to the attention of the social services or the health services, could they be satisfied? As mentioned,

TABLE 5. Provision of different kinds of public care for the old-old (80+) in the municipality of Jönköping, 1988. (in percentages)

Receipt of Home Help	Place of Residence	
	Long-Term Care (Nursing Home)	6
	Old Age Home	12
Home Help, Lives at Home	Service Apartment (Municipal)	7
	Private Dwelling	35
No Home Help, Lives at Home	Private Dwelling, No Home Help but Home Health Care	2
	No Service Use at all	38
Total		100%

Source: Adapted from Sundström and Cronholm 1988.

unmet needs are still small. Cutbacks in social services now taking place may well change that, and closer monitoring of service provision might be needed in the future.

Actual service patterns in Tierp are shown in Table 6. Approximately one-third of the group aged 75 to 84 and just over half of the oldest age group received at least one hour of Home Help in 1986. One-third of the 75 to 84 age group and approximately one-half of the 85 and over age group received home visits from the District or Assistant Nurse. Almost half of the 75 to 84 age group and four-fifths of the oldest group received Home Help from the social services and/or a home visit from the District/Assistant Nurse.

Local contact with care services varied considerably within the municipality. The proportion of the very oldest age group (85+) who received Home Help during the year ranged from 36 percent to 91 percent among the different parishes. The chance of having received a home visit from the District/Assistant Nurse also differed

TABLE 6. Proportion of elderly who received some type of home visit, Tierp 1986. Non-institutionalized elderly.

Age	75-85 (N=1.448) %	85+ (N=260) %
Visit from:		
Home Help	37	56
*District/Assistant Nurse	32	51
Evening/Night patrol	4	10
Some form of home visit	47	79

* Home Health Care is provided by District and/or Assistant Nurses

Source: The Tierp Data Base (Thorslund 1991,a)

greatly; the likelihood of having had at least one visit in 1986 was twice as great in one parish as in another. However, some of the discrepancy disappears when all types of visits are taken into account. For example, a low number of visits by the District/Assistant Nurse tends to be offset by a high number of visits from the Home Help services, and vice versa. It was also found that most of the needy elderly had some form of contact with a doctor, usually at the local health center. A few minor, untreated medical problems were detected in systematic home visits to all elderly persons, but all major problems were already under "supervision" (Thorslund 1991a.).

In terms of actual service provision, the rural municipality of Tierp conforms to the national pattern. A majority of those elderly age 75 and over who require assistance with activities such as shopping, cooking, cleaning, and outdoor mobility receive Home Help. For example, 74 percent of those elderly age 75 to 84 incapable of shopping by themselves, and 88 percent of those age 85 and over, rely on Home Help for some aid. Thus, most of the needy elderly do receive practical help with homemaking from the welfare state (Thorslund 1991a).

WHO ARE THE CAREGIVERS?

This section will provide a more comprehensive picture of the pattern of caregiving in Sweden. Table 7, which uses recent data from nationwide surveys describing the frail elderly, shows the types of help the elderly receive for specific tasks. In particular, such assistance is broken down into formal services (Home Help), informal sources (spouse, adult children, other family members), and a combination of the two.

The most extensive formal input is with house cleaning and bathing (45 percent and 41 percent, respectively); help with these tasks is almost evenly balanced between formal and informal care. Aid for other Activities of Daily Living (ADL)-needs, on the other hand, is two to three times more likely to be provided informally than through Home Help. Combined efforts, which occur less than 15 percent of the time for all activities, are most frequent for shopping and dressing/undressing, cooking and getting out of bed. One

TABLE 7. Help received by frail elderly, by activity and primary caregiver.
Non-institutionalized elderly (65+) in Sweden, 1988.

Carer, primary

Activity	Formal	Infor-mal	Com-bined	Other	No Answer	Total	(N)
Instru-mental ADL							
Shopping	22	61	11	6	—	100%	361
Cooking	21	59	8	12	0.4	100	202
Cleaning	45	45	6	3	1.4	100	469
Laundry	19	70	4	7	0.3	100	417
Basic ADL							
Getting out of bed	32	59	7	2	—	100	37
Dress/ Undress	25	61	12	2	—	100	52
Toilet visits	33	60	4	4	—	100	23
Bath/ Shower	41	52	3	2	1.6	100	146

Source: Statistics Sweden, Undersökningen av Levnadsförnhållanden (ULF) 1988.
Reproduced from Johansson, Thorslund, Smedby, and Wernberg 1991.

implication is that the welfare state has only "taken over" marginal aspects of the frail elderly's everyday needs.

Even if illustrative, these figures do not provide information on the volume of care efforts, an extremely difficult factor to assess. Typically, the amount of time spent on care has been used as the yardstick. Previous estimates have placed the ratio between formal and informal care in the Nordic countries between 1:4 and 1:3 (Tid för omsorg 1982; Lingsom 1985).

Swedish data both from the nationwide survey and from the more closely observed local cases such as Tierp indicate that about a third of all care provided to the frail elderly living in their own homes is formal. Two-thirds is provided by family and other informal care-givers (Johansson and Thorslund 1991). Data for public service provision is more reliable than that for informal care; it is likely that informal caregivers do even more than estimated here. Moreover, formal care tends to be used primarily by those frail elderly who either lack family and/or who live alone.

When family is available, a lesser percentage of older people use Home Help, and when they do, they benefit from fewer hours. Even so, the formal care may have great symbolic importance and give needed relief to caregivers.

In this context we may also mention the Swedish programs for support to caring family members. Though they encompass only minor fractions of these caregiver–between 1 and 10 percent in various communities–they are still significant. Support for caring families is an official objective of elder care.

The largest program allows a family member the option of employment as a Home Helper for his or her frail kin. Initiated in the 1960s, mainly to ameliorate conditions for unmarried women caring for their parents, it has declined in scope; currently the program utilizes 7,000 helpers, and covers 2 percent of all Home Help clients (Sundström 1986).

A second program, which was put into effect at the end of 1989, provides up to 30 days of paid leave (based on sick pay through the National Health Insurance) to care for someone "near" (not necessarily a blood relative). In practice it has been limited in scope and used primarily for terminal care patients, who stay in their own homes.

Finally, we need to address more specifically the issue of who are the caregivers. We know, for example, that at any given time about 4 percent of all adults in Sweden are caring for about 8 percent of the adult population who are functionally impaired in some way. About half of these recipients are elderly.

Supplementing this information with a longitudinal, local study, we estimate that about one-fifth of the oldest population had, at one time, provided care to at least one parent. A nationwide survey in Norway has indicated similar conclusions. More recently, we asked similar questions about caregiving to a sample of very old people in Jönköping, shown in Table 8. Since requirements for who was counted as a caregiver were stricter than for previous studies, the percentages responding positively are lower. However, the patterns remain constant. Among women, 31 percent provided care at some time during their adult life, usually to a parent or a spouse. Moreover, a fifth of these women cared for more than one person. Only 17 percent of older men reported a similar experience of caregiving to at least one person. Overall, a quarter of all older people provided care at some time, many of them in very demanding situations. There is a paucity of solid research on the consequences of this for caregivers. In any case, we warn against exaggerating the negative outcomes.

Available studies clearly indicate that women have been caregivers more frequently than men. Yet, when it comes to marital relationships, men may attend to spouses in need nearly as often as women. To be sure, women take on such caregiving responsibilities twice as often as men (14 percent and 8 percent, respectively). Yet, this may be more a matter of demography than of anything else. In Sweden, the statistical risk of a married person becoming widowed is three times higher for women than for men at any age. Prior to the spouse's death there is likely to be a period of frailty. As there are more married elderly men than women, the actual number of the former engaging in caregiving for a spouse is somewhat equivalent to that of the latter. These factors may explain much of the gender difference in spousal care, rather than significant disparities in care "morale" (Sundström 1992; Arber and Gilbert 1989).

INSTITUTIONAL CARE

In earlier decades, an institutional approach dominated public care for the aged who could not cope for themselves in their own

TABLE 8. Caregiving experience among those elderly 84 to 90 years old, Jönköping, 1987 (in percentages)

Caregiving experience	Women	Men	Total
No extensive caregiving experience	69%	83%	74%
Caregiving experience	31	17	26
Cared for			
Mother/father	16	8	13
Parents in law	4	1	3
Spouse	14	8	11
Handicapped offspring	3	1	2
Other person(s)	8	2	6
Number of people cared for			
One	24	15	21
Two	3	2	3
Three	—	—	—
Four	1	—	1
Five	2	—	1
Total experience of care	31	17	26
(N)	(161)	(93)	254)

Source: The OCTO-Project 1992, Institute of Gerontology, Jönköping.

homes. Even during the 1950s and 1960s, due to government subsidies and policies, the number and proportion of the elderly Swedish population living in institutions rose.

Since the late 1970s, public policies have come to stress the importance of older people staying in their own homes, this being the most humane and also the most economical approach. There is general agreement among those agencies responsible for social welfare and care that the majority of institutions for the old (and also for other groups) should be closed down and replaced by more help in a home environment.

Institutional old-age care is the responsibility of both municipalities and county councils. Municipalities operate old-age homes for healthy elderly people who nevertheless have a hard time managing autonomously in their own homes. The construction of old age homes started to decline during the 1970s and almost completely ceased during the following decade. Part of the resulting loss of beds is being replaced by service apartments. By 1988 there were some 900 municipal institutions with 44,000 places.

The function of these facilities has changed as well, from literally "a home" to a provider of short-term care at the very end of life; more and more people live their last days in old-age homes, but they begin doing so later and later in life and live in them for shorter and shorter average periods. In fact, every year the average age of the residents rises. Simultaneously, these facilities are now trying to become more homelike.

The care of elderly people with illnesses, on the other hand, is provided by county council nursing homes and geriatric departments; these are referred to collectively as the long-term care system. The aim of geriatric departments, which are often linked to hospitals, is to rehabilitate and allow the elderly patient to return home as soon as possible. Such departments also offer opportunity for relief care, whereby the patient is admitted for a certain time to allow the family taking care of the patient at home to have some relief. They also provide respite care, when patients spend certain regular fixed periods in the department.

Nursing home residents tend to be older people with incurable illnesses or those who have undergone complete treatment and whose physical and/or mental capacity is reduced. These facilities are more anonymous than the old-age homes and offer less privacy. However, in many places there are efforts underway to make long-term care facilities more homelike such as letting people bring their own furniture.

In Sweden, as in the rest of the Nordic region, virtually all institutional care of the elderly takes place in publicly owned and operated facilities, unlike the situation in many other countries. This has been the case for centuries, although privately owned institutions used to be a little more common (mainly operated by charitable and religious organizations). The monthly fees charged by old-age homes are income-related.

It should be noted that a significant number of institutionalized older people have very weak family ties, are childless, or have never married. Moreover, the same percentage of the elderly (regardless of age category) live in institutions in Sweden and the United States, as well as other Western countries. One would expect otherwise: that the expansion of Home Helper services and other support for independent living in Sweden would mean that fewer people moved into institutions. Of those aged 65 and above in Sweden, 5 percent live in institutions. Of those aged 80 or more, the figure is about 25 percent. One interpretation of this might be that noninstitutionalized old-age care has not significantly increased the number of elderly people who remain in their own homes, but instead has improved their living conditions during the period while they still live at home.

THE FUTURE OF CARING FOR FRAIL ELDERS

The evidence strongly suggests that informal and formal caregivers manage to provide more care for the frail elderly today than ever before. Even if the expansion of public services shows that more old persons receive some aid, most of the care, past and present, is still undertaken by family members.

The expenditure levels for public services such as elder care tend to be dependent on taxes and economic growth. Since the latter continues to be relatively slow, and tax rates are impossible to raise politically, there is little possibility that the public provision of care in Sweden will expand. At best, we may expect to maintain social services at current levels.

However, the total service and care needs of the elderly are going to increase more quickly than the resources of the welfare state's services for the elderly. What are some of the possible consequences? More relatives than today will provide care as it becomes harder to obtain services from the public sector. Although many relatives had not been planning to become caregivers, they may adapt naturally to the new situation. On the other hand, others will experience this new and unexpected role at least partly as a burden. Women will be particularly encumbered, hindering many of them from gainful employment (Thorslund 1991b). We foresee that the actual responsibility for an elderly person in need of help and supervision will be shouldered even more than today by informal caregivers.

It also will be necessary to make tougher decisions about priorities within the public sector. Already certain groups, namely the single elderly, are given precedence (Sundström 1983, Thorslund 1991b; Thorslund, Norström, and Wernberg 1991). It can be expected that this trend will strengthen. Efforts should be made by the public sector to encourage and support families who are willing and able to give help rather than to focus predominantly on elderly persons without families.

In addition, the privately organized sector can be expected to expand. For example, construction companies are at present showing considerable interest in building private "service houses." (There are also a number of cooperative "service houses" under construction.) Desperate staff in overcrowded hospital wards are undoubtedly going to encourage those patients with sufficient financial resources to apply for private care in order to be able to concentrate on or give priority to those patients who cannot afford such alternative forms of aid.

Because of the strong expansion of public sector services and care hitherto, the demand for private alternatives has not been particularly great. Over recent years, however, long waiting lists have begun to form in many parts of the country, both for various kinds of institutions such as service houses and nursing homes, and for surgery using the latest medical technology, such as hip replacement, cataract, and heart by-pass operations. Private alternatives for those patients who are prepared to pay are starting to appear. This is, of course, a development which will be accompanied by increasing inequities between society's "haves" and "have nots."

The expansion of the private sector does not necessarily mean that total care resources will increase. Staff availability will continue to be restricted, at least for the near future. The development of private sector care will, to a large extent, be achieved by recruiting staff from the public sector. Consequently, even harsher priority decisions will have to be made in the public sector. This, in turn, can lead to increased demand for private alternatives.

Home Help service jobs (as well as those in institutions) in Sweden, as elsewhere, are nearly exclusively women's work. They are also on the lowest rungs of the pay scale and low-status positions. Work conditions are perceived as unattractive (though there are contrasting opinions) and most Helpers work part-time by choice. Usually the service is short of staff, only lately improved through the slight rise in unemployment presently faced by Sweden. Another factor influencing the scarcity of personnel is the relatively small birth cohorts in the age groups that tend to work as Home Helpers.

Some analysts are arguing for the development of nonfamily and nonpublic forms of care such as elders providing help to each other, collectives, and self-help groups (Berglind et al. 1991). These initiatives may well postpone some dependency on family and public resources, and provide other kinds of very significant support, but in our opinion they will not sufficiently care for the very frail population.

To sum, as in other nations, there is a growing number of very old people in Sweden. The frail among them will be a growing challenge especially to the formal system of care and to their families. We will also see a growth of alternatives that up to now have been relatively uncommon in the Swedish welfare state. We foresee, as well, that families will have to take on greater tasks in the future. If they cannot do so, there is a very real risk of misery on the part of frail elders, a suffering unknown among contemporary older people.

REFERENCES

Arber, Sarah, and Gilbert, Nigel. 1989. Transitions in caring: Gender, life course and care of the elderly. In *Becoming and Being Old. Sociological Approaches to Later Life*, edited by Bytheway, Bill; Keil, Teresa; Allat, Patricia; and Bryman, Alan. Sage, London, 72-92.

Berg, Stig, and Sundström, Gerdt. 1989. *Kommunal och regional variation inom äldreomsorgen.* Rapport 70, Institutet för gerontologi, Jönköping.

Berglind, Hans; Harriman, Siv; Jansson, Kjell; and Sohlberg, Sune. 1991. Gentjänstenen–möjlighet för svensk älde-omsorg! Socialförvaltningen, Lidingö. Mimeo.

Fried, Robert. 1979. *De äldres levnadsförhållanden i Stockholm*, USK 1979:8, Stockholmskommun, Stockholm.

Habib, Jack, and Sundström, Gerdt. 1990. *Understanding the Pattern of Support for the Elderly: A Comparison Between Israel and Sweden*. Manuscript.

Hokenstad, Merl C., and Johansson, Lennarth. 1990. Caregiving for the elderly in Sweden: Program challenges and policy initiatives. In *Aging and Caregiving: Theory, Research and Policy*, edited by Biegel, David E. and Blum, Arthur. Sage, CA.

Hunt, Audrey. 1970. The Home Help Service in England and Wales, Her Majesty's Stationery Office, London.

Johansson, Lennarth, and Thorslund, Mats. 1991. Care Needs and Sources of Support in a Nationwide Sample of Elderly in Sweden. *Zeitschrift för Gerontologie*. In press.

Johansson, Lennarth; Thorslund, Mats; Smedby, Björn; and Wernberg, Kerstin. 1991. Formal and informal support among elderly in a rural setting in Sweden. *Journal of Gerontological Social Work*. In press.

Jonsson, Janne, and Lundberg, Olle. 1984. *De äldre i välfärden*. Institutet för social forskning, Stockholm.

Lingsom, Susan. 1985. *Uformell omsorg for syke og eldre*. Statistisk sentralbyrå. Samfunnsekonomiske Studier 57, Oslo.

Octo-project. 1992. Tabulations from the first waves of the OCTO-Data Base, Institute of Gerontology Jönköping, unpublished mimeo.

Rinell Hermansson, Alice. 1990. *Det sista året*. Uppsala, Diss.

Samuelsson, Gillis and Sundström, Gerdt 1988. Ending one's life in a nursing home. A note on Swedish findings. *International Journal of Aging & Human Development*, Vol 27 (2),81-88.

SCB (Statistics Sweden). 1990. *Statistiska Meddelanden* SM S 9001, Social hemtjänst 1989.

Shanas, Ethel, ed. 1968. *Old People in Three Industrial Societies*. London.

Sjöberg, Ingrid. 1988. Statistics Sweden, Undersökningen av Levnadsförhållanden (ULF), Stockholm.

Sjöberg, Ingrid. 1985. *Pensionärer*, Rapport 43, Undersökningen av Levnadsförhållanden (ULF), SCB, Stockholm.

Sundström, Gerdt. 1983. *Caring for the aged in welfare society*. Stockholms Studies in Social Work 1. Stockholm.

Sundström, Gerdt. 1986. Family and state: Recent trends in the care of the aged in Sweden. *Aging and Society*, 6, 169-196.

Sundström, Gerdt. 1987. A haven in a heartless world? Living with parents in Sweden and the United States 1880-1982. *Continuity and Change*, Vol. 2, No. 1, 145-187.

Sundström, Gerdt, and Cronholm, Inger. 1988. *Hemtjänsten: de äldsta vårdta-

garna och omsorgsapparaten, Rapport 68, Institutet för gerontologi, Jönköping.

Sundström, Gerdt, and Berg, Stig. 1990. Ensamboende bland äldre: en analys av kommunala variationer och deras effekter på äldreomsorgen, PM till Äldredelegationen, Socialdeparte mentet.

Sundström, Gerdt. 1991. Psykisk ohälsa på ålderdomen inte bara demens, *Läkartidningen* 10, 863-866.

Sundström, Gerdt. 1992. Omsorgsmönster bland äldre kvinnor och män i Norden. In *Gamle Kuinner,* edited by Helset, Anne. Nordenderes liv i tekst og tall. Nordic Council of Ministers and Institute of Gerontology, Oslo.

Swedish Government Bill. 1990/1991: 14.

Thorslund, Mats. 1991a. Are special health visits for the elderly needed? Tierp Data Base, unpublished.

Thorslund, Mats. 1991b. The increasing number of very old people will change the Swedish model of the welfare state. *Social Science and Medicine,* 32, 455-464.

Thorslund, Mats, and Johansson, Lennarth. 1987. Elderly people in Sweden: Current realities and future plans. *Aging and Society,* 7, 345-355.

Thorslund, Mats; Norström, Thor, and Wernberg, Kerstin. 1991. The utilization of home help: A multivariate analysis. *The Gerontologist,* 31, 116-119.

Tid för omsorg. 1982. Slutrapport från projektet Omsorgen i samhället, Stockholm.

Wall, Richard. 1988. The living arrangements of the elderly in Europe in the 1980s. In *Becoming and Being Old. Sociological Approaches to Later Life,* edited by Bytheray, Bill; Keil, Teresa; Allat, Patricia; and Bryman, Alan. Sage, London.

Chapter 4

New Challenges for Elder Care in Finland

Riitta-Liisa Heikkinen

INTRODUCTION

One of the chief goals of the Western welfare state is to enhance the well-being of its citizens and to promote justice and equality in society. These objectives are pursued by aiming to reduce income differentials and to provide basic security for all citizens through social welfare and health care services (Julkunen 1990).

In Finland, which today ranks among one of the most affluent western states, social welfare and health care are administered at the national level by the Ministry of Social Affairs and Health. The Ministry's chief responsibility is to promote the social, psychic, and physical well-being of all citizens, and in this way to guarantee them a decent human existence. It also bears responsibility for the preparation of legislative reforms, for resource policy, and for the administration of social security. Assisting the Ministry in these tasks are a number of central offices and various organizations with specific areas of expertise. Two central offices, the National Board of Health and the National Board of Social Welfare, were united on the first of March 1991.

For the purpose of regional administration, Finland is divided into twelve provinces. The provincial administrations, and their social and health departments, guide and supervise welfare and health services within their respective areas. Local government is in the hands of 460 communes (towns or rural communes) which provide most of the social and health care services. Small communes form federations to run health care jointly. The state subsidizes approximately half of all social and health costs borne by the communes. Currently, the Gross Domestic Product (GDP) ratio of public and social expenditure in Finland approximates the average level of Western European countries.

One of the most important target groups for welfare services in Finland is the elderly. All older people are provided with basic income security through the national pension scheme, while the aim of social services is to help the aged cope independently in the community. The focus of health care is on maintaining their health and functional ability.

From the mid-nineteenth century until 1950, the relative size of the elderly population (65 years and over) remained more or less unchanged in Finland; during this period the growth of the elderly population was only marginally faster than the growth rate for the whole population. Since 1950, the number of older people has been increasing at an accelerating rate, reaching 12.7 percent of the total population of some five million in 1988. Current prognoses are that by the year 2030, the aged will represent 25 percent of the Finnish populace, which is almost four times higher than in 1950 (Valkonen and Nikander 1990). These predictions mean that in 2030 there will be around 1.1 million elderly people in Finland, up from just over 660,000 in 1989; people in the age group 75-84 numbered around 230,000 and those 85 or over 50,000. Since mortality among men is higher than among women, the proportion of men in the oldest age groups is markedly lower than the proportion of women: in 1985, for instance, men represented less than one-third of the age group 80-84 years. However, it is expected that this imbalance will be somewhat reduced in the future because of the growing number of males who reach a high age (Valkonen and Nikander 1990), chiefly as a result of lowered mortality through the reduction of cardiovascular diseases. In 1988, life expectancy at birth was 78.7 years for Finnish women and 70.7 years for men.

A crucial factor related to the coping ability and quality of life of elderly people is whether they live alone or with their spouse, children, or others. In 1985, 34 percent of the aged population in Finland lived alone (Valkonen and Nikander 1990). This figure has gradually increased since 1960, when only one-fifth of the population aged 65 and over lived alone. There are two main reasons for this development: first, the changing age structure within the oldest age groups and, second, the fact that fewer and fewer people live with their adult children (Valkonen and Nikander 1990), particularly in urban areas.

It is difficult to say exactly how the needs for care and treatment of the elderly population are going to develop over the next 25 years. For instance, while the growing number of old people living alone has increased the need for outside help and care, it is hard to tell whether this trend will continue in the future. What we can predict with reasonable certainty is a continuing increase in the proportion of divorced people. At the same time, the number of widowed women living alone may begin to decline with the increasing mean age of men.

In 1989, over 30 percent of the aged female population was married; the figure for men age 65 and over was a considerably higher 71 percent. Approximately half of the women in this age group were widows, while among men 16.5 percent had lost their spouse. Eight percent of the males in this age group had never married, as opposed to approximately 13 percent of women. Among aged males about 5 percent and among aged females approximately 6.5 percent were divorced. (Väestö 1990).

Following a sharp increase in divorce rates in the mid-1960s, every third marriage in Finland now results in divorce. No changes are expected in overall divorce rates in the near future. However, in the older age groups we will probably see quite dramatic changes: while the elderly of today do not belong to what is commonly known as the "divorce generation," the future elderly do; therefore, the number of divorced elderly people is bound to increase. On the other hand, remarriage as well as open marriage are becoming increasingly common even among the elderly.

Developments over the last several years suggest that there might be some improvement in the health and functional ability of the elderly, indicating that the demand for care by the youngest older people will be somewhat reduced. (Heikkinen 1987). Services may be needed mostly by those at the more advanced ages. On the other hand, detrimental health habits such as smoking and alcohol consumption have recently been increasing, especially among women, and this may lead to increased morbidity (Svanborg 1988a, 1988b). It is also difficult to predict the future course of cancer morbidity in the elderly; one rather disturbing factor is the growth of new environmental hazards. In any event, although the aging of the population will increase the need for care and treatment, it is going to become more difficult to evaluate the precise requirements for future care.

CURRENT USE OF HEALTH CARE SERVICES BY THE ELDERLY

The health care system in Finland is hierarchically organized. The patient must first apply to a local health center or private doctor for examination and treatment. Patients who cannot be treated at this level will be referred to the outpatient department of a hospital and, if necessary, admitted to a hospital. In acute cases, patients apply directly to a hospital policlinic. Community health centers mainly provide general practice (GP) services, though they are additionally responsible for preventive health care and for the provision of home nursing services. Communes and federations of communes also run their own hospitals.

Finland has 21 central hospital districts for specialist treatment. In each district there is a central hospital, a mental hospital, and other hospital beds. In 1986 the total number of hospital beds in Finland per 1,000 inhabitants was 13.9. In comparison with other western countries, this ratio is roughly the same as in Sweden and lower than that in Norway and Japan.

Often suffering from multiple illnesses and impaired functional ability, elderly people are frequent users of health care services. In 1988, the costs of treatment for elderly people aged 65 and over represented 47.1 percent of total health care expenditure. Of all patients admitted to the hospital in 1988, 62.9 percent were in this age group; the respective figure for the use of outpatient services was 14.8 percent. In cost terms, the elderly population accounted for 59.3 percent of hospital treatment and for 16.8 percent of outpatient care.

Most clients of home nursing services are old people. According to a recent report by the National Board of Health (Sosiaali-ja terveydenhuollon kertomus 1988), supervised outpatient services are provided for 70,000 patients. Altogether, outpatient care personnel made 2.7 million visits, of which 88.5 percent were to people aged 65 or over (the figure for the age group 65-74 was 22.4 percent, and for people aged 75 or over about 66 percent). During the 1980s, there was a marked increase in the use of home nursing services, and with the continuing growth of the aged population both the need for and the use of these services will also continue to increase. Another factor which will contribute to increased use of these services is the current emphasis on outpatient care instead of institutional treatment (Mäkinen 1991).

In the 65 to 69 age group, the average stay in the hospital is two weeks. For men and women aged 85 and over it is about five weeks and ten weeks, respectively (Virjo and Kivelä 1985). About 8 percent of the elderly Finnish population is in permanent institutional care: 5 percent live in old people's homes and around 3 percent is hospitalized.

OLD PEOPLE'S HOMES

In 1960, there were over 27,000 places in old people's homes in Finland. The figure for 1988 was roughly the same. However, during the past three decades the number has varied somewhat from year to year, peaking at around 31,000 in the late 1970s. The declining number of places in old-age homes during the 1980s was due, in part, to an administrative reorganization which placed some homes under the health care sector. In addition, some privately owned old people's homes were transformed into service homes (Arajärvi and Parkkinen 1989).

The reasons for institutionalization lie both in the living conditions and in the health status and functional ability of elderly people. Permanent institutionalization is more common among old people who are over 75 years of age, who have been diagnosed as suffering from dementia, and who are unable to cope with activities of daily living. Illness and disability are the two most common reasons why elderly people are admitted to institutional care. A recent study among an elderly rural population indicated that all elderly patients of health-center hospitals and over 80 percent of the residents of old people's homes were admitted because of some illness or disability (Anttila 1989).

The research evidence suggests that the majority of old people would want to live in their own homes as long as possible (Arajärvi 1981). If ongoing efforts to upgrade institutions and create more homelike settings are successful, then in the future it should be easier for people to move in.

In communal-owned old people's homes there are a total of some 25,000 places. Private old-age homes, which are mostly run by associations and nonprofit organizations, currently have around 3,000 places. They are small, homelike settings with facilities to make one's own household. Residents are generally in comparatively good health and, accordingly, less emphasis is given to medical treatment than in communal-owned old people's homes. This is one important reason why private homes have fewer staff and therefore lower operating costs. In private old people's homes, clients pay the fees themselves. However, elders who are without means can apply to the commune for housing subsidies. Communes also contribute to the operating costs of private old people's homes by paying a certain monthly sum to the association or organization, based on the number of beds they operate.

Communal-owned old people's homes vary considerably in size. In the biggest communes there are still a number of large institutions where residents have little choice over such things as when to eat or go to sleep. Generally, the aim in current development efforts is to give increasing freedom and independence to residents in old-age homes by improving the flexibility of services. Traditionally, these institutions have tended to be "preservative" rather than "rehabilitative," and inclined to rather heavy drug use. Today, increasing emphasis is placed on rehabilitation.

Old people's homes currently have places for one in ten people aged 75 and over. Three decades ago this figure was one in twenty. The reduced need for placement in old people's homes is primarily due to the improved functional ability of elderly people and to the better availability of outpatient services (Arajärvi and Parkkinen 1989). The following table describes the percentages of the Finnish population living in old people's homes by age groups in 1965 and 1986 (Arajärvi and Parkkinen 1989):

Age (years)	1965	1986
65-74	2.8	1.2
75-84	11.0	6.1
85 and over	27.2	23.5

Compared to many other nations, the Finnish social welfare and, in particular, the health care system have favored institutional care. In most cases, however, outpatient care is far more economical than treatment in an institution, and most people who are in need of care prefer to stay at home. It is indeed for both financial and human-itarian reasons that priority is now given to the development of outpatient care in Finland.

According to the national program adopted by the Cabinet in 1988, the number of places for elderly people in old people's homes and in community health centers must not exceed 18 percent of the total population aged 75 and over. Furthermore, the aim in old people's homes is to give more space to short-term and part-time treatment. Short-term in this context means treatment provided reg-ularly, or according to the client's needs, over a period of no more than three months; the purpose is to help the elderly client cope independently at home. In part-time care, elderly clients visit the old people's home during the day but go home at night–although sometimes they prefer to stay the night and spend their day at home. Different types of day care services are currently available in approximately 40 percent of the communes.

There remain a large number of people in Finland who continue to live in old people's homes even though they could be cared for in their own houses. At the same time, there are certain areas where there are not enough institutional places for the elderly. Part-time treatment in particular is in short supply, and therefore a program has been launched to make this service available to at least every tenth person aged 65 and over by the year 2000 (Arajärvi and Parkkinen 1989). In order to check the growth of placement in old people's homes, communes are required to provide service homes for people who need help and support on a daily basis. Elderly people living in service homes have access to a wide range of support services: meals, hygiene, cleaning, etc. The goal of the Ministry of Social Affairs and Health is to increase the number of places in service homes so that by the year 2000 three percent of the elderly population will be living in such homes (Arajärvi and Parkkinen 1989). By the year 2030, the need for places in service homes will approach 34,000, which is approximately seven times the number of places that were available in 1988 (Arajärvi and Parkkinen 1989).

In Finland, the elderly resident of a service home pays the full rate for accommodation plus a certain proportion of the services he or she uses. It is estimated that the Gross Domestic Product (GDP) ratio of expenditure on institutional care and housing services used by the elderly will increase by over 1 percent from 1988 to 2030.

The fee for institutional care depends on the resident's personal income; neither the spouse's nor the children's income levels are relevant. In cases where the elderly patient cannot afford to pay for services, the commune will cover the expenses. There is also a law which guarantees a monthly cash flow for people living in institutions.

In 1988, expenditure on old people's homes amounted to FIM 2,300 million, or 2 percent of total social security expenditures and 0.5 percent of the GDP (Arajärvi and Parkkinen 1989). This figure includes care and treatment provided in old people's homes, part-time care, and housing services for the elderly. It is assumed that the number of places in old people's homes for the population aged 75 and over can be reduced in Finland by one-fifth. However, given that this age group is estimated to double in size by the year 2030, the need for those places will actually be one and a half times greater than in 1988 (Arajärvi and Parkkinen 1989).

In terms of staffing, the situation in old people's homes has continued to improve since 1960, when there was one staff member for every four clients. Today, the ratio is 1:2, and current plans are to increase staff numbers to a level where there are seven staff members to ten clients.

In staff training, the emphasis is on medical care. Three-quarters of the staff are nurses and the remaining one-quarter are auxiliary workers who have completed at least a nine-month basic training course. Unqualified staff is occasionally used to meet temporary shortages of workers. Ward sisters in old people's homes are specially trained nurses, who typically have specialized in internal medicine, psychiatry, or geriatric nursing. In view of the qualification requirements in this job and the fact that nurses have to work in three shifts, pay levels are currently unsatisfactory. As long as there are other options open to nurses, old people's homes will continue to have difficulty recruiting competent staff for this demanding job, in which turnover rates have long been comparatively high.

DOMICILIARY HELP AND CARE

Home Help services were originally launched in Finland by voluntary organizations. Today, the bulk of these services are provided by communal authorities. In 1987, a total of 11,581 Home Helpers served some 200,000 households. Currently, the Home Help system is suffering from a rather acute shortage of staff resources, especially in larger towns and cities. Therefore, it is unable to provide adequate support to all the people who need help in their daily activities. The National Board of Social Welfare has recently estimated that, in order to fully meet the present demand for help and assistance, the Home Help system would need an additional 500 full-time homemakers or Home Helpers (Metsola 1990).

Home Helper training involves two years of full-time studies, while training courses for homemakers last three months. Home Help services consist of cooking, cleaning, and help in various activities of daily living. In 1987, every fifth aged person in Finland received Home Help services. There are also various support services to help elderly people, such as meals-on-wheels and transportation services.

Home Help services are also provided by voluntary organizations. In 1987, such organizations were active in 20 different localities, with a total staff of 14 homemakers and 127 Home Helpers (Metsola 1990).

In the absence of any statistics, it is very difficult to estimate the exact amount of caring work that is done by relatives and family members. We know that in 1980 (Metsola 1990) there were some 70,000 households in Finland (representing about 4 percent of the total household number) where one or more family members were caring for an elderly person, a disabled person, or a chronically ill patient. There were 75,000 people being cared for, 42,000 of whom were aged 65 and over. According to the population survey conducted by the National Board of Social Welfare (Sihvo 1988), 67 percent of the people needing help received assistance through the services provided by social welfare. Over 100,000 people turned to other sources of help. The Catholic Church is also involved in the effort to help elderly people living at home, although parish nurses do not actually do Home Help work. Nevertheless, their regular visits to aged people and their assistance in various day-to-day errands is an invaluable service.

All in all, the burden for the care of the elderly remains very much with the society rather than relatives. Older people who do have family caregivers are nevertheless eligible for public services.

Home Help is mainly financed by communes and the state. In 1987, fees collected from clients covered 8 percent of the total expenditure on Home Help services and 26 percent of the costs of support services. As in the case of institutional care, fees are determined on the basis of the recipient's income.

DEMENTIA: A SPECIAL PROBLEM OF ELDERLY PEOPLE

One of the most serious illnesses requiring systematic care and treatment of the elderly is dementia. In Finland about 7 percent of the population aged 65 and over suffer from moderate or serious dementia; the figure for the population over 85 is much higher, 17 percent (Erkinjuntti 1990). If we include in these statistics elderly people with mild dementia, the figures are twice as high. Given the continuing tendency for the proportion of the very old to increase in the population, it is now feared that without a breakthrough discovery of preventive and curative methods we are going to see a dramatic increase in the number of dementia patients (Sulkava 1990).

In 1980, there were around 44,000 people in Finland suffering from serious or moderate dementia; the prognosis for 1990 is 58,000 and for 2030 as much as 95,000 (Erkinjuntti 1990). Currently, more than half of these patients are in institutional care, and if this situation continues, dementia will indeed become a very serious challenge for the future development of social welfare and health care services (Sulkava 1990).

With the growing number of dementia patients, new forms of treatment will be required that can help to reduce the need for permanent hospitalization. Recently, there has been some experimentation with two new types of care which serve as extensions to Home Help, i.e., day care and short-term care. The experience so far suggests that it is indeed possible even for serious cases to be treated at home, provided that relatives are periodically able to get some rest. A few weeks' "holiday treatment" in an institution, for instance, gives relatives a welcome opportunity to get away for a while and take a complete break (Sulkava 1990).

Dementia patients can retain their independence and functional ability even in institutions, but this requires a suitable environment and a competent nursing staff to create a secure, homelike atmosphere (Sulkava 1990). Even rehabilitation is possible. The most urgent need at the moment, however, is for new hospices and places of treatment where relatives can leave their kin in good conscience. These homes for demented patients do not need full medical equipment, but they must be able to monitor their patients. A couple of years ago the Central Union for the Welfare of the Aged and the Alzheimer Association in Finland established the first day home for dementia patients in Helsinki. Since then, a number of new homes have been opened throughout the country by communes and by private organizations. There are also several homes for short-term care (Sulkava 1990).

THE CARE OF THE ELDERLY IN THE FUTURE

The demographic prognoses on the use of and need for health care services among the elderly in Finland suggest that the continuing growth of the elderly population is going to have some dramatic consequences in society. These impacts will be felt in production, in the labor markets, and in investments. By the turn of the century, the number of people aged 75 or over will be twice as high as today, and that in itself is bound to generate a growing need for care and treatment in Finland.

According to forecasts issued by the Ministry of Social Affairs and Health, the communal social and health care sector will continue to expand quite significantly during the next decade. The estimate is that the number of people working in this sector will increase by around 57,000 by the year 2000, with two-thirds of the new jobs accruing from social welfare. According to the ministry's report, the continued growth of social and health care services over the next ten years seems both justified and possible (Rauhala 1990).

According to Rauhala (1990), these optimistic estimates are based on assumptions of linear development. This, he argues, is a problematic premise, particularly given the element of surprise inherent in such predictions. Rauhala also points out that the profound changes that are now taking place in the European economic system are bound to affect the Finnish economy, although it is unclear exactly how they will do so.

The aging of the population will also be reflected in the availability of labor power. Already the growth of the work force has come to a halt, and this situation is going to continue into the future. By the year 2000, the estimated turnover rate in the work force will reach 10 percent (Rauhala 1990). The number of jobs in the service sector will continue to increase, and there will be a growing shortage of female labor in occupations which are traditionally female dominated.

Throughout the twentieth century, all caring occupations in Finland either have remained strongly female dominated (health work) or have become female dominated (social welfare and the medical profession). Care has always been and still is a woman's occupation, whether in the context of the family, voluntary associations, the neighborhood, or in public and professional services (Julkunen and Rantalaiho 1990).

There is now some indication that women are moving into new types of jobs (Julkunen 1990). Partly as a consequence of this tendency, there are growing fears in Finland that the field of caring is approaching a major crisis. The most visible symptom of this crisis is currently in the Helsinki region, where there is an acute shortage of workers in the social welfare and health care sector. One of the reasons why women are now moving out of the social and health care sector is the low level of pay in relation to their level of education.

Although frequently criticized for red tape and for their failure to respond flexibly to changing conditions and individual needs, the public services provided by the welfare state enjoy rather widespread popular support in Finland. They seem to give people a general sense of security, and there is also confidence in the quality of those services (Julkunen 1990). People know that training in the field of both social welfare and health care is of a very high standard, and that the physical welfare of the aged is in competent hands. The aim of development efforts is to encourage a more comprehensive and at the same time a "softer" approach. Institutions in particular are seeking to raise their profile, to adopt an "open doors" policy in relation to the surrounding community, and to increase social interaction among residents.

In order to guarantee the continuity of both institutional care and care provided at home, it has been suggested that pay levels in the social and health care sector should be raised. Greater attention also must be paid to the working conditions of Home Help, including shorter working hours and more part-time employment options (Arajärvi and Parkkinen 1989). An interesting question for the future is whether men can be encouraged to take a greater interest in the caring professions. If there was an inflow of men in these jobs, then the future outlook would be altered considerably.

In spite of repeated calls for an increased role of relatives in elder care, there seems to be no return to the old world. Women have joined the active labor force in large numbers; they currently represent over 50 percent of wage and salary earners and are no longer willing to return home, nor indeed would that now be possible.

A serious problem at the moment is that the high interest rate, stagnating national economy, and low level of investment will make it increasingly difficult for society to respond to the challenges posed by the aging of the population during the twenty-first century (SUOMI 1990). In any event, one of the major questions for the near future is going to be the organization of care for the elderly: who is going to take care of them and under what social conditions? Julkunen and Rantalaiho (1990) also raise the issue of whether care will be a natural basic right for the elderly of the future or whether it will become a privilege for those who can afford to pay for it. Recently, there has been increasing public debate in Finland on the use of (old) age as a criterion for caring. Opinions tend to clash most particularly in situations where resources are inadequate to provide expensive treatments for all patients and, consequently, where different groups must be ranked in some sort of order; a good example is by-pass operations.

The configuration of all caring systems is shaped by the social structure and political, economic, historical, and environmental determinants (Heikkinen 1989). The use of age as a criterion for treatment is not based on medical arguments; instead the debate that is now unfolding refers primarily to socioeconomic considerations. According to the dominant view in Finland today, the aged have a natural right to receive all kinds of care. However, attitudes may well be changing now, especially in response to the deteriorating economic situation in the country.

Regardless of what kind of changes we will see in the service systems, it is already clear that in the very near future the elderly users of those services will differ in important respects from the users of today. The material resources of elderly people are improving all the time. For instance, by 2010, the employee pension scheme will be fully in effect and everyone who has performed a reasonable amount of work will be able to retire with a decent pension (Rauhala 1990). However, the full implementation of this scheme requires a continuous 2 percent annual growth in GDP (Rauhala 1990).

There has also been a significant improvement in the educational level in Finland; the difference is particularly outstanding between prewar and postwar generations. In addition, people now have far better opportunities to maintain their health and functional ability, a central concern in current gerontological research (Heikkinen et al. 1984; Heikkinen et al. 1990). The elderly of the future will also be used to leading an independent life; they probably will expect a wider range of quality public services than do older people today.

In recent years, there have been a number of major projects in Finland concerned with the development of service systems for the elderly. These have been undertaken by individual communes, communal central organizations, the Ministry of Social Affairs and Health, and various organizations in the health sector. The scope of these projects and experiments is rather extensive, although in most cases the emphasis is on the development of outpatient services.

In Jyväskylä, central Finland, a research program, the EVER-GREEN project (see Heikkinen et al. 1990), has been initiated for the purpose of improving the physical, psychic, and social well-being of the elderly as well as enhancing the quality of both institutional and outpatient services. The project is strongly focused on prevention, revolving around the key concept of functional ability. To implement the development interventions, the researchers from the University of Jyväskylä are working in close collaboration with the local authorities.

In terms of the plans for the future development of old-age policy both at the national and communal level, Finland intends to place a strong emphasis on intensifying cooperation and coordination between health care and social welfare, particularly between specific services provided by the two sectors.

In our attempt to respond to the challenges of the future, and to guarantee the continuity and quality of care, we need to make critical use of the growing body of research which is being produced in the field, and, importantly, to work closely with the elderly themselves in the effort to promote their well-being.

REFERENCES

Anttila, S. Maaseudun vanhusten terveydentila, sosiaali- ja terveyspalvelujen käyttö ja kuolleisuus, *Acta Universitatis Tamperensis* ser A vol 277, Tampereen yliopisto, Tampere 1989 (English summary).

Arajärvi, E., and Parkkinen, P. Hoiva-Suomi 2030, Sosiaalimenot vuosina 1960-2030. *Taloudellinen suunnittelukeskus, Valtion painatuskeskus,* Helsinki 1989.

Arajärvi, R-L. Asuminen, Eläkeikäiset Tampereella. Haastattelututkimus 60-89-vuotiaiden tamperelaisten terveydentilasta, toimintakykyisyydestä, palvelujen käytöstä ja elintavoista, edited by E. Heikkinen, R-L Arajärvi, M. Jylhä, S. Koskinen, M. Pekurinen and P. Pohjolainen. Kansanterveystieteen julkaisuja M 65/81 Tampere 1981: 86-95.

Erkinjuntti, T. Aivojen ikääntymismuutokset luultua vähäisempiä, *Vanhustyö* 2/90, 4-8, 1990.

Heikkinen, E. Health implications of population aging in Europe. *World Health Statistics Quarterly,* vol. 40, No. 1, 22-39, 1987.

Heikkinen, E.; Arajärvi, R-L.; and Era, P. Functional capacity of men born in 1906-10, 1926-30, and 1946-50. A basic report. *Scand J Soc Med. Suppl* 33, 1984.

Heikkinen, R-L. Primary care services for the elderly in six European areas at the beginning of the 1980s. In *Health, Lifestyles and Services for the Elderly*, edited by W.E. Waters, E. Heikkinen, and A.S. Dontas. Public Health in Europe 29, World Health Organization Regional Office for Europe, Copenhagen 1989, 75-98.

Heikkinen, E.; Heikkinen, R-L.; Kauppinen, M.; Laukkanen, P.; Ruoppila, I.; and Suutama, T. Iäkkäiden henkilöiden toimintakyky, Ikivihreät-projekti Osa I, Sosiaali-ja terveysministeriö, *Suunnitteluosasto Helsinki* 1990 (English summary).

Julkunen, R. Suomalainen hyvinvointivaltio–naisten liittolainen? Department of social policy, University of Jyväskylä, Working papers o. 58, 1990.

Julkunen, R., and Rantalaiho, L. (toim). Hyvinvointivaltion sukupuolijärjestelmä, Tutkimussuunnitelma. Department of social policy, University of Jyväskylä, Working papers o. 56, 1990.

Mäkinen, E. Classifying disability in supervised out-patient care. A comparative study with Joensuu classification and four other methods. University of Helsinki, Department of General Practice and Primary Health Care 1:1991, Thesis (M.D.), Helsinki 1991.

Metsola, A. Kotipalvelun mahdollisuudet ja rajat, Kotipalvelun nykytilaa ja kehittämistä selvittävän työryhmän muistio. *Sosiaalihallituksen julkaisuja* 10/1990.

Rauhala, U. Apua tarvitsevat ja auttaminen, *Sosiaalinen aikakauskirja* 1:1990.

Sihvo, T. Arki ja apu, sosiaalihallituksen väestötiedustelun raportti 1. *Sosiaalihallituksen julkaisuja* 14/1988.

Sosiaali- ja terveydenhuollon kertomus OSA: kansanterveys. Sosiaali-terveyministeriö. 1988. Annual Statistics. National Board of Health.

Sulkava, R. Dementiapotilaiden uudet hoitomuodot. *Vanhustyö* 2:1-3, 1990.

SUOMI 1990-2005. Haasteiden ja varautumisen aikaa, Taloudellinen suunnittelukeskus, Valtion painatuskeskus. Helsinki 1990.

Svanborg, A. The health of the elderly population: Results from longitudinal studies with age-cohort comparisons. In *Research and the Aging Population*. Ciba Foundation Symposium 134, 3-11. John Wiley and Sons, Chichester 1988a.

Svanborg, A. Cohort differences in the Göteborg studies of Swedish 70-year-olds. In *Epidemiology and Aging in an International Perspective*, edited by Brody, J.A., and Maddox, G.L. Sringler Publishing Company, New York 1988b, 27-35.

Väestörakenne. 1989., Väestö 1990:12.

Valkonen, T., and ja Nikander, T. Vanhojen ikäluokkien koon ja rakenteen muutokset. In *Vanheneminen ja elämänkulku, Sosiaaligerontologian Perusteita*, edited by M. Jylhä, and P. Pohjolainen. Weilin ja Göös, Mänttä 1990, 60-79.

Virjo, I., and Kivelä, S-L. 65 vuotta täyttäneiden keskimääräiset hoitoajat yleissairaaloissa 1978-1981. *Suomen lääkärilehti* 40: 2322-2327, 1985.

Chapter 5

The "Graying" of Israel

David Guttmann
Ariela Lowenstein

INTRODUCTION

David Ben Gurion, the first prime minister and the founder of the State of Israel, used to say: "He who does not believe in miracles is not a realist." Indeed, when it comes to aging, Israel has experienced not one but five miracles. The first miracle is the tremendous growth of the elderly population. From a meager 40,000 to 50,000 in 1948, when the State of Israel was created, to approximately 420,000 in 1991, the country has experienced a shocking 1,000 percent increase in its aged population (65 years and older) in less than two generations' time. Moreover, from a country of the young, in which only 3 percent were elderly in 1948, Israel has become a country of the old, with close to 10 percent of its inhabitants in advanced age. The 90,000 people aged 80+ compose close to 20 percent of all elderly 65 years old and older (Be'er and Factor 1990).

The second miracle is the seemingly unbelievable fact of these elderly living together rather amicably. In a country in which the Biblical prophecy of gathering the exiles from all corners of the earth has become a reality, the some 100 different ethnic and cultural subgroups within the aged population exhibit a remarkable ability to live together and share in the joys and the vicissitudes of life. A short visit to any of the social clubs or day care centers for the elderly would attest to this miracle.

Closely connected to the second, the third miracle is in the composition of the aged population. Israel is a country where the great majority of the elderly are not native born. At present the "sabras," or native born and raised elderly, compose a meager 6 percent of all the aged, while the majority are from European countries, especially Poland, which accounts for over 20 percent of all the aged living in Israel (*Israel Statistical Yearbook* 1990). At the same time, among the European-born elderly are tens of thousands of survivors of the Holocaust, but their numbers are quickly dwindling; in less than two decades they all will be dead.

Thus, the concept of aging for the present generation of elderly in Israel is different from what is commonly expected elsewhere. That is, for the native born, whose parents came as young pioneers and who were the founding fathers and mothers of the cities and the kibbutzim and villages, the whole idea of aging and caring for the elderly was totally "foreign;" it did not fit the prevailing ideology of the time, well before the creation of the State. As for the survivors of the Holocaust, many of them were young people who never experienced the aging of their grandparents and who subsequently had to learn this role without the benefit of role models.

Given this situation, the fourth miracle is even more remarkable. In Israel, as in the United States, less than 5 percent of all the elderly are living in institutions. The strength of Jewish tradition in filial responsibility seems to be a major cause in this miracle (Guttmann 1990). For, despite the lack of role models, the elderly are not abandoned, warehoused, or shipped to nursing and old-age homes unless there is no other choice. Several cultural groups within the general population, including the ethnic-religious minorities, such as the Arabs (both Moslem and Christian), the Druz, the Cherkes (of Caucasian origin), the Ultra-Orthodox, and the Oriental Jews, in particular, have strong traditions against institutionalizing elderly parents.

The last of the miracles is reflected in the rapid growth of services to the aged. Known by the world as a people who rely on improvisation more than on planning, the system of services to the aged population has grown by leaps and bounds and encompasses the majority of the elderly, irrespective of their financial and social standing. For example, day care centers for the frail and largely homebound aged have grown from a total of nine in 1982 to well over 60 in 1989, and all but 5 percent of the aged are covered by the main Sick Fund for health care services. While both the Ministry of Health and the Sick Fund of the Labor Union maintain a network of hospitals and clinics under different eligibility coverage and under different quality in services provision, the miracle still holds in terms of cooperation, especially at the municipal and community levels. With this background in mind, let us consider the demographic composition and trends that characterize the aged population in Israel.

DEMOGRAPHIC TRENDS

Bergman (1980, 208) has noted that

immigration is the central phenomenon of Israel's existence. Without it, Israel could never have come into existence, nor can it sustain itself without its continuation. In it lies the nation's historical raison d'etre as the haven for those in need and as the spiritual, cultural, and historical center it can offer to Jews in other countries.

In 1990, a total of 23,699 new immigrants aged 65 and over arrived in Israel. Of these people, 8,005 were aged 75 and older, boosting the total elderly population of the country by some 5 percent (*Israel Statistical Yearbook* 1990). It is interesting to note that of the 23,699 new immigrants, 22,869 are from the Soviet Union and 357 from Ethiopia. Demographic forecasts predict an even greater influx of elderly immigrants in this decade. Thus, the 1990s and the first decade of the next century will be characterized, among other things, by some major demographic changes in the composition of the aged population of Israel.

At present, according to the *Statistical Abstracts* of the country (*Israel Statistical Yearbook* 1989), the number of aged can be summarized as the following:

	Aged 65-74 (in thousands)	**Aged 75 and over** (in thousands)
Jews	220.4	159.0
Christians	3.6	2.7
Moslims	9.5	7.0
Druz and others	1.7	1.3

In other words, 94 percent of those aged 65 and over are Jews, while the remaining 6 percent are non-Jews. The majority of the aged in Israel reside in the three largest cities: Tel Aviv, Haifa, and Jerusalem. Close to 30,000 elderly live in small towns and in various rural settlements, while those living in kibbutzim number over 13,000 people.

Israel is distinguished from European countries by its much lower proportion of persons living alone and by a higher proportion of couples. Among the elderly, couples without children and single females are predominant, especially among those aged 65 to 74 (Achdut and Tamir 1986). Forty-seven percent of couples in Israel do not have children. Only 23 percent of households in the 75 and over age group consist of single females, compared to 50 percent in the Scandinavian countries and 45 percent in the U.S. and Canada. This difference apparently stems from the relatively low rate of divorce and separation in Israel where matters of divorce are controlled by the Rabbinical courts. Furthermore, Israeli families are larger than in other Western countries. Of course, living alone does not in and of itself constitute a high risk factor for the elderly (Taylor 1988) unless accompanied by other economic, social, health, psychological, and support risks.

As a result of the aging of the immigrants from the late 1940s and 1950s, when Israel experienced massive waves of immigrations, there will be a substantial increase in the number of people aged 65 and over by the end of this century (*Israel Statistical Yearbook* 1989). Elderly people 75 years old and older will constitute 50 percent of the entire aged population, and by the year 2025 there will be a significant increase in the number of people aged 80 and over, as well (Habib 1988; Morginstin 1990).

These last two groups of elderly in Israel are the "population at risk" of institutionalization. At the same time, they constitute the main consumers of health and social welfare services (Habib, Factor and Shmueli 1987). These forecasted demographic changes will result in a large increase in the number of the frail elderly. Consequently, there will be a need to expand the institutional and community-based services to this population.

The next decade will bring an entirely different aged population. There will be a tremendous increase in native-born aged and considerable growth among Asian- and African- born elderly who, in 1989, numbered a total of 104,000 (*Israel Statistical Yearbook,* 1990). Demographic forecasts predict an increase in level of education and standard of living for these groups. As a result, they will demand different treatment in every sphere of life and a much greater involvement in the planning of services (Guttmann and Lowenstein 1991). The pioneer generation will disappear, along with the last remnants of Holocaust survivors.

The ability of the informal system of support to provide assistance to needy elderly will undergo important changes due to three factors: (1) the size of the nuclear family will be smaller due to a decrease in fertility patterns and behaviors of Israeli women; (2) there will be a greater flow of women into the labor market. Today, 80 percent of the disabled and/or frail elderly are assisted by their families. Women, either daughters or daughters-in-law, are the main caregivers, as determined from studies in other developed countries (Morginstin 1987); and (3) in the coming decades the country will experience four- and even five-generation families in growing numbers. Four- and five-generation families may include two generations of elderly parents (Shanas 1984).

Demographers such as Della Pergola (1989) predict that as a result of the above, the "syndrome of the lonely elderly" will become one of the central problems of aging in the twenty-first century.

An analysis of the elderly's living arrangements in Israel during the past decade shows that, as in the Western Hemisphere, a sharp decline occurred in the proportion of multi-generational housing from 33% in 1972 to 20% in 1982. This decline in the course of time is to be attributed to the modernization process: a rise in living standards, a change in preferences and norms, and a drop in the birthrate. (Shmueli 1989, ix)

Among the other predictions regarding the coming 20 years are increased urbanization of the religious and ethnic minorities in Israel.

THE "GRAYING" OF THE MINORITY POPULATION IN ISRAEL

The aged within the Arab population in Israel present a relatively new phenomenon in terms of numbers and problems. Under the British Mandate, which preceded the creation of the State of Israel, Arab aged were few and did not constitute any particular problem. A tradition of filial ties and honor for the parent enabled most of these people to be cared for within the family and the village. In 1948, there were only a couple thousand Arab elderly citizens aged 65 and older in the newly created State of Israel. Today they number 25,000 and comprise 3 percent of the non-Jewish population in the country (*Israel Statistical Yearbook* 1989). One estimate puts the number of Arab elderly aged 65 and over by the turn of the century at 38,000, or a growth of 58 percent in a decade. The largest increase in numbers of Arab aged is expected to be among the Moslems, while the smallest increase is expected among the Christians.

Twenty-two percent of the Arab elderly and 18 percent of the Jewish elderly are aged 80 and over. Moreover, there is a more extensive need for services among the Arab aged since they tend to have greater physical and mental disabilities than those who are Jewish (Weil 1991). For example, the 1985 survey of the elderly population (60 years old and over) found that the rate of homebound Arab elderly is higher than among the Jewish elderly (*Sixty + Survey* 1985).

The minority elderly in Israel can be divided into three groups: Moslems (77.6 percent); Christians (12.8 percent), and Druz (9.6 percent). The aged within these three religious and ethnic groups vary. In the Moslem minority they comprise only 2.6 percent; Christian aged constitute the highest percentage (4.7 percent), while the Druz are in the middle with 3.5 percent elderly. Well over two-thirds of all minority aged are illiterate, women more than men, but within one generation this will dramatically change, due to the mandatory education of all children in Israel.

The standard of living of the Arab elderly is closely tied to its household composition. As a rule, with the exception of the elders in East Jerusalem, those who live in one-generation households, i.e., alone or with a spouse or relative, have a considerably lower standard of living (measured in terms of available or not available items, such as bathroom or shower, heating appliance, refrigerator, radio and television, etc.) than the elderly who live within households of the extended family (*Israel Statistical Yearbook* 1983). However, among the latter, the standard of living of Christian elders is better than that of their fellow Moslem and Druz elders, largely due to the fact that the Christian Arabs are mainly congregated in the cities, whereas the Moslem and Druz reside in villages (Weil 1991).

In Israel,where fertility is high and attention is largely focused on the welfare of the children, the elderly increasingly find themselves in a more difficult situation. Urbanization and modernization have eroded the traditional commitment of the family to the welfare of the aged, and these people have to rely more and more on the formal system (i.e., governmental and public services) for survival and support (Weil 1991). Today,over 5 percent of all three religious groups of elderly Arabs maintain separate households, and this trend is growing rapidly. In ten years, close to two-thirds of the Arab aged in Israel will live independently of their children. This change in household composition will affect the quality and availability of care for the homebound elderly and for the disabled, in particular, who traditionally have relied on the assistance provided by their adult children. The role formerly fulfilled by adult children will place a tremendous burden on the State, especially since the law connects eligibility for services to the aged to the household composition and living arrangements of the elderly. That is, elderly living in one-generation households are entitled to homemaking and personal services, heating, and hot meals.

OCCUPATIONAL AND ECONOMIC OUTLOOK

The question of how the older new immigrants from the Soviet Union will be absorbed into Israeli society has been raised ever since the first waves of immigration from that country to Israel became a reality in the early 1970s. Of special concern was, and still is, their potential for employment and economic contribution. Many of these older immigrants were employed in their native country in occupations not in demand in Israel, or were pensioners according to the Soviet system in which men retire at age 60 and women at age 55. Therefore, these elderly not only have to reenter the labor market, but a substantial number must undergo occupational change as well.

Based on previous experience with those immigrants who came during the first waves of the 1970s and early 1980s, the evidence suggests that such older people tend to make the necessary adjustments to the prevailing market economy. As Matras (1991) has pointed out, well over half of those aged 55 to 64 were employed five years after their settlement, 59 percent of whom successfully underwent occupational changes. Matras (1991) relates this success to their educational level and background, a level that is higher than that of native-born and other immigrant elderly. For example, of the 22,869 new immigrants aged 65 and over who arrived from the Soviet Union in 1990, one-third, or 7,411, had 13 or more years of education. Among these immigrants, the majority were employed in engineering as well as in scientific and academic professions. In addition, many were in managerial and administrative positions. Common to all of these immigrants is a high level of motivation to find and maintain employment, even when such work means a serious drop in their former socioeconomic status. They are also willing to undergo the necessary training, despite all the difficulties inherent in mastering a new language and new skills.

Today there is a high rate of unemployment in Israel, over 10 percent (*Israel Statistical Yearbook* 1990). The competition with younger workers, native born and immigrants, is keen. How unemployment will impact on the mental health of the older immigrants is not known at present. But there are indications that it will be severe. Already the country has been shocked by cases of suicide among the new elderly immigrants, many of whom were depressed because of their inability to be absorbed via the labor market into Israeli society. Nevertheless, one thing is clear: these immigrants represent a potentially active and productive labor force that is willing and able to support itself and to contribute to Israel's economy.

DISABILITY AND MENTAL HEALTH

Life expectancy in the U.S. is 71 years for men and 79 for women; in Israel it is 73 for men and 77 for women. Comparative statistics on the eradication of contagious diseases indicate other similarities between the two countries as well. Such equivalence is surprising considering that the U.S. spends 11 percent of its GNP on the health of its citizens, whereas Israel commits 7 percent of its GNP for the same purpose. America's annual per capita expenditure on health was $1,290 in 1984 as compared to Israel's $472 (Goell 1991). Yet, Israel's performance on measures of cumulative health care delivered over time compares more than favorably with that of the U.S.

Moreover, in Israel over 95 percent of the population is covered by some form of comprehensive medical insurance–despite the rising cost of health services delivery to a population which harbors large numbers of destitute immigrants from Third World countries, such as the Ethiopians. In contrast, over 40 million citizens in the U.S., or well over 15 percent of the entire population, are not covered by any health insurance, and millions of those with health care policies do not have sufficient protection, especially for catastrophic illness, including mental diseases (Goell 1991).

While the elderly compose only 10 percent of Israel's population, they occupy 35 percent of all beds in hospitals and consume 50 percent of all medications administered in such institutions. The public expenditure for keeping the aged in hospitals is estimated at $63 million a year. The medical problems of the old cause significant increases in chronic, infectious, and acute diseases. Coupled with their psychological problems and ailments, the elderly require new approaches in the delivery of medical services. The present system of health care is largely geared to a much younger population, one whose physical and mental health is significantly different from that of the elderly.

In Israel, the definition of frailty is similar to that used by McCuan, Hooyman, and Fortune (1985). These gerontologists claim that four conditions of mental and physical impairments combine to make an elderly person frail and in need of support from social networks. The elderly are viewed as frail if (1) their living situation is unsafe without significant and regular assistance from others; (2) if their condition is subject to rapid and unpredictable functional setbacks or (3) is not reversible to any significant extent because of chronic conditions; and (4) if they are unmanageable in the community without some extensive support from informal, nonpaid sources.

The arrival during the past two years of large numbers of elderly Jews from the Soviet Union, Ethiopia, and South America necessitates a reassessment of the population with various disabilities and mental health problems for whom services will have to be provided by the existing network of clinics, hospitals, mental health centers, and other curative, preventative, and protective services. The last assessment was provided by the Central Bureau of Statistics in a national survey performed in 1985 (Factor and Primak 1991), and its results are already dated. According to this survey, the rate of disability among the elderly Jewish population in 1985 was about 8 percent in ADL (Activities of Daily Living), and about 38 percent in IADL (Instrumental Activities of Daily Living). Among the elderly non-Jewish population, the rate of disability was higher: 22 percent in ADL and 42 percent in IADL. The researchers found that disability proportions rise with age; that is, the older the person, the higher the likelihood for an increase in disability. Women were found to be more disabled than men. It was projected that these figures would increase by 29 percent for the Jewish elderly and by 44 percent for the non-Jewish elderly by the year 2,000.

It is important to note that these rates of disability are based on demographic conditions that existed prior to the massive waves of immigration to Israel by Jews from the Soviet Union during the past three years. Changes in the composition of the elderly population will have a major impact on the capacity of the existing health, education, and social welfare services (along with housing and employment) to provide for the needs of the newcomers.

Disability among all minority elders in Israel is higher for women than for men, and significantly increases after age 80. Eligibility figures for benefits and entitlements included in the Nursing Act of 1988 show that in the Jewish sector 5.66 percent are eligible for the entitlement, whereas in the Arab sector the figure is 9.7

percent. Thus, in planning services for the disabled elderly who are limited in their performance of daily activities, attention will have to be paid to the growing gap between the two sectors and its implication for the resources of the National Insurance that pays, by law, for services rendered to those eligible under that Act. The Nursing Act of 1988 has created rapid development of social services to the elderly, and especially to the homebound and the disabled who "surfaced" when that law was put into effect.

Medical and health care equipment to needy aged are under the auspices of Yad Sara, which is a unique voluntary charitable organization which loans, free of charge, a variety of medical and rehabilitative instruments after hospitalization discharge, as well as after treatment in the health clinics. It is a universal service without any eligibility criteria, and was developed to respond to a need for such equipment which is not provided for by the hospitals or the sick funds.

SENILE DEMENTIA

Closely tied to the subject of disability among the elderly population of Israel is the prevalence of senile dementia. Alzheimer's disease and senile dementia are the most severe mental disturbances in the elderly, and their incidence and prevalence rises with advancing age (Heinik 1987). In various countries, between 10 and 15 percent of the elderly 65 years and older suffer from senile dementia, while 6 percent are diagnosed as severe cases. These people are in need of constant supervision and care. At the same time, they constitute the main consumers of health and social care services. Available information points to a "blatant gap" in knowledge about the extent of this phenomenon (Haber-Schaim 1987).

One estimate, based on prevalence rates found abroad (and applicable to Israel) with respect to severe dementias, is that close to 20,000 elderly belong in this category. Such older people exhibit symptoms of deteriorating intellect in memory, learning, orientation, concentration, communication, and cognitive functioning, changes in personality, and an inability to perform daily activities. Seventy-eight percent of people with severe dementia live in the community, 5 percent are in mental hospitals, and the remaining 17 percent are in long-term care institutions. Of all the elderly found in the latter, 26 percent were diagnosed as suffering from organic senile dementia, while those found in mental hospitals constitute over one half of the entire population residing in these hospitals (Haber-Schaim 1987).

Public mental health and welfare services are unable to meet the needs of the demented and their families. In addition, primary care physicians rarely refer suspected cases for diagnosis to geriatricians, psychiatrists, or neurologists. Nor do families caring for elderly individuals exhibiting cognitive or mental symptoms of dementia procure such professional assessments (Haber-Schaim 1987).

Social workers could play an important role in referring demented elderly people for diagnosis to any of the psycho-geriatric screening units that have been established in the country during the past decade. They could provide direct services to the families of the demented as well. Yet, there are many obstacles that prevent them from fulfilling their professional roles. Chief among these is the relationship between social welfare agencies and the public health services and clinics. The latter, it seems, are reluctant to engage in the psycho-geriatric problems of the elderly. Moreover, the existing community services are not adequately staffed or equipped to treat diagnosed cases of senile dementia. Few programs engage in community outreach programs to identify people in need of psycho-geriatric care. There is a need, therefore, to strengthen teamwork and coordination among the various professionals and to identify the common goals for intervention: the reduction of the severity of suffering by the elderly demented and their caretakers; postponement of the need for institutionalization; and assistance to the families who carry the major burden of care. As is known from gerontological and geriatric literature, of all types of care for home-bound elderly, caring for the demented is the most difficult for the family (Krulik, Hirschfeld, and Sharon 1984).

In the day-care centers for the frail and disabled elderly, which have grown during the past decade from a handful to well over sixty, there are some provisions for serving the demented elderly as well as the nondemented. However, the programs can accommodate only a small fraction of those in need. Although there have been recent attempts to develop self-help groups among the families of the demented elderly, such endeavors are only beginnings. Much greater effort by both the formal and the informal systems is needed to ease the burden of care for the demented elderly in Israel and to deal with this complex problem—which gets worse with each passing year.

THE LONG-TERM CARE INSURANCE LAW

In response to demographic trends, the inadequacy of existing programs in meeting needs, the growing burden of care of the elderly and their families (Lowenstein 1983), and the political will of legislators, the Israeli Parliament finalized a law in April 1986 (originally passed in 1980) which created the framework for Long-Term Care Insurance within Israel's existing social security system. The law was implemented in two stages. The first started, as soon as the law was approved in 1986, on an experimental basis in four locations. The initial intent was to develop and extend the infrastructure of the services, and to complete all the professional, legal and administrative preparations necessary for ensuring a smooth operation of the system. The second stage began in 1988 and constituted the main part of the law: granting a personal right to long-term care benefits.

By September, 1990, 70,000 applications were submitted, from which 27,000 were approved for severely dependent elderly. About 1,500 of the latter were entitled to care within day-care centers (Friedman 1990), while the rest received aid in their homes. Prior to the enactment of the law, long-term care services to homebound elderly were provided by the health and welfare institutions under various administrative arrangements. The scope of such services, however, was rather limited and only about 5,000 elderly benefitted from them.

The 1986 long-term care act is without parallel in the social security legislation of the Western world. It also is one of the most complex pieces of social legislation ever passed in Israel (Habib, Factor, and Be'er 1987). The law determines the rights to nursing care of old people on a national basis within an insurance scheme (Schnitt 1988). It's primary aim is to formalize the concept of personal entitlement to state-provided long-term care services for an older person who is seriously disabled. The law does so through clearly defined eligibility criteria that intend both to meet individual needs and to enhance the family's role as a primary caregiver. In fact, an important contribution of the bill is that it specifies the role of the family in providing care. It links the informal care system with the formal service structures, and delineates the role of private and public agencies in service development and provision (Morginstin 1987).

Services and benefits to the disabled elderly are paid through contributions from the working population. Services include personal assistance in the home or in organized community facilities, Home Help, personal attendance, laundry, meal preparation and delivery, and the supply of absorbent undergarments for the incontinent. The care plan also indicates which agencies will provide assistance. An essential goal of the law is to increase the availability and accessibility of quality services in the community, as well as of personnel who provide care at home and in day-care centers. The measure also provides funds for increasing the number of elderly in nursing homes.

The main element in the implementation of the act is the integration of all State agencies operating in the sphere of long-term care of the aged, particularly the Ministry of Health and the Ministry of Labor and Social Welfare, as well as the Sick Funds. Overall responsibility for the law's operation and monitoring is vested in the National Insurance Institute, though it shares administrative and service responsibility with local professional committees.

THE SERVICE NETWORK

The aim of the service network is to promote a continuity of life style for the elderly in their normal environment, enabling them to maintain maximum self-sufficiency and to participate as actively as possible in society. The focus of services ranges from the older person's home at one end of the scale, to the community in which he or she resides, and to institutions at the other end of the scale (Bergman and Lowenstein 1988).

The current long-term care network in Israel must be analyzed within the special historical context of the pre-state period (prior to

1948), when three separate and different welfare systems were developed: that of the British Mandatory Government, that of the Jewish community of Palestine, and that of the General Federation of Labor–Histadrut. In the first years after the creation of Israel as an independent state, and as a result of the mass influx of immigrants and urgent problems related to the absorption of elderly arrivals, the government assumed responsibility for service provision to the elderly through a specially created voluntary national organization called "Malben." This organization, which was established and funded by the Jewish Distribution Committee, initially emphasized institutional care. This was perceived at that time as a quick, effective solution to the most pressing needs of the aged newcomers.

During the 1960s there was a gradual shift in the orientation of services to the aged, with increased attention to noninstitutional, community-based services (Bergman and Lowenstein 1988). Leaders of Malben and other providers for the aged initiated these changes primarily in reaction to the rapid demographic changes the country was experiencing. At the same time, the government of Israel assumed greater responsibility for the welfare of its aged citizens.

Services to the elderly in Israel are not based on age-specific legislation; they are covered through the General Welfare Services Law of 1958, under which each local authority is charged with the establishment of a local welfare service office to extend services to those in need, including the aged. In addition to local government services, there are a considerable number of voluntary agencies (national or local). In the last few years there has been proprietary involvement as well, especially in the area of institutional care. Services operated by the voluntary sector, which is based on the Jewish tradition of mutual aid and collective responsibility, have a long history in Israel.

In 1969, the National Association for Planning and Development of Services for the Aged in Israel (ESHEL) was established. This is a unique partnership between a voluntary agency, the American Jewish Distribution Committee, and government (the Ministries of Welfare, Health, and Finance). It is jointly funded, on a matching basis. In the first decade of its operation, ESHEL developed a variety of programs and services for different groups of aged in the community and in institutional settings. However, in the 1980s the emphasis changed, with the group focusing on the handicapped and dependent elderly. This was reflected in massive investments in the construction of new residential facilities and day-care centers, as well as in the development of a variety of training programs (Rotem 1991).

A basic policy goal in the current service network is to develop a broadly diversified system of benefits and services to meet a continuum of changing needs. The long-term objective is to assist the family and to develop services so as to enable the elderly, even disabled dependent individuals, to remain in the community as long as feasible. The intent is to confine the use of institutional services which currently constitute an important part of the long-term care system.

In recent years there has been a growing awareness in Israel of the gaps between needs and services, especially for the disabled elderly. The first estimates were made at the end of the 1970s when the population of individuals aged 75 and over was forecast to rise by 52 percent (from 119,000 to 181,000) between 1983 and 1995 (Habib, Factor, and Be'er 1987). As a result, efforts have been made to expand public investment in services for the elderly. The service network encompasses home-based services (which are similar to those in other countries), community-based (open care) services, and institutional (closed care) facilities.

COMMUNITY SERVICES

Day-Care Centers

Day-care centers, which have been developed mainly during the past decade, are unique services for the physically handicapped and the cognitively impaired elderly. Their main goals are to prevent or postpone institutionalization and to help caregivers. About 60 day-care centers operate today in Israel–50 in the communities and 10 in conjunction with old age homes. Together, these centers serve close to 11,000 elderly. Their growth during the 1980s was primarily due to the efforts of ESHEL, in cooperation with the appropriate governmental ministries and local authorities.

Various models of day-care centers were developed–some exclusively for the handicapped, some for the cognitively impaired, and others for integrating these two populations. The guiding principle was "community-environment fit," i.e., to fit the operation and services offered both to the unique needs of the target population in the area served and to the existing network of health and welfare services in that community.

The day-care center provides a combination of health and social services, including personal care services (bathing, meals, etc.) and professional services (social worker, nurse, physiotherapist, etc.), as well as social-recreational activities. In addition, day-care centers provide services, such as meals, protected workshops, counselling, and referral, to older people's homes.

According to a recent evaluation of day-care centers in Israel by Korazim, Trachtenberg, and Habib (1990), about 77 percent of the elderly served are physically and emotionally impaired. The remainder suffer from such problems as depression and loneliness, as well as from a variety of health problems. The study found great variability among the centers. These findings prompted ESHEL to develop guidelines for the future planning of and standards for day-care centers (Day Care Center for the Aged 1990).

In the Arab sector, the emphasis since the early 1980s has shifted from the independent aged to service provision for the frail elderly. Accordingly, several day-care centers have been created in the large villages. Other regional programs focusing on the frail aged were developed by ESHEL, as well (ESHEL 1989).

Social Clubs

Social clubs provide an important universal community service, mainly for the well and independent elderly. They serve as social-recreational frameworks, as well as bases for volunteer work. Although many of the clubs operating today provide similar services as those available at day-care centers, they attempt to focus their efforts on the needs of particular target populations. In addition to a great variety of social, cultural, recreational, and educational activities, many of the clubs offer health prevention services, hot meals, social work counselling, and even occupational therapy.

Most of the clubs are neighborhood-based and geared to the specific needs of different ethnic and cultural groups. The main agencies operating such clubs are: the welfare departments of the local authorities, some with the cooperation of Mishan (a branch of the Labor Federation); the Community Centers Association; and various voluntary associations, such as B'nai B'rith, Wizo, etc. Some clubs are integrated into existing community centers. In the main cities there are a few larger "regional" clubs with membership between 300 and 1,500. These offer a greater variety of activities and services, and usually operate during the whole day. The clubs are administered by professional managers who work with representatives of the elderly users and with volunteers. With the cooperation of ESHEL, the clubs developed special programs to absorb the new Russian immigrant elderly, providing an array of services for this population, such as Hebrew lessons and social work services.

In the big cities such as Tel Aviv or Haifa, some fifty clubs operate, serving about 15 percent of the independent elderly. The Sixty+ Survey of the Central Bureau of Statistics (1985) revealed that 12 percent of the elderly not using the clubs would be interested in doing so. Therefore more publicity should be provided, as well as more outreach, especially to identify the lonely elderly. In addition, more older people of Eastern origin should be encouraged to participate in the clubs, to equal their proportion within the elderly population (*Masters Program for Services for the Aged*, Tel Aviv 1986; Haifa 1989).

Volunteer Services to the Elderly

Programs geared to alleviate loneliness in old age, which involve a large array of social and religious organizations, provide opportunities for a variety of social activities, volunteer roles, and the creation of new and meaningful social relationships (Guttmann and Lowenstein 1991). Volunteer programs developed by the Ministry of Social Welfare and by ESHEL, the Association for Planning and Development of Services for the Aged in Israel, foster enhanced self-esteem and a sense of usefulness among the elders (Adelson, Kaminsky, and Cohen 1979). In 1972, the National Institute of Social Insurance opened its first Counseling Center for the Aged administered by volunteers. Since then, these centers have become standard features throughout the country. "Young-old" volunteers, 60-70 years of age and older, attempt to alleviate the loneliness of the recently widowed and homebound elderly through friendly home visits. Other organizations on behalf of the elderly use similar approaches. Such visits ensure support for those confronting the painful changes widowhood brings (Lopata 1978) or for those experiencing social isolation.

Volunteers also assist the regular staff in day-care centers. Their roles are particularly significant for survivors of the Holocaust, as many survivors are themselves volunteers. Kahana, Harel, and Kahana (1988), in analyzing stress-related mental and physical health indicators and the ability to cope with the effects of Holocaust experiences, point to the value of sharing and disclosing these traumatic events with interested parties. The researchers found that those able to talk to other family members and friends consistently portrayed more positive effect than those unable to do so. Thus, the availability of social support for and communication among Holocaust survivors are important contributors to higher levels of psychological well-being.

The importance of religion in late life has been recognized by gerontologists. Berman (1981), among others, has demonstrated the correlation between life satisfaction and religious activities. For example, he argues that Orthodox Jews adjust better to aging than the nonorthodox. The former's strong belief and faith in God help them to overcome grief, loneliness, and despair. Consequently, each year volunteers in Israel organize such activities as Passover seders in hotels around the city for the lonely elderly (Kerem and Zweig 1990). Volunteers also aid synagogues in their social activities and educational programs offered to older members of the congregation. For many, the synagogue is the reflection of the Jewish spiritual self (Olitzky 1985). Volunteers assist with efforts such as transportation and escort services, enabling frail and disabled elderly to attend synagogue on a regular basis.

Interaction among the generations also relies heavily on volunteer services. Studies show that the more frequent the contacts, the less stereotypical are attitudes among all generations, resulting in reduction of loneliness among the elderly (Isaacs 1986; Roseman and Rosen 1984). On the other hand, older people are important for linking the past to the present and the future, and for molding the identity of children. Mentally and physically capable lonely older people have been encouraged to act as foster grandparents to children from "broken homes" and to orphans. Many of these young-sters benefit considerably from warm and caring relationships with a grandparent figure. One particularly innovative and successful program is called "a grandparent for the kindergarten." Elderly persons "adopt" a kindergarten in their neighborhood and help with various chores and supervision of the children. They also serve as surrogate grandparents to children with special needs.

Local Associations for the Aged

One by-product of day-care centers in Israel has been the establish-ment of Local Associations for the Aged. Today, ninety-one such groups operate throughout Israel. ESHEL, which was instrumental in creating seventy of these, has developed training programs for their members. The latter include professionals from the various health and welfare agencies in the community, public leaders, and representatives of the elderly population. The main goal of the Local Associations is to help in the development of new community services, as well as to serve as a "meeting ground" for professionals from different agencies and organizations on behalf of the aged.

LONG-TERM CARE INSTITUTIONS

Historically, institutional care was the first type of service devel-oped in Israel, preceding community-based services by some 50 years. There were six notable stages in institutional development: the first toward the end of the last century, when the first home was created in Jerusalem (in 1879) for independent but lonely aged; the second, until the creation of the State of Israel, when various *lan-desmanshaft* organizations, especially of German origin, estab-lished similar homes; the third during the first years of the State of Israel–through the creation of "Malben"; the fourth when the Hista-drut instituted its "individual" sheltered housing and collective homes for independent elderly; the fifth with the entry of the private sector; and the sixth during the 1970s with the establishment of regional homes by ESHEL. These facilities provided a continuum of care for the frail population, ranging from the independent el-derly to those in need of skilled nursing facilities (Bergman 1981).

By 1989, there were 187 long-term care institutions in Israel, operating 18,000 beds. Of these, about a third were for the semi-independent (independent in ADL, and usually limited in homemaking capacity), about 25 percent for the frail, another third for those in need of skilled nursing, and the rest for the mentally infirm. There are approximately 48 beds per 1,000 Jewish elderly in the population. About 38 percent of the total beds belong to the private sector, and another 38 percent to the voluntary sector. The rest are divided between the public sector (14 percent) and ESHEL (10 percent). Close to half, or 8,320 elderly, were referred to institutions by the health or welfare agencies; their institutional costs were partially or fully subsidized through public sources.

One indicator of unmet needs is the number of elderly on waiting lists for placement after assessment and approval of the regional health of social service bureau. In 1989, there were 1,600 such elderly; about 60 percent of them required facilities for nursing care or were mentally infirm (Be'er and Factor 1990).

The overall rate of institutional placement in Israel, however, is relatively low–only about 5 percent of the elderly aged 65 and over are in institutional settings. This percentage, of course, increases with age. Of those aged 85 and over, about 20 percent are in residential care.

Changes in the size and composition of the elderly population, and especially the recent large waves of immigration, continue to dictate a rapid increase in the need for long-term care beds. Approximately 1,000 additional beds will be built by 1993.

In the period from 1983 to 1989, the institutional system increased by 30 percent. All of the growth took place in beds for disabled elderly, and especially for the frail elderly, whereas there was a decrease in beds for those who are independent. This reflects the philosophy of providing for independent older people in the community. Further, the major expansion was in the private sector, which contributed almost two-thirds of the total between 1987 and 1989, mainly in beds for nursing care and the mentally infirm.

The institutions for well and frail elderly are under the supervision of the Ministry of Labor and Welfare, and licensing is based on the 1955 Supervision of Homes Law. Nursing homes are under the supervision of the Ministry of Health, and their licensing is based on the 1940 National Health Ordinance. Institutions differ along four dimensions: quality of care, admission criteria, openness, and cost (Bergman, Factor, and Kaplan 1985). Quality of care varies by sponsorship. Usually the commercial sector ranks lower than the others with regard to the range of professional services offered, the education and training of personnel, and the patient/staff ratios. Eligibility criteria have been laid down by the Ministries, but they allow for a great deal of discretion. Some institutions have their own criteria, ranging from ethnic-cultural to purely economic considerations.

SHELTERED HOUSING

Sheltered housing is a recent development in Israel, emerging largely since the early 1980s. In the years 1985 to 1989, it grew by 29 percent (Be'er and Factor 1990). By 1989, there were 73 programs, operating 6,314 units for elderly singles and couples. This represented about 16.8 units per 1,000 elderly. Approximately half belong to the public sector and to "Amigur," a governmental agency, 36 percent to the voluntary sector (primarily Mishan), and 17 percent to the private sector. Two target populations are served through sheltered housing: the well elderly, mainly through the private sector, whereby people can finance their own stay; and the economically needy elderly, for whom there is no requirement for a security deposit.

Sheltered housing programs differ in certain characteristics: the size of the program, contact and integration with community or institutional services, eligibility criteria, and the basket of services offered. In most of them there are housing managers, emergency facilities, and various social services. In some of the new programs a nursing unit is also added. No governmental licensing or supervision exists.

TOWARD THE TWENTY-FIRST CENTURY

In planning for the twenty-first century, Israel needs to be guided by both continuity and change in its existing services network. The major question entails priorities in resource allocation, especially now that the State is confronted with massive waves of elderly immigrants.

Two main target populations should be addressed: the first is the well aged, many of whom will be native born, with more resources and expectations for services than the elderly of the 1990s. For this group, we foresee the development of new types of community services such as neighborhood service centers, programs focusing on prevention of illnesses and health promotion, local information centers, and a single entry point for services. There will be a need to develop a variety of volunteer activities and encourage more active participation by the elderly in the decision-making process. Moreover, the supply of sheltered housing will have to be increased, as will the development of alternative housing models. According to one source, a high priority will be placed on loans to the elderly for renovating their apartments (Rotem 1991).

The second target group is the "old-old" (80+) and the frail elderly who, discounting further immigration, will grow by 36 percent by the year 2,000, and represent 40,000 people (Factor and Primak 1991). For these elderly, there will be a need to increase the scope of home-based and community-based services. These include respite care, home-care services, day-care centers, services for the mentally impaired, and support to family caregivers.

In addition, there will be a need to develop more institutional beds for the frail and handicapped elderly by enlarging existing facilities and promoting further investment by the private sector. Some of the kibbutzim today are beginning to cooperate with private agencies to build new models of residential facilities within the framework of the kibbutz, both for members and for outsiders.

These developments should be closely tied with training and educating new professionals in aging services, with emphasis on interdisciplinary work, such as family doctors in community clinics, field level managers and semi-professional workers. There also will be a need to improve the quality of care, physical standards, nutrition, and client participation in decision making, and to strengthen the links between institutions and the community (Rotem 1991). In addition, service coordination, especially at the local level, should be emphasized with the support and encouragement of the local associations for the aged.

A special target group will be the frail and the disabled among the Russian immigrants for whom housing and institutional beds will have to be developed. Also, more public funds should be allocated for the frail elderly of Sephardic origin, for their resources are more limited than those elderly of Ashkenazi origin.

CONCLUSION

Israel's commitment to the welfare of its aged citizens has been documented not only by its progressive laws, but through the many innovative and creative networks of social and health care services. In recent years, priorities in services development and provision have shifted in favor of children, who constitute perhaps the most deprived group among the poor and the needy of the country (Guttmann and Cohen, in press). However, the aged still maintain a certain political leverage, which, in combination with age-old Jewish tradition, ensure heightened awareness of their needs, and a national interest in their well-being. Despite this generally positive attitude, serious gaps remain in home-based and institutional care, as well as in personnel development. Moreover, the recent trend toward privatization of hospitals, nursing homes, sheltered housing, and health care will enlarge the growing gap between the "haves" and the "have nots" among the aged, and will create a situation which may run counter to the existing goal of quality care for all those in need. The prevailing ideology of "Honor thy father and thy mother" may well be in jeopardy.

REFERENCES

Achdut, L., and Tamir, Y. 1986. *Retirement and Well-Being among the Elderly.* National Insurance Institute, Jerusalem.

Adelson, G.; Kaminsky, P.; and Cohen, C. 1979. Volunteers can help patients adjust. *Health and Social Work* 4(1): 184-199.

Be'er, S., and Factor, H. 1990. *Long-Term Care Institutions and Sheltered Housing: The Situation in 1989 and Changes Over Time.* Brookdale Institute, Jerusalem (Hebrew).

Bergman, S. 1980. Israel. In *International Handbook on Aging,* edited by E. Palmore. Greenwood Press, 208-233.

Bergman, S. 1981. Introduction. In *ESHEL Guidelines for Planning Old Age Homes in Israel.* Jerusalem (Hebrew).

Bergman, S.; Factor, H.; and Kaplan, A. 1985. *Census of Institutions for Long Term Care in Israel, 1983.* Brookdale Institute, Jerusalem.

Bergman S., and Lowenstein, A. 1988. Care of the aging in Israel: Social service delivery. *Journal of Gerontological Social Work,* 12(1/2): 97-116.

Berman, R.U. 1981. A Judaic journey creates communication: In-service education of staff of a Jewish home for the aged. *Journal of Jewish Communal Services* 58(1): 61-66.

Day Care Center for the Aged–Guidelines for Management and Operation (1990). ESHEL–The Association for Planning and Development of Services to the Aged in Israel, Jerusalem (Hebrew).

Della Pergola, S. 1989. *Conference on Aging in the Jewish World.* Jerusalem.

ESHEL–Association for the Planning and Development of Services for the Aged in Israel. 1989. Jerusalem (Hebrew).

Factor, H., and Primak, H. 1991. Disability among the elderly Jewish population and projections of its extent expected by the year 2,000. *Gerontology,* 53:28-38 (Hebrew).

Friedman, S. 1990. *The Services for the Aged–A General Review.* Ministry of Labour and Social Welfare. Jerusalem (Hebrew).

Goell, Y. 1991. Not so sick as all that. *The Jerusalem Post,* Friday, July 26: 11.

Guttmann, D. 1990. Filial Responsibility–A Logo Therapeutic View. *The Journal of Aging and Judaism,* 3(4): 173-187.

Guttmann, D., and Cohen, B.Z. In press. Teaching about poverty in Israeli Schools of Social Work. *International Social Work.*

Guttmann, D., and Lowenstein, A. 1991. Demographic changes in Israel and their implications for professional education in aging for the 21st century. *The Journal of Aging and Judaism,* 5(3): 215-226.

Haber-Shaim, N. 1987. Senile dementia in Israel: A first assessment. *Gerontology,* 36-37: 3-15 (Hebrew).

Habib, J. 1988. Population aging and Israeli society. *Journal of Aging and Judaism,* 1(2):7-28.

Habib, J.; Factor, H.; and Be'er, S. 1987. Evaluating the needs for long-term care services and their cost. *Social Security,* 30 (Hebrew).

Habib, J.; Factor, H.; and Shmueli, A. 1987. *The Need for Community Services and Their Cost.* D-142. Brookdale Institute, Jerusalem (Hebrew).

Heinik, J. 1987. Alzheimer's disease and psychosis. *Gerontology,* 36-37:16-20 (Hebrew).

Isaacs, L.W. 1986. With our young and with our old. *The Journal of Aging and Judaism,* 1(1): 57-67.

Israel Statistical Yearbook, Statistical Abstracts. 1983, 1987, 1989, 1990. The Central Bureau of Statistics. Jerusalem, Israel.

Kahana, B.; Harel, Z.; and Kahana, E. 1988. Predictors of psychological well-being among survivors of the Holocaust. In *Human Adaptation to Extreme Stress,* edited by P. Wilson, Z. Harel, and B. Kahana. New York: Plenum Press, 171-192.

Kerem, B.Z., and Zweig, H. 1990. *Special Programs in the Field of Aging.* Szold Institute, ESHEL, and Ministry of Labour and Social Welfare, Jerusalem (Hebrew).

Korazim, M.; Trachtenberg, S.; and Habib, J. 1990. *Day Care Centers Overall Research Approach and Findings on Target Populations and Models.* Brookdale Institute. Jerusalem. (Report No. 1, Hebrew).

Krulik, T.; Hirschfeld, M.; and Sharon, R. 1984. *Family Care for the Severely Handicapped Children and Aged in Israel.* Dept. of Nursing, Sachler School of Medicine, Tel Aviv University.

Lopata, H.Z. 1978. The absence of community resources in support systems of urban widows. *The Family Coordinator,* 27(4): 383-388.

Lowenstein, A. 1983. The Nursing Insurance Law. *Gerontology,* 3-8 (Hebrew).

Master Program for Services for the Aged in Haifa. 1989. Haifa Municipality, Haifa (Hebrew).

Master Program for Services for the Aged in Tel Aviv-Yaffo. 1986. Tel Aviv Municipality, Tel Aviv (Hebrew).

Matras, J. 1991. The absorption of older immigrants into the labor force. *Gerontology,* 53:20-27 (Hebrew).

McCuan, E.E.; Hooyman, N.; and Fortune, A.E. 1985. Social support for the frail elderly. In *Social Support Networks and the Care of the Elderly,* edited by W.J. Sauer and R.T. Coward. New York: Springer Publishing Company, 234-248.

Morginstin, B. 1987. Response of formal support to social changes and patterns of caring for the elderly. *Social Security,* 30, 78-97 (Hebrew).

Morginstin, B. 1990. *The Impact of Demographic and Socio-Economic Factors on the Changing Needs of the Very Old.* National Insurance Institute. Jerusalem (Discussion Paper 3).

Olitzky, K.M. (1985). Synagogue: A new concept for a new age. *Journal of Jewish Communal Service,* 62(1): 8-10.

Ordinance of the Nation's Health, 1940. Ministry of Health, Jerusalem.

Roseman, Y., and Rosen, G., eds. 1984. *Jewish Grandparenting and the Intergenerational Connection.* Summary of Proceedings. The American Jewish Committee, New York: Institute of Human Relations.

Rotem, D. 1991. *ESHEL's Five Year Plan 1991-1995.* ESHEL. Jerusalem (Hebrew).

Schnitt, D. 1988. The Long-Term Care Insurance Law–the legal aspect. *Social Security,* Special English Edition, 84-102.

Shanas, E. 1984. Old parents and middle-aged children: The four and five generation family. *Journal of Geriatric Psychiatry,* 17(1):19.

Shmueli, A. 1989. Single and multi-generational living arrangements of elderly persons in Israel, 1972-1982. *Social Security,* 33:32-43 (Hebrew).

Sixty + Survey. 1985. Central Bureau of Statistics. Jerusalem, Israel (in Hebrew).

Taylor, R. 1988. The elderly as members of society: An examination of social differences in an elderly population. In *The Aging Population, Burden or Challenge,* edited by N. Wells and C. Freer. The Macmillan Press Ltd., London.

Weil, H. 1991. *Welfare Services in the Arab Sector in Israel.* ESHEL. Jerusalem (Hebrew).

Chapter 6

The Care of Frail Older People in Britain: Current Policies and Future Prospects

Alan Walker
Lorna Warren

INTRODUCTION

This chapter has three main aims. First, we outline the extent of the need for care among older people in Britain. As in other countries, this need is primarily confined to periods of frailty associated with advanced old age rather than evenly distributed across the population of older people. Therefore, our analysis concentrates on those aged 75 and over. Second, the main forms of care provision in Britain are described as a prelude to a discussion of recent changes in service provision and their implications for older people and their caregivers. Third, we summarize the main deficiencies of the existing pattern of care for frail older people and examine some of the recent innovations in this field to see whether they would offer improved prospects for both older people and their caregivers.

THE GROWING NEED FOR CARE

Britain, like other industrial societies, has experienced a significant growth in the need for care over the course of this century. This is a trend, moreover, that is likely to continue well into the next century. The major source of this growth is the expansion in the numbers of older people and especially the numbers in the oldest age group. The causes of this population aging–a long-term decline in fertility coupled with declining mortality among all age groups–are also a common feature among industrial societies (Ermisch 1983), hence the widespread concern on the part of national governments and international economic agencies about the so-called economic "burden" of aging (Walker 1990).

In the past 50 years, the number of people aged 65 and over has more than doubled to just over 9 million (15.8 percent of the population), while those aged 75 and over tripled to 4 million (7 percent). This is a continuing trend: apart from a slight decline between 1991 and 2001, the population aged 65 and over is projected to continue to increase steadily well into the next century, to over 11 million (18 percent of the population) in 2021. The largest rises between now and 2021 are expected in the numbers of those aged 75 and over and 85 and over: 30 percent and 98 percent respectively. By 2021, women will outnumber men in the 85 and over age group by approximately 2.5 to 1, so the world of advanced old age is predominantly a women's world.

As age increases, the incidence of ill-health and disability rises, hence the consumption of both informal care and formal health and social services also increases. This is not to imply that age itself is the cause of need and demand for care. On the contrary, the relationship between age and need is not so straightforward. Many 80 year-olds remain active and interdependent with their families and friends while others require varying levels of physical help and support. But as age increases beyond 50, there is a marked rise in the incidence of disability in successively older age groups–particularly at the lower levels of severity. There is a very rapid increase in severe incapacity beyond the age of 70 (Townsend 1981; Martin, Meltzer and Elliott 1988, 19). For example, the prevalence of very severe disability in Britain is as follows[1]:

Age Group Cumulative Prevalence Rate
     (per 1000 population)
     40-49   11
     50-59   23
     60-69   47

70-79	100
80+	388
Total population	40

The prevalence of very severe disability among women aged 75 and over is more than three times greater than the rate for men in the same age group (240 per thousand compared with 76 per thousand).

All of the major causes of physical ill-health and disability in old age–arthritis, cardiac and pulmonary conditions, blindness and failing sight, deafness, circulatory conditions–are more likely to occur in successively older age groups and often do so concurrently. The situation is similar with mental deterioration: around 6 percent of all persons aged 65 and over suffer from some form of dementia but, among those aged 80 and over, this increases to 22 percent (Family Policy Studies Centre 1986). Moreover, women aged 80 and over are more than 40 times as likely as those aged 59-65 to suffer from an organic brain syndrome, while men in the oldest age group are twice as likely as their younger counterparts to experience organic mental impairment (Royal College of Physicians Committee on Geriatrics 1981).

The positive association between old age and the prevalence of disability means that population aging automatically entails a growth in the need for care. However, it is important not to assume that these needs are necessarily commensurate or permanent because there are good reasons to expect that future generations of older people will be healthier than present ones (Manton 1986; Butler, Oberlink, and Schechter 1990). Predictions based on current levels of disability among older people indicate a substantial rise in the need for care over the next 30 years. For instance, between 1991 and 2021 there will be a rise of 26 percent in the number of older people unable to bathe or shower alone–that is an average of an extra 20 people per day for the next 30 years (Phillipson and Walker 1986, 7).

While they indicate the scale of the challenge facing informal and formal caregivers, statistics such as these demonstrate, paradoxically, that the most important source of care in old age is self-care. In other words, the vast majority of older people are not in need of care from others and are able to look after themselves with either very little or no assistance. Even among those aged 75 and over, only a minority suffer from severe disablement (less than one-fifth) and, as a result, the need for major inputs of care also stems from a minority. For example, in a random sample of people aged 75 and over living in Sheffield, England, Qureshi and Walker (1989, 75) found that three out of five (62.6 percent) needed either no or only very minor assistance with personal care and household management tasks. At the other end of the severity scale, one in five (21 percent) required substantial care and tending. The ratio of those needing substantial physical assistance between the 75 to 79 and 85-plus age groups was one to six.

Not surprisingly, the supply of both informal and formal care varies in line with this picture of increasing need in advanced old age. A national survey of informal caregivers in 1985 found that over half (54 percent) were caring for someone aged 75 and over (three-quarters of the 75 year-olds and over were women) compared with 36 percent in the 45 to 74 years age range (Green 1988, 18). Furthermore, within the population aged 75 and over, those aged 85 or over are more than four times as likely as those aged 75 to 79 to be receiving high levels of care and tending (Qureshi and Walker 1989, 82). As far as care is concerned, the average expenditure per head of public hospital and community health services on those aged 75 and over is two and a half times that spent on the 65 to 74 age group and ten times the spending on the 16 to 64 age group. In the personal social services,[2] the ratio of public expenditure per head between the 75-plus and 65 to 74 age groups is four to one (Ermisch 1990, 42).

The Future Supply of Informal Care

While policymakers are primarily concerned with the growing need for care from the perspective of expenditure on the health and social services, the fact is that, for those older people in need of it, the main source of care is the family. Thus the numbers of very frail people aged 80 or more living in private households is some two-thirds higher than the number living in all hospitals, nursing and residential homes put together (219,000 compared with 133,000). Among those aged 70 to 79, there are more than three times as many very frail older people living in their own or their relatives' homes than in all communal establishments (183,000 compared with 54,000).[3] Qureshi and Walker (1989, 119) confirmed the importance of the family as the primary source of informal care: only 9 percent of those aged 75 and over in their survey received regular help from nonrelatives.

The main providers of informal care within the family are female kin (Land 1978; Finch and Groves 1983), even though a substantial number of caregivers nowadays are men (Arber and Gilbert 1989; Evandrou 1990). In the Sheffield study of family care, daughters were the most common source of help: over half (52 percent) of older people receiving assistance had at least one daughter helping, while one in four of them was being helped by a lone daughter (Qureshi and Walker 1989, 120). In addition, women bear the main burden of guilt and worry that caring relationships usually entail (Graham 1983; Ungerson 1987; Lewis and Meredith 1988). The crucial importance of the family, and female kin in particular, as the mainstay of care for older people has been demonstrated in a long series of studies in North America as well as Britain (see, for example, Shanas et al. 1968; Block 1985; Shapiro 1985; Qureshi and Walker 1989).

To a very great extent, the future supply of informal care for frail older people and, in turn, the demand for health and social services, rests on the question of how far the family, and especially female kin, will be willing or able to continue shouldering the main responsibility. Certainly, there are powerful normative pressures at work compelling women into caring roles–especially the ideology of "familism" (Dalley 1988; Qureshi and Walker 1989). These pressures are buttressed by social policies–particularly the norm of "non-intervention" in the family practiced by successive British governments (Moroney 1976; Walker 1991a). Equally, however, the caring relationship is likely to be subjected to increasing strains in the future as a result of socio-demographic changes. There are five main changes to be considered briefly.

First, the ratio of potential family caregivers per person aged 75 and over has declined steadily over the course of this century (Eversley 1982) and can be expected to continue to do so. Moreover, as a result of the decline in fertility in the 1920s and its slow recovery, the generation currently in advanced old age has fewer children than any previous generation in Britain. Population projections suggest that the number of women not having any children is rising slightly while the number having two or more children is falling slightly (Central Statistical Office 1990, 44).

Second, the growth in the proportion of people surviving into advanced old age means that more and more older people, particularly women, are outliving their relatives. Women aged 80 and over experience the highest rate of widowhood and are the most likely to be living alone (61 percent do so compared with 36 percent of all those aged 65 and over) (Kiernan and Wicks 1990, 23). In the Sheffield study of family care, 63 percent of women aged 75 and over were living alone compared with 28 percent of men; nine out of ten single-person households were the result of bereavement (Qureshi and Walker 1989, 36).

As in other industrial societies, the proportion of older people in Britain sharing the same residence as their children is small and has declined over the post-war period (Fengler, Danigelis, and Little 1983; Qureshi and Walker 1989). This does not mean, of course, that the family is breaking up or less willing to care for older people than in the past–as the evidence on the active caring role of the family quoted earlier shows–but merely that both sides of the caring relationship prefer "intimacy at a distance" (Rosenmayer and Kockeis 1963).

The fact remains, however, that an increasing proportion of older people has no surviving relatives. Thus, over the next 30 years it is predicted that the numbers of people aged 85 and over living alone will increase by 55 percent (the overall predicted rise for those aged 65 and over is 19 percent). In Britain there are, in addition, special problems facing older people from racial minorities who emigrated to this country in their later years, leaving most of their adult relatives behind. They form a very small but potentially vulnerable group.

Third, increasing longevity means that the aged caregiver is becoming a more and more common phenomenon. Nationally, 8 percent of people aged 75 years or over are caregivers–a significant figure given the relatively high prevalence of disability in this age group.

Fourth, family breakdown is likely to have some impact on the future supply of informal care. Over the last 20 years the divorce rate has more than doubled and, largely as a result, lone-parent families now comprise 16 percent of all families with children compared to 8 percent in 1971 (Kiernan and Wicks 1990, 14). Britain has one of the highest proportions of lone-parent families in the European Community (EC), though no EC country matches the US, where the rate is around 25 percent. Even though the rate of remarriage in Britain is high, the impact of family breakdown and reconstitution is likely to have some, as yet unknown, influence on patterns of obligation within the family.

Fifth, economic change may affect the supply of informal care. For example, the growth of poverty during the post-war period, mainly associated with the rise of unemployment, has weakened the ability of some families to care for their relatives (Walker and Walker 1987). Moreover, there is evidence from the Sheffield research on family care that unemployed sons had less contact with their older parents than working sons and were less likely to give them any practical assistance (Qureshi and Walker 1989, 115).

Finally, there is the continuing upward trend in female labor force participation: from 52 percent of 25-44 year olds in 1961, to 74 percent in 1991, to an estimated 80 percent in 2000. This may have some impact on the ability and willingness of women to care for their older relatives though, remarkably, there are no signs as yet of it doing so. Indeed, many of the physical and mental costs associated with caring result from the fact that women are often sustaining two or three separate sets of responsibilities–caring for the nuclear family, caring for older relatives, and paid employment–with predictably deleterious consequences for their own health. Today, 3 million of the estimated 6 million caregivers are also in paid employment.

This brings us to what is, perhaps, the major question concerning the future supply of informal care to frail older people in Britain and indeed other industrial societies: whether or not women will be prepared to go on bearing the multiple burdens of caregiving in the face of rising need (in terms of both the scale of help required and the time period over which it must be sustained); the various constraints on their ability to provide care; and their own growing opposition to the unequal division of domestic labor.

THE CHANGING ROLE OF THE STATE
IN THE PROVISION OF CARE

The future of care for frail older people rests primarily on the outcome of developments in the informal sector because the state has always played a relatively minor role in direct care provision, though it has exerted a powerful covert influence in maintaining the primacy of the family (Walker 1991a). As far as the formal sector is concerned, the state has dominated both direct care provision and funding for the whole of the post-war period, with the private (for profit) and voluntary (nonprofit) organizations occupying very minor roles. However, in recent years this pattern of formal care has begun to change dramatically under the steam of neo-liberal ideology.[4]

Responsibility for social care in Britain has rested primarily with local authorities (funded by a mixture of central grant and local taxation) while the national health service (NHS) is concerned with medical treatment (funded entirely from general taxation and administered by central government). Of course, the distinction between care and treatment is not always easy to make–especially when, as in Britain, there is a system of community-based general practitioners and allied services. This administrative distinction may be one reason why the proportion of older people living in institutions is relatively low in Britain compared to North America. Thus, only about 6 percent of older people live in hospitals or residential and nursing homes compared with 10 percent in Canada. The involvement of institutional care increases markedly at the upper end of the age and severity of disability continua and especially when frailty and advanced old age are combined. So, among very frail older people aged 80 and over, nearly two-fifths (38 percent) are in communal establishments compared with only 5 percent of those with minor disabilities. Among those aged 70-79, the figures are 23 percent and 2 percent, respectively (Martin, Meltzer, and Elliot 1988, 18).

In Britain, the favored option of successive post-war governments of different political persuasions has been "community care." This political consensus was sustained, in part, by the ambiguous and largely symbolic nature of the term "community care," but, more importantly, it enabled the state to both promote the primacy of the family in caregiving and minimize its own role to that of a casualty or last-resort service (Walker 1991a). Moreover, the consensus existed solely at the policy level; there never was consensus between service providers and service users or potential users. In fact, the relationship between people in need of care and their caregivers, on the one hand, and the state, on the other, in community care policy is best analyzed in terms of conflict rather than consensus (Walker 1983). Also, paradoxically, even though institutions have played a small part in the care of older people, they have dominated the budgets of both health and social services for the whole of the post-war period. As a consequence, community services are often referred to as the "Cinderella" services. In the personal social services, these typically comprise Home Helps or home caregivers, home wardens, meals-on-wheels, personal mobility aids, and telephones. In addition, most social service departments (SSDs) provide or fund day centers for older people (see Table 1).

Not surprisingly, the political consensus on community care was a precarious one. It relied on ambiguity and uncertainty of purpose in policy and the absence of strategic planning; the maintenance of the family as the main provider of care with local SSDs in a very minor role; and the subordination of the funding of community care services to institutional interests in both the health and social services. Thus, to paraphrase Edelman (1977), the words "community care" have succeeded magnificently but the policy itself is a miserable failure.

Such consensus as there was between the two main political parties was confined to the assumption of the secondary role of the formal sector to the informal sector and on the premise that when services were provided in the community the most appropriate location for the planning, organization, and delivery of these services was SSDs. Beyond this general support for a value-laden and idealistic concept, the primacy of the family and the leading role of SSDs in service provision, there was no deeper consensus among policy-

TABLE 1. Health and Social Services Provision for Older People (England and Wales)

	1974		1979		1984	
	Nos	Nos. per 1000 75+	Nos	Nos. per 1000 75+	Nos	Nos. per 1000 75+
Average daily number of occupied geriatric beds	54,600	22.1	54,500	19.6	54,100	17.1
SSD Homes (occupied places)	98,600	40.0	109,100	39.3	109,200	34.5
Nursing Homes (long-stay occupied beds)	11,900	4.8	13,800	5.0	24,100	7.6
Voluntary Homes (occupied places)	22,300	9.5	25,600	9.2	26,900	8.5
Private Homes (occupied places)	19,300	7.8	26,800	9.7	55,000	17.4
Day Patient (attendances/day)	4,100	1.7	5,000	1.8	7,000	2.2
SSD Day Centre (places)	13,800	5.6	29,100	10.5	34,400	10.9
Home Help staff (wtes)*	45,200	18.3	49,600	17.9	56,700	17.9
Meals (100 per year)*	35,200	14.3	43,300	15.6	45,000	14.2

Note: * Numbers of home help staff (whole-time equivalents) and meals served to all client groups but are predominantly for older people.

Source: Audit Commission (1986) p. 19.

makers (Titmuss 1968; Walker 1986a). For example, over the whole of the post-war period there was (and remains) a wide divergence among local authorities in the levels of their service provision (see, for example, Webb and Wistow 1987, 160-185). Moreover, the failure to extend social services provision in response to rising need has resulted in a growing "care gap" between the need for care and the provision of domiciliary services (Walker 1985).

The End of the Consensus on Community Care

Since the election of the first Thatcher government in 1979, the assumptions underlying policy in the personal social services have changed dramatically. In contrast to its post-war predecessors, this government was characterised by an overt neo-liberal ideology which remained the driving force behind policy throughout the 1980s. So it was new ideologically inspired pressures–budgetary and resource constraints and the cost-effectiveness imperative– combined with a major expansion of need for care, particularly among older people, that produced the political will to overcome both the policy inertia and power struggle between sectional inter- ests that had lain behind the precarious consensus on community care. But the policy itself departs significantly from the previous consensus. Thus, the emphasis has been shifted away from care in the community largely by local authority personnel toward a con- fusing mixture of care by the community itself and private care, regardless of whether in domiciliary or institutional settings. There are three main dimensions to this change in policy (Walker 1981).

In the first place, while the primary intention of community care policy over the past 12 years appears to have been the negative one of reducing the role of health and social services authorities in the provision of care, the 1980s also witnessed for the first time the active official encouragement of the private sector. This new policy direction was signalled early in the life of the first Thatcher govern- ment when, soon after coming to power, the Department of Health and Social Security (DHSS)[5] moved to encourage a switch in the provision of residential care from the public sector to the private sector.

It did so by employing two complementary policies. On the one hand, the resources available to local authority SSDs were cut while, on the other, the private sector was offered a substantial financial inducement. The DHSS agreed not only to meet the full cost of care in private residential and nursing homes for those living on income support,[6] but it also allowed its local offices to set limits on such payments as were deemed appropriate for their area. As a result, the number of places in private residential homes for older people and people with physical and mental disabilities nearly doubled (97 percent) between 1979 and 1984, and by 1990 had risen by 130 percent since 1979. Between 1989 and 1990 alone the proportion of beds in private residential homes for older people rose by 9 percent while beds in private nursing homes increased by 27 percent. At the same time, the number of beds in local authority homes declined slightly during the 1980s (see Table 2).

The parallel story of expenditure on both residential and nursing homes was that of a rapid increase from £6 million ($10.2 million) in 1978, to £460 million ($782 million) in 1988, and to £1.3 billion ($2.21 billion) in 1991. The proportion of older people in private residential homes receiving help with their fees through income support payments increased from 14 percent in 1979 to 35 percent in 1984 and, by 1988, had reached 56 percent (Bradshaw and Gibbs 1988, 4; NACAB 1991, 6). Since this growth in spending conflicted with the government's policy of reducing public expenditure, the DHSS acted to stem the flow of resources first by freezing local limits and then by imposing national ceilings for residential and nursing home payments. These limits are currently £150 ($255) for residential and £200 ($340) for nursing homes for older people and, therefore, still represent a major source of income to the private sector. In addition, many local authorities use private homes on an agency basis to house some of their residents. This action had a relatively minor impact on the growth of social security subsidies, and this proved to be the fastest growing element of public expenditure in the 1980s.

Secondly, at the same time that it imposed severe resource constraints on local authorities and encouraged the rapid growth of private residential and nursing homes, the government embarked on a radical program of mental health hospital closure. The policy of hospital rundown, particularly of mental illness facilities, dates back to the late 1950s. However, prior to 1987 no major hospital had been closed (Social Services Committee 1985, xix). The government achieved this breakthrough by exerting considerable pressure on health authorities to close hospitals within specified time limits.

TABLE 2. Numbers of people aged 65 and over in residential care (England)

	1980	1989	% Change 1980-1989
All residents 65 and over			
LA homes	102,890	95,335	−7
Voluntary homes	25,449	25,801	+1
Private homes	28,854	111,391	+286
All homes	157,193	232,527	+48
All residents 75 and over			
LA homes	76,078	83,573	+10
Voluntary homes	21,626	22,832	+6
Private homes	25,220	100,266	+298
All homes	122,924	206,671	+68
All residents 85 and over			
LA homes	35,938	43,763	+22
Voluntary homes	10,761	13,109	+22
Private homes	12,467	53,954	+333
All homes	59,166	110,826	+87

Note: LA = Local Authority
Source: DH (1989b) Table B.

This radical Conservative policy succeeded in promoting community care whereas previous consensus policies had failed to overcome both institutional inertia and professional interests. However, the main motivation for doing so has been cost-efficiency, with the effectiveness of care received in the community taking second place. This was the main thrust of the trenchant critique of the government's community care policy toward people with mental disabilities by the all-party House of Commons Social Services Committee (1985), one of the most authoritative among several similarly critical reports to be issued over the last 10 years. The

Social Services Committee focused attention on the disaster course that had been set by forcing a closure program without sufficient planning, preparation, and consultation and, furthermore, without any agreed understanding of what the intended community care would actually entail. It was especially mindful of the danger that community care is perceived as a cheap option.

The official rhetoric surrounding the government's policy may be community care, but the reality is actually more like decanting and dehospitalization, coupled with an increase in both public and private residential placements. Thus, while the numbers in long stay hospitals have declined, there has been a commensurate increase in people with mental disabilities living in both public and private homes. The result of hurried dehospitalization in the face of the underfunding of community-based services is that many people with mental disabilities are merely being shifted from one large institution to another, smaller one. People are ending up in residential homes that they do not need because there is no realistic alternative and private sector homes are subsidized by social security payments.

The Social Services Committee summed up the irresponsible nature of the government's care in the community policy in a famous sentence: "Any fool can close a long stay hospital: it takes more time and trouble to do it properly and compassionately" (Social Services Committee 1985, xxii). In trying to bring some sense to bear, the Committee attempted to establish the basic principles of a community care policy and insisted that statutory health and social services are central to the provision of community care. Both suggestions fell on deaf ears because they harked back to the pre-1980s consensus, though the government did act in response to the Committee's criticisms and ordered the slowing of the discharge program (DHSS 1985).

Thirdly, the government has been gradually residualizing the role of local authority social services, that is, reducing them from the main provider of formal care into the provider of those services for which no one else will take responsibility. A series of what seemed, as they occurred, to be separate policy developments over the past 12 years may, with the benefit of hindsight, be seen as part of this evolving residualization strategy.

In 1980, in a speech to directors, the then Secretary of State for Social Services, Patrick Jenkin, outlined a supportive and decidedly residual role for the social services: "a long-stop for the very special needs going beyond the range of voluntary services" (Jenkin 1980). In 1981, the White Paper on services for older people asserted, in a widely quoted phrase, "care in the community must increasingly mean care by the community" (DHSS 1981, 3). The previous year, when giving evidence before the House of Commons Social Services Committee, the Secretary of State justified the cuts in PSS expenditure and the closure of long-stay hospitals (outlined above) on the unsubstantiated assumption that the informal and voluntary sectors would expand:

> When one is comparing where one can make savings one protects the Health Service because there is no alternative, whereas in personal social services there is a substantial possibility and, indeed, probability of continuing growth in the amount of voluntary care, of neighbourhood care, of self help. (Social Services Committee 1980, 99-100)

This aim of placing greater reliance on quasi-formal voluntary help and informal support was reflected in the Care in the Community (1981) and the Helping the Community to Care (1984) initiatives by the DHSS.

But it was the second Thatcherite Secretary of State for Social Services who in 1984 provided the clearest and most detailed outline of the new residual role proposed for social services. He argued that there are "three paramount responsibilities" of SSDs: to take a comprehensive strategic view of all the sources of care available in the area; to recognize that the direct provision of services is only part of the local pattern and that in many cases other forms of provision are available; and to see a major part of their function as promoting and supporting the fullest possible participation of the other different sources of care. The fundamental role of the state, according to this view, was "to back up and develop the assistance which is given by private and voluntary support" (Fowler 1984, 13).

This policy of residualization itself comprises three main elements (Walker 1981). In the first place, the provision of community care is deliberately fragmented. Though sometimes presented as promoting a more mixed economy of welfare, the main motivations here have been to curtail the monopoly role of local authorities in the delivery of formal care–an aim that, as we have seen, has already been achieved in several parts of the country with regard to the residential care of older people–and to encourage the growth of cheaper sources of informal and quasi-formal care. To aid the development of voluntary help, self-help, and informal care (see p.132 above) a series of special initiatives, including the Care in the Community and the Helping the Community to Care programs, were introduced. One result of this policy of fragmentation was the advent, in the 1980s, of a wide range of precarious, often short-lived, projects relying on grant aid and government training schemes.

Secondly, there is marketization. As we have seen, while finances for local authority services have been tightly controlled, the private sector has been encouraged to expand by the open-ended provision of social security subsidies. Contracting out, or the purchase of service contracting, has a long history in the personal social services but it has been used primarily in relation to the voluntary sector (Webb and Wistow 1987, 89). So far, direct privatization has not affected the social services to the same extent as the NHS. But the Local Government Act (1988) gave the Secretary of State for the Environment powers to add to the list of services which must be contracted out.

Thirdly, the government has pursued a twin-track policy of decentralizing administration and operations, while centralizing control over resources. This is one manifestation of the general new right strategy of rolling back the frontiers of the state while centralizing state control (Gamble 1987). The process of centralizing control over social services resources began early in the life of the first Thatcher administration with the introduction of a new system of providing central government grant income to local authorities and, within it, detailed assessments for the different elements of personal social services spending (Walker 1985, 27). But responsibility for the operation of social services within centrally determined budgets remains with local authorities.

The cumulative impact of these three sets of policy developments is a strategy aimed at further residualizing the role of local authorities providing community care. Although some aspects of these policies were to be found under former governments, a concerted strategy of this sort has not been previously identifiable. Of course, in relation to the totality of care, both formal and informal, the social services have never been anything other than residual. The essence of the Thatcher and, since November 1990, the Major governments' approach toward community care, however, is that it is attempting, with some success, to reduce the role of local authorities as providers within the formal sector. Furthermore, it is intended to fill this artificially created care gap with a mixture of private, voluntary, and informal care.

A Mixed Economy of Welfare?

Some policy analysts (see, for example, Day and Klein 1987) have viewed the government's policy of boosting the growth of the private sector of residential care for older people as beneficial in terms of increasing choice in an expanding "mixed economy or welfare." Indeed, the appeal to increased choice has proved an important source of popular legitimation for the very fast expansion of the private sector. However, while it is true that there has been a rapid multiplication of private homes–estimated by the Audit Commission[7] (1986) to have been doubling in size each year for the first part of the 1980s–genuine choice requires a range of alternatives: public sector homes, day care, and the chance to remain in an ordinary home with community support. But, ironically, this latter choice has been restricted by the "perverse incentive" (Audit Commission 1986) for older people to enter residential care rather than stay in their own homes provided by social security. Furthermore, when it comes to entering a residential home, the concept of "choice" is rarely appropriate. The need for residential care usually arises because of a crisis of care in the informal sector, leaving little time to "shop around" for alternatives. Thus, as Bradshaw and Gibbs (1988) have confirmed, the promise of choice held by the supporters of the private sector is often illusory.

A study of the private sector by the Center for Policy in Aging found that only a quarter of residents exercised any choice about the home to which they were admitted, while nearly a quarter said that their admission resulted from unsolicited arrangements by a third party (Bradshaw and Gibbs 1988, 18). Choice between private homes is severely restricted by factors such as geographical location, waiting lists, and ability to pay. There is, for example, a clear north-south divide in the public/private mix of welfare. Private nursing home beds in the southwest outnumber those in the northern region by seven times. In two regions, South East and South West Thames, the private sector was providing more than half of the total unit health care for older people by the mid-1980s (Larder, Day, and Klein 1986). According to the Audit Commission (1986), a more equitable spatial distribution of resources for health and social services, which has been one aim of central allocation policies in the funding of the NHS and local government since the late 1970s, is being counteracted by the distribution of social security payments for private nursing and residential homes.

Within local areas, choice is restricted by the admission criteria applied by private homes, often excluding confused or demented people or those who are difficult to control. Thus, one survey found that there is a tendency for private homes to select the less severely disabled older people, leaving the more severely disabled for the public sector (ADSS 1986). Also, private homes often levy charges above the social security limits, requiring top-up payments, or make supplementary charges for single rooms or items such as laundry. This problem has been worsening since the government imposed national limits on social security payments in 1985 and subsequently failed to raise the benefit ceilings in line with increases in residential and nursing home charges. As a consequence, and despite the high cost of these payments to the Exchequer, more and more older residents are finding that their benefits are inadequate to cover the fees they are charged. According to the latest DSS figures, in August 1988, 42 percent of private residents in income support were paying fees above the national limits (Social Services Committee 1990).

The evidence suggests that older residents are not able to exercise much choice once they are inside private homes. A recent study of homes in North Yorkshire found that 21 percent had undergone a change of ownership in the previous 18 months (Bradshaw and Gibbs 1988, 19). Residents have no say in such changes and are not always informed before they happen. Nor do they have any choice about other changes in the character of their home:

> Residents entering small homely homes may find them enlarged. Residents have no control over the mix of residents or who shares their bedroom. As charges move ahead of (income support) limits residents may find themselves shifted into double or treble rooms, required to commit their pocket money to supplement the (income support) allowance or being subsidised by relatives–often without their knowledge. (Bradshaw and Gibbs 1988, 19-20).

Questions have been raised not only about the distributional consequences of the government's policy of promoting the private sector; considerable doubts have also been raised about the quality of the care provided. As the private residential sector has mushroomed, evidence has been mounting of abuse, misuse of drugs, fraud, lack of hygiene, and fire hazards in some homes (Harman and Lowe 1986; Holmes and Johnson 1988). Some of the worst cases of abuse have been documented by the media, such as Yorkshire Television's 1987 program "The Granny Business." Evidence of abuse in the private sector inevitably invites comparison with the public sector. Although there are similar instances of ill-treatment to be found there (see, for example, Gibbs, Evans, and Rodway 1987), they do not appear to be on the same scale as those in the private sector. However, concentrating on this sort of comparison of worst practices diverts attention from the two key issues: the operation of power in a residential setting, regardless of whether it is publicly or privately run, and which of the two sectors can be sufficiently regulated to ensure that no abuse of power occurs.

Unfortunately, those who argue that a reduced role for the public sector in the direct provision of care can be balanced by an increased regulatory role (see, for example, Day and Klein 1987) overlook the ideological imperative behind the expansion of the market in the care of older people in Britain. Marketization may be seen as one among many examples of the Thatcher and Major governments' neo-liberal inspired antagonism toward the decommodifying aspects of the welfare state. It is intended to challenge the extent, albeit limited, to which the social services intrude on market values and threaten their reproduction by promoting citizenship rights and needs-based priorities. Within this sort of ideological context, regulation is never likely to be given a prominent place. Regulation hinders the efficient operation of the market and this might endanger the government's primary goal of expanding private provision.

Community Care in the 1990s

In 1987, the government instituted a review of community care provision by Sir Roy Griffiths, a director of one of the country's largest supermarket chains. The Griffiths Report was published in March 1988 and a White Paper, "Caring for People," followed in November 1989. The proposals in the White Paper were enacted by the NHS and Community Care Act (1990) though the implementation of the main elements of the Act was recently postponed from April first, 1991 to April first, 1993 (until after the next general election).

What are the main changes in policy that will flow from the implementation of the Act? The White Paper defined four key components of community care which together reflect the emphasis on the promotion of choice in policy developments over the previous decade, cast in the language of consumerism. They are: services that respond flexibly and sensitively to the needs of individuals and their caregivers; services that intervene no more than is necessary to foster independence; services that allow a range of options for consumers; and services that concentrate on those with the greatest needs (DH 1989a, 5). In the White Paper, "choice" is defined as "giving people a greater individual say in how they live their lives and the services they need to help them" (DH 1989a, 4). This is to be achieved in two main ways: a comprehensive process of assessment and care management, which "where possible should induce [the] active participation of the individual and his or her caregiver," and a more diverse range of nonstatutory providers among whose benefits is held to be "a wider range of choice of services for the consumer" (DH 1989a, 19, 22).

The main changes affecting older people and others in need of care are as follows: local authorities will have "lead agency" responsibility for assessing need, designing packages of care, and ensuring services are delivered. Local authorities will also have to produce and publish plans for the development of community care services. There will be a unified community care budget in the control of local authorities comprising resources transferred from social security to augment social services finances (this will end the practice of social security subsidizing the private sector in an open-ended way because, after April 1993, such payments will depend on assessments of need by local authority social services personnel). Some controversy surrounded the award of "lead agency" status to local SSDs. This policy is in line with the Griffiths Report (1988) but at odds with the government's residualization strategy. However, as Griffiths (1988, vii) states, "the role of the public sector is essentially to ensure that care is provided. How it is provided is an important but secondary consideration." In other words, the policy is entirely consistent with the residualization of local authorities as direct service providers.

What are the likely implications for frail older people of this radical change in the organization and delivery of services? In theory this new policy offers the prospect of wider choice and the opportunity for service users to exercise some influence over the care packages they receive. In practice, however, these goals are unlikely to be realised.

In the first place, the reorganization of services is being conducted in the context of neo-liberal ideological hegemony. Thus, the measures being implemented (like the Griffiths review that inspired them) are primarily management oriented, with an overriding concern for cost containment rather than meeting need or promoting quality. As a result, the policy enacted by the government does not contain any concrete proposals for directly involving older people or their caregivers in decision making. In the absence of clear guidelines for such involvement, it is likely that professional opinions will continue to dominate. This is evident in the language employed: "managers of care packages," "case managers" and "caring for people." Thus, instead of determining their own packages of care, service users are still seen as passive recipients.

Secondly, also as a result of the ideological context of change, a premium is placed on nonstate forms of provision. Local authorities will be expected to employ competitive tendering or other means of marketizing the production of welfare. This gives a rather slanted meaning to the "mixed economy of care." For example, the White Paper suggested that one of the ways social services departments could promote a mixed economy of care is by "determining clear specifications of service requirements, and arrangements for tenders and contracts" (DH 1989a, 23). But evidence from the U.S. indicates that competitive tendering may actually reduce the choice available by driving small producers out of contention (Demone and Gibelman 1989).

Thirdly, the government's professed aims of increasing choice, and sensitivity to the requirements of older people and others needing care, will be inevitably compromised by the process of assessment which is required to ration resources. Thus no one will receive public funding for residential care after April 1993 unless they have been assessed and recommended by case managers. This process is bound to limit individual choice and user influence while, conversely, enhancing the power of bureau-professionals. Moreover, users do not have a right to elect to be assessed and there are no safeguards for those who disagree with professional assessments.

Fourthly, despite the rhetoric concerning the needs of caregivers, there are no proposals designed to ensure that their needs are taken into account. In the absence of such guarantees, of course, there is a danger that, under financial pressure, they will be ignored. Furthermore, the fact that there might be a conflict of interest between caregivers and receivers is not recognized by the government. This is a very real problem facing frail older people, their caregivers and service providers. The failure to address this dilemma stems from the assumption underlying both these proposals and the Griffiths Report, namely, that the family should in all circumstances be the primary source of care. However, research has shown that this confidence in familism is sometimes misplaced; family care can be both the best and the worst form of support (Qureshi and Walker 1989). If policymakers continue to assume that the family is always the soundest basis for care, they will overlook inherent conflicts in the caring relationship and be guilty of imposing some destructive relationships on both caregivers and receivers.

The Limitations of Consumerism

Underlying these deficiencies in the new community care arrangements–especially when viewed from the perspective of service users–are the legacy of antagonism toward public welfare provision discussed earlier and a very restricted concept of user involvement (Walker 1991b).

The Griffiths Report, White Paper, and NHS and Community Care Act all derive from the limited form of supermarket-style consumerism which assumes that if there is a choice between "products" service users will automatically have the power of exit. Of course, even if this is true in markets for consumer goods, in the field of social care many older people are mentally disabled, frail, and vulnerable; they are not in a position to "shop around" and have no realistic prospect of market exit (Walker 1991b).

Two questionable assumptions are fundamental to the consumerist model of social care. On the one hand, it is assumed that monopolies only operate in the public sector. On the other hand, it is assumed that the private sector can adequately substitute for the public sector. But, for example, as far as older residents in either a public or a private home are concerned, the provider is the monopoly power because they have no alternative. Having a range of theoretical alternatives will not make the consumers sovereign if they cannot exercise effective choice. A financial transaction does not necessarily mean the bestowal on the purchaser of either influence or control over the provider. Furthermore, unlike markets for consumer durables, in the field of social care if the private producer goes out of business this will not only have immense human consequences, but the public sector will be expected to pick up the pieces. In other words, the private sector exercises equivalent power over older people as do public providers, but it does not necessarily carry the same responsibility.

The only way that frail and vulnerable older people can be assured of influence and power over service provision is if they or their advocates are guaranteed a "voice" in the organization and management of services. This would, in turn, ensure that services actually reflect their needs. In practice, the weak form of consumer consultation that is being pursued under the 1990 Act could consist of no more than an occasional survey among older people together with minimal individual consultation at the point of assessment. Thus, despite the rhetoric about making services more responsive to users, in practice the government's proposals are silent on how frail older people and their caregivers can be guaranteed some influence over the services they receive.

On the basis of the strategy that has been pursued by the British government over the last 12 years and embodied in the legislation due to be implemented in April 1993, the prospect facing frail older people and their carergivers is bleak. The government has already made it clear that there will not be any additional resources for community care and, indeed, that it is looking for efficiency savings. There is no prospect that care gap will be bridged. In fact, the government expects increased inputs from family members, friends, and neighbors. Delay in the implementation of the NHS and Community Care Act will mean that more older people will enter private residential and nursing homes which they do not necessarily need and, as a consequence, even larger sums of money will be spent for such care.

RECENT INNOVATIONS IN SOCIAL CARE

The strategy being pursued by the government has not addressed the longstanding deficiencies of the British system of care for older people: excessive concentration of resources on a minority in institutional care; a minimum casualty service that relies heavily on the unpaid domestic labor of mainly female kin and low paid, mainly female social services workers; wide territorial variations in levels of provision; lack of responsiveness to the needs and preferences of older people and their caregivers and the virtual absence of any rights to services; lack of user involvement in the management and operation of services; underfunding and, therefore, a growing care gap as resources fail to keep pace with need; and a rigid separation between health and social services. While the government has failed to tackle these defects in a concerted way, various small scale local initiatives attempted over the last decade provided some more optimistic signs of the possible alternative ways of caring for frail older people in the community (for reviews of such schemes, see

Durward and Morton 1980; Ferlie 1983; Isaacs and Evers 1984; Salvage 1985).

Despite sharing the aim of assisting older people to live in their own homes, the specific nature of community care schemes has varied quite widely. Early projects tended to be concerned with the extension of the Home Help role from one which was mainly devoted to cleaning tasks to one which involved a greater element of care, for example, assisting older people with rising and retiring, washing and dressing (Hedley and Norman 1982). Commonly, schemes offer more intensive, augmented, extended, or special support–especially in terms of flexibility of tasks and availability of time (Lovelock 1985)–with the aim of obviating or postponing the need for residential or hospital care. A number have rehabilitation as a core focus, concentrating on older people who have been discharged from the hospital. Such schemes are more likely to use joint health and social services money and therefore to be associated with health and/or voluntary agencies in providing combined packages of care. Finally, there are projects concerned with supporting the caregivers of frail older people. They provide a few hours or occasionally weekend respite for caregivers, taking over their usual tasks of housework, shopping, personal care, drug supervision, escorting, companionship, and so on. They may be restricted to certain groups, for example, caregivers of older people who are suffering from Alzheimer's disease. Within some districts a combination of different services may be found (Cloke 1984).

One example of an innovation that extended the range and intensity of services provided is the Coventry Project (Latto 1980). Essentially, it was created to discover the effects of a planned doubling of Home Help provision. The range of Home Help hours increased (to include regular daily and weekend care and, for a small number of older people, late evening and early morning visits). Specialist skills were encouraged and rewarded (for example, working with stroke victims, the deaf, and people with senile dementia), and a hairdresser and full-time male Help/handyman joined the team. A mobile home Help provided a free "rapid response and surveillance" service for up to a month for people being discharged from the hospital with sudden and severe illness, or experiencing some other crisis. The outcome was that the proportion of time spent on cleaning tasks fell by a quarter while that spent on personal care increased from one-twentieth to one-fifth. In turn, the roles of Home Help organizer and Home Help were affected: while the organizer's role extended largely in the interface with the social work team, the Home Help role intruded more into the area of the community nursing service.

An increasing number of innovative projects have been based on the community care model devised during the mid-1970s by the Personal Social Services Research Unit (PSSRU) at the University of Kent (Davies and Challis 1980, 1986; Challis, Chessum, and Luckett 1982). This approach "concentrates the responsibility for case management to enable and encourage the workers to organise more efficient care" (Davies and Challis 1986, 227). The projects have differed in terms of their organization: for example, in East Kent, community care staff have been placed in area teams; in North Wales, the scheme social worker has been a member of a specialist team for older people; and in Gateshead, the scheme is run as a separate small team. In each case, however, the philosophy and techniques have been similar (Challis and Davies 1984).

The Darlington Community Care project has been built on the case management approach of the Kent and Gateshead projects, though with a different aim: to maintain at home frail older people who would have otherwise remained in long-stay hospital care. It therefore sought to extend activities into a joint health and social services model of provision based upon a multidisciplinary geriatric team to use multi-purpose care workers to reduce overlap between personnel (Challis, Darton, Johnson, Stone, Traske, and Wall 1989).

In Mid Glamorgan, a special care scheme providing more intensive Home Help was created for the benefit of older people "felt to be at risk of delayed discharge from hospital" (Victor, Holtermann, and Vetter 1986). Other similar "home from hospital" projects have been established which aim to prevent the necessity for readmissions and to assist the older person in becoming independent in the community (Russell and Brenton 1989).

Schemes like the Neighbourhood Services Project in Dinnington (Seyd, Tennant, and Bayley 1984), as well as the Kent project, have sought to organize informal or quasi-formal helpers into a support network or to sustain existing networks. There are also a growing number of projects whose object is primarily to support the informal caregivers of older people living at home. Perhaps the best known of these are the volunteer-run, but local authority funded, Crossroads Care Attendant schemes which aim to relieve stress in families or persons responsible for the care of people with disabilities. These initiatives can be found nationwide (Phillips 1982). Elsewhere, there exist collaborative schemes between health, social services, and the voluntary sector (see Cloke 1984; Lovelock 1985).

In general, then, these innovatory schemes, which show sensitivity toward and use of informal caregivers and informal care networks by the formal sector, have aided in delaying the need for residential care (Qureshi, Challis, and Davies 1983). They have also proved that it is possible to provide care in their own homes, at no extra cost to the social services departments to older people who might have been admitted to hospital or residential care (Davies and Challis 1980). Nevertheless, in spite of the wide range of such schemes, there is little evidence of a significant change in the structure of social services departments themselves, particularly between residential and field staff, outside of the experimental projects (Goldberg and Connelly 1982). In practice, furthermore, there have been very few attempts to provide a full substitute for residential care for frail older people.

This is one reason why the Neighbourhood Support Units (NSUs) initiative by Sheffield's SSD is a potentially important and radical departure. The Units aim to provide the whole range of services required by older people, from routine domiciliary assistance through to comprehensive care, at the same level as that which should be available in a residential setting. Home Helps and wardens have been replaced by teams of support workers whose jobs also encompass duties fulfilled by staff in day centers and undertaken by social work assistants. NSUs attempt to enable both older people and their informal caregivers to have more control over the definition of their needs and the way in which local resources are used to meet them. This innovation represents one of the few examples of an attempt to enhance the SSDs role in caring for frail older people and, therefore, it has not been funded or promoted by central government, in contrast to the Kent Community Care Scheme. The effectiveness of NSUs is currently being evaluated by a team based at the University of Sheffield (Warren and Walker 1991).

While innovations such as those briefly described here do provide some suggestions as to how care for frail older people could be improved, there are few signs of change in traditional roles within either the family or the health and social services. Moreover, the majority of innovatory schemes are not only based on the assumption that women will continue to be the primary unpaid or low paid caregivers, but some, such as the Kent Scheme, actively legitimate this subordination (Walker 1986b, Qureshi and Walker 1989, 270; Ungerson 1990). Finally, it must be remembered that many initiatives in social care never get past the pilot stage of being "demonstration" projects. They remain as pilot projects,

> a device that enables government to get away with short bursts of highly visible action, without tackling the more complex, underlying problems of the organization of care for vulnerable, marginal groups such as frail elderly people. (Russell and Brenton 1989, 227).

CONCLUSION

Britain, like other industrial societies, is faced with a continued expansion in the need for care. Research evidence shows that the limits to family care have been reached (Qureshi and Walker 1989) and it may well be that various social, economic, and demographic pressures on families, and especially female kin, will reduce their ability and even their willingness to provide care. In the face of these major socio-demographic developments, social care policy has been dominated by neo-liberal ideology over the last 12 years, which has favored nonstate forms of care, traditional family roles, and self-help. The outcome has been a bizarre coupling of reductions in the capacity of local authorities to provide community care services with a massive expansion in the private residential and nursing home sector. Therefore, because of the perverse financial incentive, many frail older people live in institutions which they do not necessarily need and when there is no evidence that this reflects their own preferences.

A range of innovative schemes have shown that it is possible to care for frail older people in their own homes at significantly lower cost than in residential or nursing homes. But most of them suffer from the limitations associated with attempting to formalize the informal sector, especially the confirmation of women in caring roles, and from the fact that some of them originate from a concern with cost efficiency rather than care effectiveness. At the time of this writing, policy is in the doldrums, waiting for the implementation of legislation in April 1993 which will significantly alter the role of local authority SSDs. However, frail older people and their caregivers cannot expect to see major improvements in their circumstances. There will be a reduction in the rate of admissions to private residential and nursing homes but, unless additional resources are made available, the infrastructure of supportive community services they require will not be forthcoming. So, for the foreseeable future, the main burden of care for increasing numbers of frail older people will continue to fall on older people themselves—either directly or indirectly through the payment of fees to private providers—or on their families.

NOTES

1. National estimates based on an Office of Population Censuses (OPCS) sample of disabled adults. Includes those living in communal establishments as well as private households in the two highest severity categories: 8/10, 9/10 and 10/10. Source: Martin, Meltzer, and Elliot 1988, 19.

2. The personal social services in Britain are financed and administered separately from the health service. They are public services, run by locally elected authorities, covering social work, residential, day care and domiciliary care for children, older people, and people with physical and mental disabilities.

3. "Very frail" is defined by the same severity categories as in note 1. Severity was defined in functional terms according to the following areas of disability: locomotion; reaching and stretching; dexterity; personal care; continence; seeing; hearing; communication; behaviour; intellectual functioning; consciousness; eating, drinking and digestion; and disfigurement, with only the three highest scores counting toward the overall score. See Martin, Meltzer, and Elliot 1988.

4. Neo-conservative in U.S. terminology or "new right."

5. The DHSS was split into two departments: Health (DH) and Social Security (DSS) on 25 July 1988.

6. Income support is the means-tested "safety net" minimum income scheme. In 1991/92 a single pensioner aged 75-79 would receive £55.20 ($93.84) per week

plus housing costs and a pensioner couple £85.60 ($145.52) plus housing costs. The sums for single persons and couples aged 80 and over are £58.10 ($98.77) and £88.45 ($150.37), respectively.

7. The Audit Commission is a quasi-autonomous body responsible for examining the cost efficiency of local government spending.

REFERENCES

ADSS. 1986. Who Goes Where? London. ADSS.

Arber, S., and Gilbert, G.N. 1989. Men: The forgotten carers. Sociology, vol. 23, no. 1:111-118.

Audit Commission. 1986. *Making a Reality of Community Care*. London. PSI.

Block, J. 1985. Utilization of informal networks within a universal home care program: Care planning for elderly patients in a Canadian hospital. Paper presented at XIII International Congress of Gerontology. New York, July.

Bradshaw, J., and Gibbs, I. 1988. *Public Support for Private Residential Care*. Aldershot, England, Avebury.

Butler, R.; Oberlink, M.; and Schechter, M., eds. 1990. *The Promise of Productive Aging*. New York, Springer.

Central Statistical Office. 1990. *Family Change and Future Policy*. York, Joseph Rowntree Foundation.

Challis, D.; Chessum, R; and Luckett, R. 1982. The gateshead community care scheme: A new life for the elderly at home. Discussion Paper 247, Personal Social Services Research Unit, University of Kent, Canterbury.

Challis, D.; Darton, R.; Johnson, L.; Stone, M.; Traske, K; and Wall, B. 1989. Supporting frail elderly people at home: The Darlington community care project. University of Kent, PSSRU.

Challis, D., and Davies, B. 1984. Community care schemes: A development in the home care of the elderly. In F. J. Caird and J. Grimley Evans, *Advanced Geriatric Medicine*, vol. 4:35-44.

Cloke, C. 1984. *Intensive Home Help and Home Care Services: A Directory*, London, Age Concern.

DH. 1989a. *Caring for People*, Cmnd 849, London, HMSO.

DH. 1989b. Personal Social Services, Local Authority Statistics, Residential Accomodation for Elderly and for Younger Physically Handicapped People: All Residents in Local Authority, Voluntary and Private Homes, England, London, DH.

DHSS. 1981. *Growing Older*, Cmnd 8173, London, HMSO.

DHSS. 1985. *Response to Second Report from the Social Services Committee*, Cmnd 9674, London, HMSO.

Dalley, G. 1988. *Ideologies of Caring*. London, Macmillan.

Davies, B., and Challis, D. 1980. Experimenting with new roles in domiciliary service: the Kent Community Care Project. *The Gerontologist*, vol. 20, No.3, pp. 288-99.

Davies, B., and Challis, D. 1986. *Matching Resources to Needs in Community Care*. Aldershot, Gower.

Day, P., and Klein, R. 1987. The business of welfare. *New Society*, 19 June, 11-13.

Demone, H., and Gibelman, M., eds. 1989. *Services for Sale: Purchasing Health and Human Services*. Princeton, NJ, Rutgers University Press.

Durward, L., and Morton, J. 1980. Catalogue of developments in the care of old people. London, Personal Social Services Council.

Edelman, M. 1977. *Political Language*. New York, Academic Press.

Ermisch, J. 1983. *The Political Economy of Demographic Change*. London, Heinemann.

Ermisch, J. 1990. *Fewer Babies, Longer Lives*. York, Joseph Rowntree Foundation.

Evandrou, M. 1990. Challenging the invisibility of careers: Helping informal care nationally. Discussion Paper WSP/49, The Welfare State Programme, LSE, London.

Eversley, D. 1982. The demography of retirement–Prospects to the year 2030. In *Retirement Policy: The Next Fifty Years*, edited by M. Fogarty. London, Heinemann.

Family Policy Studies Center. 1986. An aging population, fact sheet 2, London, FPSC.

Fengler, A.; Danigelis, N.; and Little, V. 1983. Later life satisfaction and household structure: Living with others and living alone. *Aging and Society*, vol. 3:357-77.

Ferlie, E. 1983. *Sourcebook of Initiatives in the Community Care of the Elderly*. University of Kent, PSSRU, Canterbury.

Finch, J., and Groves, D., eds. 1983. *A Labour of Love?* London, Routledge & Kegan Paul.

Fowler, N. 1984. Speech to joint social services annual conference. 27 September, London, DHSS.

Gamble, A. 1987. *The Free Economy and the Strong State*. London, Pluto.

Gibbs, J.; Evans, M., and Rodway, S. 1987. Report of the inquiry into Nye Bevan Lodge. London, Southwark Council.

Goldberg, E. M., and Connelly, N. 1982. *The Effectiveness of Social Care for the Elderly*. London, Heinemann.

Graham, H. 1983. In *A Labour of Love?*, edited by Finch and Groves. London, Routledge & Kegan Paul, 13-30.

Green, H. 1988. *Informal Carers*. London, HMSO.

Griffiths, Sir R. 1988. *Community Care: Agenda for Action*. London, HMSO.

Harman, H., and Lowe, M. 1986. *No Place Like Home*. London, House of Commons.

Hedley, R., and Norman, A. 1982. *Home Help: Key Issues in Service Provision*. London, CPA.

Holmes, B., and Johnson, A. 1988. *Cold Comfort*. London, Souvenir Press.

Isaacs, B., and Evers, H., eds. 1984. *Innovations in the Care of the Elderly*. London, Croom Helm.

Kiernan, K., and Wicks, M. 1990. *Family Change and Future Policy.* York, England, Family Studies Centre.

Land, H. 1978. Who cares for the family? *Journal of Social Policy.* vol. 7, No.3, pp. 257-284.

Larder, D.; Day, P., and Klein, R. 1986. *Institutional Care of the Elderly: The Geographical Distribution of the Public/Private Mix in England.* University of Bath.

Latto, S. 1980 Extension of service–The coventry project. In *Report of a Conference on Research and Policy Making in the Home Help Service,* Social Services Research Group, 37-47.

Lewis, J., and Meredith, B. 1988. *Daughters Who Care: Daughters Caring for Mothers at Home.* London, Routledge.

Lovelock, R. 1985. *Against the Tide: Approaches to the Domiciliary Support of Frail Elderly People in Hampshire.* Portsmouth, Social Services Research and Intelligence Unit.

Manton, K. 1986. The linkage of morbidity and mortality: Implications of increasing life expectancy at later ages for health service demand. In *Ageing with Limited Health Resources,* edited by Economic Council of Canada. Ottawa, Canadian Government Publishing Centre, 39-49.

Martin, J.; Meltzer, H.; and Elliot, D. 1988. *The Prevalence of Disability Among Adults.* London, HMSO.

Moroney, R. M. 1976. *The Family and the State.* London, Longman.

NACAB 1991. *Beyond the Limit.* London, National Association of Citizens Advice Bureaux.

Phillips, D. 1982. The crossroads care attendant scheme. In *Care in the Community: Recent Research and Current Projects,* edited by F. Glendenning. Stoke, Staffs, Beth Johnson Foundation, 113-116.

Phillipson, C., and Walker, A., eds. 1986. *Ageing and Social Policy.* London, Gower.

Qureshi, H.; Challis, D., and Davies, B. 1983. Motivation and rewards of helpers in the Kent Community Care Project. In *Volunteers: Meanings, Patterns and Motives,* edited by S. Hatch. Berkhamsted: Volunteer Centre.

Qureshi, H., and Walker, A. 1989. *The Caring Relationship.* London, Macmillan/ Philadelphia, Temple University Press.

Rosenmayer, L., and Kockeis, E. 1963. Propositions for a sociological theory of aging and the family. *International Social Service Journal,* vol. 15, No. 3, 410-26.

Royal College of Physicians Committee on Geriatrics. 1981. Organic mental impairments in the elderly: Implications for research education and provision of services. *Journal of the Royal College of Physicians,* vol. 15, No. 3.

Russell, J., and Brenton, M. 1989. Bridging the gap between hospital and home: Two models of Der presented to the Alberta Association on Gerontology. Alberta, May.

Salvage, A. V. 1985. *Domiciliary Care Schemes for the Elderly: Provision by Local Authority Social Services Department and Recommendations for their*

Introductions, Volumes 1 and 2, Research team for the *Care of the Elderly*. Cardiff, Wales, University of Wales College of Medicine.

Seyd, R.; Tennant, A.; and Bayley, M. 1984. *The Home Help Services*, Neighborhood Services Projects-Dinnington, paper No. 6, Department of Sociological Studies, University of Sheffield, England.

Shanas, E.; Townsend, P.; Wedderburn, D.; Friis, M.; Milho, P.; and Stehouwer, J. 1968. *Old People in Three Industrial Societies*. New York, Atherton Press.

Shapiro, E. 1985. Caring about carers: What have we learned from research and experience? Paper presented to the Alberta Association on Gerontology, Alberta, Canada, May.

Social Services Committee. 1980. *The Government's White Papers on Public Expenditure: The Social Services*. Vol. II, HC 702, London, HMSO.

Social Services Committee. 1985. *Community Care*. HC 13-1, London, HMSO.

Social Services Committee. 1990. *Community Care: Services for People with a Mental Handicap and People with a Mental Illness*. HC 664, London, HMSO.

Titmuss, R. M. 1968. *Commitment to Welfare*. London, Allen & Unwin.

Townsend, P. 1981. Elderly people with disabilities. In *Disability in Britain*, edited by A. Walker with P. Townsend. Oxford, Martin Robertson, 91-118.

Ungerson, C. 1987. *Policy is Personal: Sex, Gender and Informal Care*. London, Tavistock Publications.

Ungerson, C., ed. 1990. *Gender and Caring: Work and Welfare in Britain and Scandinavia*. London, Harvester Wheatsheaf.

Victor, C. R.; Holtermann, S.; and Vetter, N. J. 1986. The effectiveness and individual costing of an augmented home care service in the Rhondda: Final report volume 1. Research Team for the care of the Elderly. Cardiff, University of Wales College of Medicine.

Walker, A. 1981. Community care and the elderly in Great Britain: Theory and practice. *International Journal of Health Services*, vol. 11, No. 4, pp. 541-557.

Walker, A. 1983. Care for elderly people: A conflict between women and the state. In *A Labour of Love?*, edited by Finch and Groves. London, Routledge & Kegan Paul, 106-128.

Walker, A. 1985. *The Care Gap*. London, Local Government Information Service.

Walker, A. 1986a. Community care, fact and fiction. In *The Debate About Community: Papers From a Seminar on 'Community' in Social Policy*, edited by P. Willmot. London, PSI, 4-15.

Walker, A. 1986b. Meeting the needs of Canada's elderly with limited health resources: Some observations based on British experience. In *Ageing with Limited Health Resources*, edited by Economic Council of Canada. Ottawa, Canadian Government Printing Centre, 27-38.

Walker, A. 1990. The economic "burden" of ageing and the prospect of intergenerational conflict. *Ageing and Society*, vol. 10, No. 3.

Walker, A. 1991a. The relationship between the family and the State in the care of older people. *Canadian Journal on Aging*, vol.10, No. 3.

Walker, A. 1991b. Increasing user involvement in the social services. In *Recent*

Advances in Psychogeriatrics 2, edited by T. Arie. London, Churchill Living-
stone.

Walker, A., and Walker, C., eds. 1987. *The Growing Divide*. London, CPAG.

Warren, L., and Walker, A. 1991. Neighbourhood support units: A new approach
to social care. Forthcoming.

Webb, A., and Wistow, G. 1987. *Social Work, Social Care and Social Planning:
The Personal Social Services Since Seebohm*. London, Longman.

Chapter 7

Canadian Long-Term Care: Its Escalating Costs for Women

Sheila Marjorie Neysmith

INTRODUCTION

Since the World Assembly on Aging was held in 1982, we have become much more conscious of aging as a worldwide phenomenon. Until that time, population aging was viewed as an issue for advanced industrialized nations only (Neysmith and Edwardh 1984). We now realize that the graying of the world will be occurring primarily in Third World countries, where two-thirds of the world's over sixty population already resides. The options available to people in these countries are far more circumscribed than those in most of the countries discussed in this volume (Neysmith 1990).

Canada is among the more fortunate nations, along with demographically similar countries like U.S. and Australia. Although there are national differences, all three enjoy high standards of living based on well-established market economies; all three worry about their "rapidly aging populations"; yet all three can look to countries such as Sweden, German, and Austria, which are already experiencing the demographic changes that we are contemplating with such trepidation over the next twenty-five years.

The use of these sets of referents is not intended to diminish the importance of decisions that Canadians face about how we will care for our frail elderly, but rather to underscore the fact that a relatively young and affluent country like Canada has the necessary human and material resources to plan for the future welfare of its elderly citizens–a possibility that does not exist for the majority of the world's elderly. Canadians thus face decisions about the allocation of resources, not issues of survival. The outcome will reflect our national assessment of the merits of competing claims by different groups within our society. On the positive side, the country's relative prosperity will allow some room to maneuver; on the negative side, Canada has entrenched structural inequities that shape the political economy within which the debate is taking place.

This chapter is both descriptive and interpretive. The first section outlines some demographic aspects of the Canadian population. Particular attention is paid to the social situation of different groups of older persons, their morbidity profiles, and patterns of service usage. Canada, as a federal state, has a central government with superior taxing powers which sets broad policy directions. However, health and social services are a provincial responsibility. Throughout the chapter, Canadian data will be used wherever it is available. However, similar issues are being discussed in Britain, Europe, and the United States. Therefore, these international debates will inform the analysis.

In the second section, several provincial long-term care strategies will be examined in order to highlight the types of issues being debated. It will be argued that, although each province has its particular regional history, there are many common themes. Current trends show that, despite the increasing volume of home care services, they continue to receive relatively few health dollars. The importance of home care is underscored in virtually all federal, provincial, and municipal documents, yet the quality and content of these services continue to be an issue; service delivery depends heavily on the labor of poorly paid female health care paraprofessionals and volunteers.

Although there is provincial variation, Canada takes a mixed market approach to long-term care services. Thus, a minimal level of public and nonprofit agencies is ensured, but the country is experiencing as well the development of an increasingly lucrative for-profit service industry. If this trend continues, in the future those elderly with financial resources will have the opportunity to purchase a range of services, while those on restricted incomes will be dependent on a shrinking public sector.

A forecast of minimal expansion in formal services means that the Canadian model of home-based care will continue to depend heavily upon the informal services provided by kin. This scenario is based on a straightforward projection of current trends. The third section of the chapter discusses the implications of this model for women who are the primary givers and receivers of care. One of the most pressing issues facing Canada is the development of community-based home-care programs on the scale now found only in traditional medical care. This chapter argues that until a serious commitment is made to redirect some of these resources, the frail elderly, as in the past, will care for themselves with support from a family member. Specifically, help with the activities of daily living will be provided by an aging spouse or female relative who lives close by, with formal services used only when informal care is not available.

The final section points to possibilities for change, but their realization will depend upon the ability of Canadian political leaders to change from the current policy track of treating illness to one of nurturing health. One strategy is to institute open-ended home-care programs combined with restrictions on hospital costs and physician fees. Only by releasing massive amounts of money from these latter sectors will there be the types of resources available to develop home care on the necessary scale. Second, an argument is put forward for detaching the nation's discussion of home care from recipients' family structure.

THE AGING CANADIAN: A SOCIAL PROFILE

At the time of the last census (1986), 10.7 percent of Canadians were over 65; of these, 8.4 percent were over 85. The latter represents about 1 percent of the total population of a country with nearly 25.5 million citizens (Statistics Canada 1986). The growth in both percentage and number of persons in the oldest cohort is of particular concern for long-term care policymakers. These patterns are not unlike those found in the U.S. and Australia.

Canada actually experienced a parallel growth spurt in its over 65 cohorts between 1951 and 1971. However, this was counterbalanced by a much more visible postwar baby boom. Issues of youth, not the elderly, constituted the social problems of the time. Today the members of this postwar cohort are still active participants in the labor force. Consequently, Canada's overall dependency ratio is predicted to actually decrease over the next 30 years and then return to current levels (McDaniel 1986, 55).

This longitudinal profile underscores the questionable validity of a demographic crisis approach to population aging. Neither rate of growth nor percent of total population over eighty-five are necessarily sufficient conditions for alarm. Obviously an aging citizenry has different needs than a youthful one, a fact which has implications for the use and distribution of resources. Of concern, however, is the connection in the public mind between population aging and rising health costs. It can result in victim blaming (Minkler 1991, 76-77). As I will argue later in the chapter, the elderly may use more health services but they are not the primary cause of rising health costs.

A prominent Canadian researcher recently analyzed data from a 1985 General Social Survey of Canadian families (Stone 1988). Although the sample was limited to persons living in private dwellings, it provided information not before available at the national level on family structure, social supports, and informal aid. Of relevance to this chapter was its analysis of family and friendship ties. It was found that by age 80, nearly one-third of respondents had two or fewer active social ties (Stone 1988, 31). Such data are important because we know that informal supports are the main sources of help amongst the elderly.

The study was limited to assistance with those types of activities for which there are available an identifiable block of services provided by service agencies (Stone 1988, 53-54). Thus, information was not sought on sources of emotional support. The data, nevertheless, do allow us to focus on a set of services that, at least theoretically, can be delivered through either formal or informal channels. For instance, by their mid-seventies even persons reporting good health were needing help with grocery shopping. The policy question is how such need will be met.

The study concluded that the majority of services were provided by informal sources. These findings are consistent with those of previous studies using less representative samples. However, this national study also showed that reliance on formal organizations rises with age for those living alone, and one-third of women over 80 live alone. The implications of these findings for the sheer quantity of future home care services that may be required is evident. The author notes that his estimates are conservative because the data set excludes people who, by census definition, do not reside in private households. At the time of the 1986 Census, 30 percent of women and 20 percent of men over 80 did not live in private households (Stone 1988, 28).

A part of any overall long-term care strategy is determining criteria for institutional care. It should be noted that in Canada there is no consistency in the nomenclature used to describe special care facilities. "Nursing homes" in one province might be called "homes for the aged" in another, "chronic care facilities" in a third. (Perhaps Quebec has the most picturesque term, "Centres d'Accueil"–meeting places!) Other than specifying certain conditions that have to be met in order to qualify for federal cost-sharing arrangements, provinces make their own decisions regarding the organization and funding of programs. Level of skilled care provided determines the per diem that is received. Upon close inspection, however, one finds inconsistencies between and within provinces.

Perhaps the most salient feature of institutional care during the 1980's was its low public profile. When long-term care policy was debated, it was community-based care that was the focus of discussion. It seems that as community-based services rose in favor, institutionally-based care fell as rapidly into disfavor. Institutional care was seen as bad, community care as good; the former as expensive, the latter as cheap. The whole discussion tends to be painted in either/or terms. Distinctly absent is the active consideration of a middle ground where people are seen as having a range of health and social service needs. For instance, Canada does not have the mix of protective housing options that one finds in the U.K. or in the Scandinavian countries. We tend to discuss care within one's own home or in an institutional setting.

Canada has about 7.5 percent of its population over 65 in some kind of institutional care; this rises to 35.6 percent for those over 85 (Forbes, Jackson, and Kraus 1987, 37). These figures are higher than those for the U.K. and the U.S. However, there is also considerable provincial variability. For example, among the 85 and over group the rate is 30 percent in Nova Scotia, 41 percent in Ontario, and 50.5 percent in Alberta (Stone and Frenken 1988). Such figures suggest that service structures, not client characteristics, are the important determinants of service usage–a theme that will be returned to repeatedly in this chapter. At the time of the 1981 census, the above percentages translated into a national average of 88.5 long-term care beds per 1000 persons over 65. However, disparate definitions of what constitutes a long-term care bed lead to some variability in estimates.

The cost of this care varies not only by province but also by the type of ownership. For example, Ontario, the largest province, is distinguished by its heavy reliance on proprietary services (Tarman 1990, 36). This is a politically contentious issue in a country officially committed to a public health care model.

Although Canadian health care costs, as a percentage of GNP, are comparable to those of other western industrialized countries, and more contained than those in the U.S., they are a constant source of public concern. The development of health care programs falls within provincial jurisdiction, but the federal government has superior taxing powers. The federal government shares the cost of provincially insured health care services, extended health care, and postsecondary education via legislation commonly known as the Established Programs Financing Act (EPF). Regularly, the provinces announce their anger with the size of federal contributions while the federal government issues figures on the escalating profile of these transfers. Editorials appear in major newspapers taking doctors to task over the size of their billings, while on the front page bed shortages in acute care hospitals and queues for elective surgery are being decried in graphic pictures.

In recent years, there have been cuts in the general EPF formula. The Finance Department has not published the losses resulting from these changes to date, but the Department does estimate that for the five years beginning in 1990 the loss will amount to about $7.4 billion. Outsiders have calculated that these sums will be considerably larger (National Council of Welfare 1990, 66-67).

Thus, the province's grievances are not unfounded. However, the federal government argues that limiting the size of transfers is its only means of controlling costs since it has no control over how these monies are used within provincial health systems. There are legitimate, and not so legitimate, claims on both sides, most of which are beyond the focus of this chapter (see Evans 1990 for a discussion of current issues). However, a focus on transfer payments does not get at the issue of reallocation *within* provincial health care budgets.

The relative dollar amounts going to various health care sectors have remained unchanged over the years. Nationally, about 50 percent of total health care expenditures is allocated for institutional care, primarily acute care hospitals; 25 percent for professional services, primarily physician fees; 10 percent for drugs and appliances; and 15 percent for all other costs (Chappell, Strain, and Blandford 1986, 107). Home care falls in the latter category. Policy statements like the following are typical:

> Community-based services will be emphasized to enhance self-reliance and to assist people to live in their own homes and communities. (*Ontario* 1990, 3)

Yet only 3 percent of the budget of the Ontario Ministry of Health goes into such services (Schwenger 1989, 215). It is this intransigence in dollar allocation that has to be weighed against rhetoric proclaiming that home-based care has become a service priority.

Moreover, data showing higher use of health services by the elderly need to be interpreted with caution. The seemingly inordinately large demands that an aging Canadian population places on the health system may actually be due to both governmental policy and the health care industry itself rather than to overuse by the elderly. It is hardly surprising that older people use more health services than younger ones. A consistent finding in Canadian data is that there is a small group of easily identified elderly persons who use health and social services intensively (Beland 1989; Roos, Shapiro, and Roos 1984). However,what they and other elderly persons use is limited to what is available. Although the Canada Health Act guarantees universal access, the types of services it covers are not determined by elderly patients but rather by policymakers in conjunction with health professionals. Not surprisingly, insured services are the traditional and costly medical ones (Neysmith 1989).

Denton, Li, and Spencer (1987) explored how population aging would affect health care costs. They concluded that it was questionable whether a crisis was imminent for two reasons: costs will rise rapidly, but not out of line with projected growth in GNP; and projections using current costs do not take into account changes in the health care delivery system to less costly alternatives, e.g., home care.

In a study of the growth in Canadian hospital costs, Auer (1987) showed that, over a twenty year period, 90 percent of the increase was due to how hospital care was delivered, not by who used the services. Despite this observation, the author's projections did not assume any changes in the health care delivery model.

A more comprehensive analysis by the Chief Statistician of Canada (Fellegi 1988, reported in Clark 1989, 130) included an overview of national trends in fertility, labor force participation of women, and incomes of the elderly. He observed that although demographic trends affect education, pensions, and health costs, social, economic, and policy developments will be more significant in the long run. These Canadian data are consistent with international comparisons showing that an aging population per se is not a significant factor in rising national health care costs (Pfaff 1990, 20; Evans 1990, 121).

A CHANGING VISION OF HEALTH

In recent years there has emerged a number of federal and provincial policy documents outlining an alternative approach to health care based on principles of prevention, the promotion of healthy life styles, and the recognition of environmental influences (Health and Welfare Canada 1986). This health promotion perspective challenges prevailing assumptions that health care (more accurately called sick care) services are the major determiners of health. It finds its clearest articulation in the concept of healthy public policy which is

> characterized by an explicit concern for health and equity in all areas of policy and an accountability for health impact. The main aim of healthy public policy is to create a supportive

environment to enable people to lead healthy lives. (World Health Organization 1988)

The principle behind healthy public policy is that the major determiners of health and disease lie outside or beyond the jurisdiction of the health sector. Thus, health programs, if they are to be effective, must be developed through a multisectoral and collaborative process which endeavors to ensure participation by the affected constituencies. Healthy public policy is chiefly concerned with creating a healthy society, dominated by low technological, holistic approaches to health; it is future oriented and questioning of the status quo (Pederson et al. 1988, 5).

These ideas, which are now finding their way into federal and provincial policy statements, as well as into the thinking of public health associations and local health care units across the country, call into question the types of health services currently available to elderly persons and their families. One of the challenges for future health policy is to determine what Canadians truly want from their health care system. Instead of treating the costs of the inputs, physicians, hospitals, etc., as the analytical end, approaches like healthy public policy can set criteria in terms of desired outcomes. This incipient discourse could be the precursor of change because, rather than being preoccupied with the state of current services, it redirects attention to the emerging needs of an aging population. One result has been an increasing awareness that a focus on age may well be a distraction when viewing health needs.

In developed countries the low socioeconomic status of certain sectors of society is seen as a crucial impediment to the attainment of national health goals. Thus, Canada has identified the reduction of inequalities as a high priority for health promotion (Health and Welfare Canada 1986; Rootman 1988). Ill health and the onset of disability as one ages are not randomly distributed in Canada. They fall disproportionately on the disadvantaged segments of the population. The rich tend to have fewer years of disability than the poor, with the average difference being 7.7 years (Wilkins and Adams 1983, 14). This disparity occurs throughout life, not just when one enters old age (McDaniel 1986, 14).

Recently, Health and Welfare Canada and Statistics Canada examined changes in mortality by income in urban areas from 1971 to 1986. The findings suggest that the disparity in all causes of mortality between income quintile in Census Metropolitan Areas (CMAs) have diminished over this time period. However, death rates among the poor are still higher than those of other Canadians for most natural and accidental causes (Wilkins, Adams, and Brancker 1989). Of particular concern is the health profile of Canada's aboriginal peoples. While there have been significant improvements recently for Status Indians living on reserves, the average life expectancy at birth for the aboriginal population in 1991 is 65.7 years for men and 73 years for women, compared to the national average of 74.1, and 81.2, respectively (Hagey, Larocque, and McBride 1989, 23). As suggested in other national studies, income differences in mortality seem to disappear among those who live into their late seventies and eighties.

Finally, Canada's stated commitment to the principle of universal access to health care seems to be continuously vulnerable to pressure to provide the "best medical care money can buy." Funding and access debates raged when universal medical care was first instituted in 1966; they emerged again when this principle was reaffirmed with the passage of the Canada Health Act in 1984. The latter, which curtailed extra billing, resulted in a doctor's strike in Ontario. Currently, in response to the decrease in federal funds discussed earlier, several provinces are threatening to institute financial penalties for persons who "overuse" hospital emergency facilities and nominal fees for each visit to "discourage" excessive visits to the doctor. Totally absent from these proposals seems to be any awareness of where and how health costs are increasing. Fiscal pressures are not caused by demographic aging or overuse of services but rather by the ways in which the health care system construes need. Over the years, analysts have consistently pointed to rapidly escalating physician supply, the fee structure, and hospital budgets as pivotal players (Roos, Shapiro, and Roos 1984; Angus 1987; Evans 1990).

Many of the dilemmas in the Canadian health care system result from the fact that a public health care system was grafted onto a private medical model where physician prescription defined the nation's health needs and how services should be developed. Consequently, the public provides the tax base but has minimal influence in determining what promotes good health. Costs, although less than in the U.S., are growing. As long as incentives that encourage traditional response remain, including uncapped physician fees, very narrow definitions of health authority, and development of hospital-based facilities, cost will continue to escalate (Evans 1987, 634). Community-based options are foreclosed because current funding patterns preclude the availability of adequate resources for alternatives. Canadian governments have always had to infuse new monies into the system when promoting initiatives in the area of community-based care. Policymakers have been decidedly unsuccessful in redirecting resources from traditional pathways. One of the results is the stunting of home care services. Not only have these services not kept up with the needs of an aging population, but they will not do so in the future unless Canada reallocates real health dollars to them.

LONG-TERM CARE

Despite some federal/provincial cost sharing arrangements, Canada does not have a national long-term care program based on legislation similar to the Canada Health Act; the latter program is able to utilize funding as a mechanism for ensuring minimum standards for certain medical services across the country. Therefore, although all provinces have extended care programs, their organization, coverage, and funding patterns differ--as does the language used to describe their various components. In the last couple of years, the larger provinces have undertaken reviews of the health and social service programs that are heavily used by elderly persons (British Columbia 1989; Alberta 1988; Price Waterhouse 1988; Ontario 1990; Quebec 1985). Despite considerable variation in the breadth and depth of these assessments, it is fair to say that the issue of cost control was a major theme in all of them.

To the outside observer, Quebec and Manitoba would seem to have the most integrated long-term care systems. Although specific organizational features differ, and many would argue that they are imbedded in differing philosophies of provincial responsibilities and community-based care, in both provinces a central authority ensures province-wide coverage while decentralized delivery structures permit considerable local variability.

Ontario, which accounts for about one-third of the country's population, has one of the most fragmented long-term care arrangements. This situation is exacerbated by the existence of separate ministries for Health, and Community and Social Services, with the latter being very much the poor cousin in terms of power and resources. Ontario has argued that the size and mix of its population warrants a "decentralized" system. Most informed sources suggest that the current system is decentralized by default, not by plan. In addition, Ontario's laissez-faire approach to long-term care has resulted in home care services remaining undeveloped while costs have escalated on the institutional side of the ledger. Even within the long-term care system, most monies go to nursing home and chronic care beds; only 23 percent of the total is spent on in-home or community services (Ontario 1990, 8).

In recent years the Ministry of Health has been facing enormous pressures to contain costs as federal transfer funds have shrunk. It was within this atmosphere of fiscal restraint that an interministerial committee was appointed to develop an integrated province-wide system of long-term care. A major policy paper has been released which outlines future directions in this area (Ontario 1990). Not surprisingly, the focus was on coordination; issues of efficiency and cost control permeate the paper.

At the other extreme is Manitoba's long-term care program, which has been in operation since the early seventies. In a national comparative assessment, it was noted that Manitoba's scheme has one of the highest per capita costs in the country. For example, in 1985 the per capita costs were: Manitoba, $20.38; Ontario, $15.05; Saskatchewan, $11.64; New Brunswick, $11.38 (Health and Welfare Canada 1987).

Shortly after the release of these figures, Manitoba engaged a group of outside consultants to conduct a thorough evaluation of home care services. This study is of interest because it captures the dilemmas facing long-term care policymakers across the country. The study revealed that clients using home care are much sicker than in earlier years. Home care is rapidly turning into a hospital replacement service, despite the fact that the program has neither the human nor financial resources to undertake this type of care. The report documents pressures for home care to assume even more of a hospital replacement function in the future (Price Waterhouse 1988, 30). These include (1) a decreasing ratio of hospital beds to population and a decrease in the length of stay and hospital utilization rates; (2) advances in medical technology which will continue to permit more people to survive in conditions where they require intensive medical support. At the same time, expanding technology makes it at least theoretically possible to implement the concept of the "hospital in the home"; and (3) public expectations that services *should* be provided at home, not in an institution.

In addition to these broad concerns about the purpose of a home care service, a specific issue raised by the consultants is whether or not the program is too expansive. There are nurse/social worker assessment teams across the province that are the access points to both home care services and chronic care facilities. Thus the system is less physician dominated than that found in several other provinces. Nevertheless, the home care budget averaged an annual growth of 19 percent over the last twelve years. This was accompanied by a growth in cases, in units of service per case, and a richer set of services than that available in other provinces (Price Waterhouse 1988, 26). On the one hand, the assessors felt that the program did not have a well-developed system of management; on the other hand, caseload and program review procedures were found to be more refined than those in other provinces.

Finally, the overall growth of costs was found to be comparable to those of other provinces. For example, Ontario and British Columbia averaged cost growths of 24 and 19 percent, respectively, during the same period. Recently instituted spending ceilings in Alberta and Saskatchewan on most components of their home care programs probably explain why their costs are now lower than in previous years. Manitoba's program administrative costs are lower than elsewhere: 17 percent as compared to 23 percent in Ontario.

Interestingly, despite the numerous financial questions raised by the evaluators, the Manitoba system is known internationally for the quality of its services (see Kane and Kane 1985 for details). It also apparently meets an accountant's and taxpayer's demand for better services at lower cost. Yet the recommendations from this evaluation endorse policy directions that are consistent with those appearing in assessments of other provincial long-term care schemes: above all, contain costs. There is not even a suggestion that home care services ought to be expanding and that this could be achieved through the diversion of resources from high cost hospital-based care. In addition, as one cost containment measure, the consultants recommended that housekeeping, meals-on-wheels, and cleaning should be provided on a fee-for-service basis under nonprofit auspice. Such a recommendation is tenable only because they examined home care in isolation from other components of the health system.

Similarly, while noting that 51 percent of the clientele live alone and 30 percent reside with an aging spouse, the evaluators point out that 75 percent of home care users have family living with them or in the same city. Specifically, they argue: "While the age of the adult relatives is unknown, it is possible that family can assume responsibility for all or part of the elderly client's needs (e.g. house cleaning, maintenance, financial management, transportation). Regions where clients lack close family proximity may need to be prepared to provide more support services than in other regions" (Price Waterhouse 1988, 72). In sum, cost savings would accrue by expanding family caregiving and instituting user fees on services. Of course, the usual caveat was inserted, namely, the provision of a sliding scale to protect those with low incomes.

Such recommendations do not reflect the fact that families *already* provide 80 to 90 percent of care. Greater family care may not be feasible or advisable. Studies have found home care users to be older and have more functional incapacities, a less positive assessment of their health, and a smaller informal network than comparable groups of non-service users. Home care users tend to receive as much or more informal help as do nonusers; however, their assistants (helpers) are less likely to be located in the home. Moreover, a greater proportion of in-home service recipients apply for senior housing (Chappell 1985; Beland 1984, 1985).

The current approach for assessing long-term care programs in Canada is only sensible in the context of a socially constructed cost crisis milieu. Perhaps most disturbing is the underlying "blaming the victim" stance which views elderly persons as overusing services. Since such individuals are the primary users of home care, these programs are particularly vulnerable to charges of overspending. In an overview of home care programs across the country, Evelyn Shapiro, a community health scientist who has tracked the Manitoba system since its inception, concluded:

> The irony of the current situation is that, although home care is more often "under the microscope" than the "big spenders," its program directors are generally further from the centre of power within the provinces' decision-making process than the high cost health sectors. (Shapiro 1988, 43)

This captures the essential contradiction that underlies long-term care policy making across the country. It tends to be based on a residualist welfare model. Namely, there are two "natural" or socially given channels through which an individual's needs are properly met: the private market and the family. Only when these break down should social welfare institutions intercede, and then only temporarily. Thus, services should be minimal.

HOME IS WHERE THE CARE IS

For every aged person in an institution there are approximately two equally impaired elderly persons living in private homes who remain there by virtue of the critical role played by informal support systems (Rowe 1985). Data from the Canadian Health and Activity Survey (Statistics Canada 1986) found that 4.5 percent of seniors over age 85 report some disability (defined as a limitation which was not alleviated by a technical aid and had lasted or was expected to last for at least six months).

Help with activities of daily living is usually provided by an aging spouse, if one is present; otherwise another family member steps in. The myth of families abandoning their elderly has been laid to rest by innumerable studies in Canada as well as the U.S. (Rosenthal 1987; Shanas 1979; Stone, Cafferata, and Sangl 1987; Brody 1985; Stolar, Hill, and Tomblin 1986; see also Connidis 1989 for a review of research in this area). In fact, the willingness of certain family members to take on enormous caring responsibilities has led to a series of studies examining the social construction of obligation within families (Finch 1989; Dalley 1988; Storm, Storm, and Strike-Schurman 1985; Fisher and Tronto 1990). Unfortunately, this research does not seem to have modified fears that kin will renege on familial care contracts if the expectation to keep them is relaxed.

Some policymakers argue that research on informal family care has been based primarily on service users; that is, there is concern that our understanding of informal care is biased toward those who approach service agencies. Thus, the "sandwiched generation" is seen as largely mythical in that it does not reflect the experience of most middle generation persons.

Indeed, in a recent study using a random sample of middle aged children in a large Canadian city, it was found that most caregivers did not score high on measures of burden. It was suggested that this was because the majority of respondents provided only minimal task support to aging parents. However, there was a subgroup with sicker parents who gave considerably more care than the others. Among these, those who scored highest on measures of burden had the lowest levels of attachment to their parents; visited and provided help most frequently; received fewer *informal* supports than the nonburdened; and had parents who received fewer *formal* supports (Bond et al. 1990, 176-77).

These data serve to position the policy debate. Namely, most families do not feel that their elderly relatives make heavy demands on them. In fact, Aronson (1990), a Canadian researcher focusing on the well-being of old women, suggests that elderly women are very concerned about placing demands on their daughters, frequently to the point of curtailing legitimate requests. However, for kin who do provide daily service, costs in terms of personal well-being and family relations can be high.

Studies in Canada, the U.K., and the U.S. show that substantial care is provided by elderly spouses, both male and female (Stone 1988; Green 1988; Stone, Cafferata, and Sangl 1987). These caregivers provide the most consistent care, and resist institutional placement longer, regardless of their spouse's level of disability. The situation of caregiving elderly spouses is qualitatively different from that of caregiving provided intergenerationally. The former are usually old themselves, but the care they give tends to be embedded within an intimate relationship which can give it a meaning not possible in other familial situations. In addition, there is mounting evidence that men and women experience conditions differently (Horowitz 1985; Brody, Dempsey, and Pruchno 1990; Pruchno and Resch 1989; Stoller 1990). Some of these differences are in the dimensions of physical and mental deterioration emphasized, assumptions about authority, task management, and the use of social supports (Miller 1990, 97).

The now considerable body of research that focuses on the costs of care to family members does not address the situation of several other subgroups of elderly. Fifteen percent of Canadians who were ever married and 9 percent of those who never married do not have children (Statistics Canada 1983). Over 80 percent of older Canadians have living siblings, but this drops to below 60 percent for those over 85 (Hays 1984). However, interaction with siblings in later life tends to be much less than that with children and grandchildren (Connidis 1989, 85). Very old people without a spouse or child have fewer options available for informal care and thus may well be the most vulnerable group of elderly. The evidence shows that among service users and institutional residents such persons are highly visible.

Several key issues for future policy making emerge from this research on informal care. First, for elderly persons requiring personal and/or instrumental assistance, most help comes from an aging spouse and/or a daughter who fits elder care in with other paid and unpaid work. To continue the current practice of referring to such persons as "the informal sector" hides the relative fragility of these arrangements while suggesting that the multi-billion dollar "format sector" is somehow an equal partner. It allow us, for instance, to suggest that families can become case managers (Seltzer, Ivry, and Litchfield 1987). Such a scenario may not be as empowering as it initially seems. An elderly spouse or a pressured daughter could be forced to take on primary responsibility for steering her way through myriad services each characterized by its own set of rules and regulations. In addition to time and energy costs, the model assumes that such a person has the knowledge, experience, and skill to perform this managerial function in a manner that maximizes benefits. Information and contacts are a form of knowledge and a source of power that professionals have to a far greater degree than elderly service recipients or their caregivers.

Second, extended family, friends, and neighbors respond to emergency situations but they do not provide the type of continuous involvement that frail persons require. Thus, it is misleading to envision them as part of the informal sector.

Third, the research outlined in the foregoing pages is an important ingredient in the formulation of policy. However, it is only one ingredient. Policy making is done in an atmosphere of competing claims. Although some voices are far louder than others, they are not necessarily those whose needs are most pressing.

THE INTERPRETATION OF NEED

The previous two sections have discussed the formal and informal organization of home care. In the case of the former, one is struck by the persistent underdevelopment of services. In all provinces, program growth has been an uphill battle; financial questions and concerns about potential misuse of services are never far from the surface. Over the last few years, Canadian policymakers have become more aware of the economic and emotional costs borne by informal caregivers, most of whom are women. However, this recognition will not necessarily lead to changes in service provisions, as the response pattern to date shows.

Efforts have been made to provide caregivers with limited help on some tasks and/or to give them a break from the daily routine. However, federal and provincial policy documents constantly reaffirm the expectation that it is the responsibility of families to provide daily care (Rosenthal and Neysmith 1990). The commitment of and burdens on families are recognized, but their need for formal supplementary care-providing services has not been linked to this acknowledgement.

It is not the specifics of programs that are important in discussions of future policy directions, but rather the assumptions that inform these dialogues. To date, policy makers have assumed that since families provide 80 to 90 percent of care, this approach is the most desirable. It is recognized that in some cases this preferred model cannot be realized because of strain on the caregiver and/or the lack of an appropriate individual in the social network of the elderly person. Services are then developed to fill in these gaps. Policy statements, however, continue to reinforce familial obligations.

Need is determined by assessment services–usually in terms of service availability. This dynamic is supported by research showing that people with similar conditions receive different services depending on where, and with whom, they happen to live (Beland 1989). Since delivery systems establish eligibility, it is not surprising that they tend to document use patterns of existing services; they are less apt to collect data indicating needs they cannot meet. Similarly, provision is based on an assessment of the person *and* the family's ability to provide service. This emphasis keeps the interpretation of need within the private realm of the household. It does, however, allow some services which supplement and support family care a definition of need that assumes family responsibility remains unchallenged. This is a quite different assumption than that posited by countries such as Sweden:

> Debate about the relationship between formal and informal care has a different point of departure in Sweden than in the United States [and Canada]. The accepted policy position is that publicly provided care is a citizen's right, and should be available to any individual or family who needs it. The decision regarding the mix of informal and formal care is a choice which rests with the family. In fact, the issue of care substitution is framed very differently in Sweden. There, the discussion is centered around the question of how much formal care is necessary so that no family is forced to substitute informal care for formal care. Families are not statutorily required to take care of the elderly, but the government does have this obligation. (Hokenstad and Johansson 1990, 254)

An unspoken corollary of the familial model of care is that caregiving should not be paid for. I would argue that, until the needs of frail elderly persons become unhooked from ideological presuppositions of family responsibility, the prognosis is poor for improving the quantity and quality of, as well as remuneration for, this type of paid labor.

The issue of wages is a real if somewhat underplayed component of the home-care discussion. One of the results of current attitudes is low wages for front line home-care providers who primarily are women. There seems to be an assumption that caring for strangers is the same as caring for family members and should be done on an altruistic basis; otherwise it will attract "the wrong kind of people." This is quite different from the criteria that we use in other skilled jobs where the dictum is to pay a decent salary in order to attract "good people." According to Leat and Gay (1987, 62) in the male-dominated service professions there is no doubt that the maxim "you get what you pay for" prevails. Most people do not question the motives of physicians or lawyers when they demand high fees. Payment and care are not antithetical–payment does not negate caring, just as nonpayment does not guarantee it.

Caring for others traditionally is women's work. This seems to be another key determinant of why it is undervalued and underpaid. However, despite such public underestimation of the job, women who provide the services view the work itself differently. In my own research on home care workers and volunteers, measures of job satisfaction were high for the intrinsic components of the job (Neysmith and Nichols 1989). However, the turnover rate was also high. Across the country it runs between 50 and 70 percent per annum primarily because of low wages. For instance, in Ontario it took a major homemaker shortage, combined with a strike by one of the larger nonprofit agencies, to push salaries beyond the minimum wage. Yet demand for this type of work is increasing as families are being expected to care for more frail persons.

The unpaid family caregiver is in an even more precarious position than the paid care provider. She does not have the option of quitting. I choose these words carefully because caring for family members is not something that women choose to do in the context of weighing alternatives. Research in Canada, Britain, and the U.S. documents how women are socialized to care, and are well aware of the costs and benefits that accrue to them. However, it has also become clear that this work is invisible when done within the family context (Baines, Evans, and Neysmith 1991; Abel and Nelson 1990; Ungerson 1990).

Competing definitions of need must be addressed in order to

understand fully the issues related to caregiving. In a market economy certain needs are seen as appropriately met in the public arena, while others are deemed to be the responsibility of the private world of the family. This "separate spheres" phenomenon has been the focus of considerable feminist analysis (Hooyman 1990). Research shows that work relegated to the private domain has fallen disproportionately on the shoulders of women. Questions of equity about the distribution of responsibilities both within families and between families and the state are increasingly being voiced, particularly since a growing number of women are affected. One of the contributions of feminist research has been in specifying how the state, the family, and a market economy interpenetrate within the lives of women (Showstack Sassoon 1987).

Ensuring that long-term care policies are just entails more than legislative guarantees that access is universal and that services are in the public sector domain. My own position is that a commitment to a long-term care system that is publicly financed, where a minimal set of services are guaranteed, similar to the medical services currently covered under The Canada Health Act, is a necessary starting point. However, I would argue even further for a long-term care system that works to change inequities within society. This means addressing the gender and class bias inherent in the current formal and informal delivery systems.

The dilemma facing Canada, and other countries with a commitment to publicly supported health care, is how to move beyond existing structures, including the medical model of care. Unless we renegotiate the types of services that we want to guarantee, reconceptualize their delivery patterns, and become more critical of the informal as well as the formal criteria that we use in rationing resources, we will continue to have an ineffective system of long-term care no matter how many dollars are poured into the health sector. To meet this challenge we will have to view elderly persons as having rights to a decent quality of life.

CONCLUSION

This chapter has assessed the current state of long-term care policy in Canada. There appears to be a chasm between policy goals and the structure of services available. Although there are few in-dications that this gap is closing, there are signs that the discourse on healthy public policy may be setting the political stage to facili-tate future change. This perspective moves the focus from individ-ual responsibility and the medical treatment of illness. Rather the health of people as they age is seen as influenced primarily by the social environment within which individuals grow old.

The development on an international scale of a feminist analysis of caring, combined with growing numbers of old people needing care, have increasingly forced the contradictions facing women into the forefront of social concern. The articulation of these contradic-tions in Canada is fostering a consideration of new options. It is no coincidence that this is occurring primarily amongst women. They are the informal caregivers, the formal care providers, and the ma-jority of care receivers. Not only have the costs to women of the status quo been documented, but new questions are now being raised. These include: Why are women ultimately *responsible* for the care of elderly persons even though some men do it? Why is caregiving undervalued work, whether at home or in the work-place? Does the low value placed on this work reflect the fact that it is done by women? What effect will current caring arrangements have on the personal, social, and financial well-being of today's young women as they move into old age?

Canadian long-term care policy will be able to meet the needs of tomorrow's elderly more equitably only if it is able to develop a viable response to these concerns. However, this will mean that we have to develop policy-making mechanisms ensuring that groups affected by services are active participants in the decision-making process.

REFERENCES

Abel, E., and M. Nelson, eds. 1990. *Circles of Care: Work and Identity in Women's Lives.* Albany: State University of New York Press.

Alberta. 1988. *A New Vision for Long-term Care: Meeting the Need.* Edmonton.

Angus, D. 1987. Health-care costs. In *Health and Canadian Society: Sociological Perspectives*, edited by D. Coburn, C. D'Arcy, G. Torrance and P. New. Second edition. Toronto: Fitzhenry and Whiteside.

Aronson, J. 1990. Women's perspectives on informal care of the elderly: Public ideology and personal experience of giving and receiving care. *Ageing and Society.* 10(1): 61-84.

Auer, L. 1987. *Canadian Hospital Costs and Productivity.* Study prepared for the Economic Council of Canada. Ottawa: Ministry of Supply and Services.

Baines, C., P. Evans, and S. Neysmith, eds. 1991. *Women's Caring: A Feminist Perspective on Social Welfare.* Toronto: McLelland and Stewart.

Beland, F. 1984. The family and adults 65 years of age and over: Co-residency and the receipt of help. *Canadian Review of Sociology and Anthropology.* 21: 302-317.

Beland, F. 1985. Who are those most likely to be institutionalized: The elderly who receive comprehensive home care services or those who do not? *Social Science and Medicine* 02:347-354.

Beland, F. 1989. Patterns of Health and Social Service Utilization. *Canadian Journal on Aging.* 8(1): 19-33.

Bond, J., M. Baril, S. Axelrod, and L. Crawford. 1990. Support to older parents by middle-aged children. *Canadian Journal of Community Mental Health.* 9(1): 163-178.

British Columbia. Minister of Health and Minister Responsible for Seniors. 1989. *Towards a Better Age: Strategies for Improving the Lives of Senior British Columbians.* Victoria.

Brody, E. 1985. Parental care as a normative family stress. *The Gerontologist.* 25(1): 19-29.

Brody, E., N. Dempsey, and R. Pruchno. 1990. Mental health of sons and daughters of the institutionalized aged. *The Gerontologist.* 30(2): 212-219.

Chappell, N. 1985. Social support and the receipt of home care services. *The Gerontologist.* 25(1): 47-54.

Chappell, N., L. Strain, and A. Blandford. 1986. *Aging and Health Care: A Social Perspective.* Toronto: Holt, Rinehart, and Winston of Canada, Limited.

Clark, P. 1989. Canadian health care policy and the elderly: Will rationing rhetoric become reality in an aging society? *Canadian Journal of Community Mental Health.* 8(2): 123-140.

Connidis, I. 1989. *Family Ties and Aging.* Toronto: Butterworths.

Dalley, G. 1988. *Ideologies of Caring: Rethinking Community and Collectivism.* Hampshire and London: MacMillan Education Ltd.

Denton, F., S. Li, and B. Spencer. 1987. How will population aging affect the future costs of maintaining health care standards? In *Aging in Canada: Social Perspectives*, edited by V. Marshall. Toronto: Fitzhenry and Whiteside.

Evans, R. 1987. Illusions of necessity: Evading responsibility for choice in health care. In *Health and Canadian Society: Sociological Perspectives*, edited by D. Cobourn, C. D'Arcy, G. Torrence and P. New. Second edition. Toronto: Fitzhenry and Whiteside: 615-636.

Evans, R. 1990. Tension, compression, and shear: Directions, stresses, and outcomes of health care cost control. *Journal of Health Politics, Policy and Law.* 15(1): 101-128.

Fellegi, I. 1988. Can we afford an aging society? *Canadian Economic Observer.* October. 4.1-4.34.

Finch, J. 1989. *Family Obligations and Social Change.* Cambridge: Polity Press.

Fisher, B., and J. Tronto. 1990. Toward a Feminist Theory of Caring. In *Circles of Care: Work and Identity in Women's Lives*, edited by E. Abel and M. Nelson. New York: SUNY Press.

Forbes, W., J. Jackson, and A. Kraus. 1987. *Institutionalization of the Elderly in Canada*. Toronto: Butterworths.

Green, H. 1988. *Informal Carers*. London: OPCS, HMSO.

Hagey, N., G. Larocque, and C. McBride. 1989. *Highlights of Aboriginal Conditions. Part I and Part II*. Ottawa: Indian and Northern Affairs Canada.

Hays, J. 1984. Aging and family resources: Availability and proximity of kin. *The Gerontologist*. 24(2): 149-153.

Health and Welfare Canada. 1986. *Achieving Health for All: A Framework for Health Promotion*. Ottawa.

Health and Welfare Canada. 1987. *National Health Expenditures in Canada 1975-1985*. Ottawa.

Hokenstad, M., and L. Johansson. 1990. Caregiving for the elderly in Sweden: Program challenges and policy initiatives. In *Aging and Caregiving: Theory, Research and Policy*, edited by D. Biegel and A. Blum. Newbury Park: Sage Publications.

Hooyman, N. 1990. Women as caregivers of the elderly: Implications for social welfare policy and practice. In *Aging and Caregiving: Theory, Research and Policy*, edited by D. Biegel and A. Blum. Newbury Park: Sage Publications.

Horowitz, A. 1985. Sons and daughters as caregivers to older parents: Differences in role performance and consequences. *The Gerontologist* 25(6): 612-617.

Kane, R., and R. Kane. 1985. *What the United States Can Learn from Canada About Caring for the Elderly: A Will and a Way*. New York: Columbia University Press.

Leat, D., and P. Gay. 1987. *Paying for Care: A study of policy and practice in paid care schemes*. London: Policy Studies Institute.

McDaniel, S. 1986. *Canada's Aging Population*. Toronto: Butterworths.

Miller, B. 1990. Gender Differences in Spouse Management of the Caregiver Role. In *Circles of Care: Work and Identity in Women's Lives*, edited by E. Abel and M. Nelson. New York: SUNY Press.

Minkler, M. 1991. "Generational equity" and the new victim blaming. In *Critical Perspectives on Aging: The Political and Moral Economy of Growing Old*, edited by M. Minkler and C. Estes. New York: Baywood Publishing Company Inc.

National Council of Welfare. 1990. *Health, Health Care and Medicare*. Ottawa: Minister of Supply and Services.

Neysmith, S. 1989. Closing the gap between health policy and the home-care needs of tomorrow's elderly. *Canadian Journal of Community Mental Health*. 8(2): 141-150.

Neysmith, S. 1990. Dependency among Third World elderly: A need for new directions in the nineties. *International Journal of Health Services*. 20(4): 681-690.

Neysmith, S., and J. Edwards. 1984. Dependency in the 1980's: Its impact on Third World elderly. *Ageing and Society.* 4(1): 21-44.

Neysmith, S., and B. Nichols. 1989. Home-help: Who pays when caregivers become care providers? Paper presented at the Annual Meetings of the Canadian Association on Gerontology. Ottawa.

Ontario, 1990. *Strategies for Change: Comprehensive Reform of Ontario's Long-Term Care Services.* Toronto: Queens's Printer for Ontario.

Pederson, A., R. Edwards, M. Kelner, V. Marshall, and K. Allison. 1988. *Coordinating Healthy Public Policy: An Analytic Literature Review and Bibliography.* Report prepared for the Health Promotion Directorate/National Health Research and Development Program Working Group on Priorities for Health Promotion/Disease Prevention Research. Ottawa.

Pfaff, M. 1990. Differences in health care spending across countries: Statistical evidence. *Journal of Health Politics, Policy and Law.* 15(1): 1-24.

Price Waterhouse. 1988. *Review of the Manitoba Continuing Care Program. Volume I. Executive Summary.*

Pruchno, R., and N. Resch. 1989. Husbands and wives as caregivers: Anticedents of depression and burden. *The Gerontologist* 29(2): 159-165.

Quebec. 1985. Ministere des Affaires Sociale. *Un Nouvel Age a Partager. Politique du ministere des affaires sociales a l'egard des personnes agees.* Les Publications du Quebec.

Roos, N., E. Shapiro, and L. Roos. 1984. Aging and the demand for health care services: Which aged and whose demand? *The Gerontologist* 24(1): 31-36.

Rootman, I. 1988. Knowledge development: A challenge for health promotion. *Health Promotion.* 27(2): 2-4.

Rosenthal, C. 1987. Aging and generational relations in Canada. In *Aging in Canada: Social Perspectives*, edited by V. Marshall. Second edition. Toronto: Fitzhenry and Whiteside.

Rosenthal, C., and S. Neysmith. 1990. *Informal Support to Older People: Conclusions, Forecasts, Recommendations and Policy Prescriptions in Recent Policy Deliberations.* A report prepared for Statistics Canada.

Rowe, J. 1985. Health care of the elderly. *The New England Journal of Medicine* 312 (13): 827-35.

Schwenger, C. 1989. Institutionalization of Elderly Canadians: Future Allocations to Non-Health Sectors. In *Aging and Health: Linking Research and Public Policy*, edited by S. Lewis. Chelsea, Michigan: Lewis Publishers.

Seltzer, M., J. Ivry, and L. Litchfield. 1987. Family members as case managers: Partnerships between the formal and informal support networks. *The Gerontologist.* 27(6): 722-28.

Shanas, E. 1979. Social myth as hypothesis: the case of family relations of old people. *The Gerontologist.* 19(1): 3-9.

Shapiro, E. 1988. *Home Care: Where is it and Where Should it be Going?* Paper prepared for a consultation of European and Canadian experts on long-term care with the Elderly Services Branch of the Ministry of Community and Social Services. Toronto.

Showstack Sassoon, A. 1987. *Women and the State: The Shifting Boundaries of Public and Private*. London: Hutchinson.

Statistics Canada. 1983. *Nuptiality and Fertility*. 1981. Census of Canada Catalogue #92-906. Ottawa: Minister of Supply and Services Canada.

Statistics Canada. 1986. *The Health and Activity Limitation Survey*. Cat # 41034. Ottawa.

Stolar, G., M. Hill, and A. Tomblin. 1986. Family disengagement–myth or reality: A follow-up study after geriatric assessment. *Canadian Journal on Aging* 5(2): 113-124.

Stoller, E. 1990. Males as helpers: The role of sons, relatives and friends. *The Gerontologist*. 30(2): 228-235.

Stone, L. 1988. *Family and Friendship Ties Among Canada's Seniors: An Introductory Report of Findings from the General Social Survey*. Ottawa: Statistics Canada.

Stone, L., and H. Frenken. 1988. *Canada's Seniors*. Statistics Canada. Cat 98-121. Ottawa.

Stone, R., G. Cafferata, and J. Sangl. 1987. Caregivers of the frail elderly: a national profile. *The Gerontologist*. 27: 616-626.

Storm, C., T. Storm, and J. Strike-Schurman. 1985. Obligations for care: Beliefs in a small Canadian town. *Canadian Journal on Aging*. 4(2) 75-85.

Tarman, V. 1990. *Privatization and Health Care: The Case of Ontario Nursing Home*. Toronto: Garamond Press.

Ungerson, C. 1990. *Gender and Caring: Work and Welfare in Britain and Scandinavia*. Hertfordshire: Harvester Wheatsheaf.

Wilkins, R. and Adams, O. 1983. Health expectancy in Canada, late 1970s: Demographic, regional and social dimensions. *American Journal of Public Health* 73(9): 1073-1083.

Wilkins, R., O. Adams, and A. Brancker. 1989. Changes in mortality by income in urban Canada from 1971 to 1986. *Health Reports*. 2(2): 137-175. Statistics Canada. Canadian Center for Health Information.

World Health Organization. 1988. *Healthy Public Policy–Strategies for Action: The Adelaide Recommendations*.

Chapter 8

French Old-Age Policies and the Frail Elderly

Michel Frossard
Anne-Marie Guillemard

Considerably longer life expectancies have transformed the composition of populations in developed nations. Everywhere in Europe, the increasing number of persons who have reached an advanced age has shed stark light on the limits and shortcomings of old-age policies. It is high time to work out new policies for providing care to people who suffer from the disabilities and loss of functional autonomy that so often come with advancing old age.

In France, this is a major point on the political agenda. During 1991, no less than two official reports were made on this topic (see Boulard 1991; Schopflin 1991). Inevitably, if France does not soon adopt new ways of handling dependence in old age, the achievements during the 20th century in lengthening the life span will result in tragedy. More and more families are facing the intractable problem of providing care, whether at home or in an institution, to aged parents whose autonomy has been impaired. At present, there are as many French families who have to care for an elderly parent as for a child less than two years old.

This chapter will be structured as follows. In the light of current and projected population trends, we shall review the shortcomings of French old-age policies. In France, the problems of the elderly

Text translated from French by Noal Mellott, CNRS, Paris.

have been raised in terms of "dependence" and the means of measuring it. Once these points have been examined, we turn our attention to the attempts to regulate and reform the various sorts of benefits and services provided to the dependent elderly.

CARE FOR THE FRAIL ELDERLY AND THE HISTORY OF FRENCH OLD AGE

Population Trends and the Characteristics of the Frail Elderly

For a long time now, France's population has been aging more rapidly than its neighboring countries. The drop in the fertility rate, which demographers have called the "demographic transition," occurred earlier in France than elsewhere. Even though the "baby boom" significantly countered this trend from 1942 until the early 1970s, this reversal ended earlier in France than in nearby lands as the fertility rate once again lowered.

A second demographic trend that has also had an impact is the longer life expectancies attained due to decisive progress in public health and hygiene. Along with Japan, Sweden, and a few other countries, France has the longest life expectancy. At birth, females and males can expect to live over eighty years and nearly seventy-three years, respectively.

The consequence of these two trends comes as no surprise: by 1950, France was one of the countries with the most aged population structure. Today, it is not alone, and the United Kingdom, Denmark, West Germany, and Belgium have aged even faster. From 1946 to 1989, the proportion of the French population at least 60 years old was rising, whereas that under 20 was falling; and this trend is expected to continue (see Table 1). Although the proportion of the middle aged has not changed much, France has never had such a low proportion of young people as nowadays. Even during the 1930s, when the birth rate was especially low, about a third of the population was under 20–far more than today.

Not only has the general population been aging, but the population over 60 has grown, as well. The percentage of persons over 75 has been rising, a trend that should be even more pronounced by the

TABLE 1. Composition of the French population by age-group, retrospectively and prospectively (in percentages).

YEAR	TOTAL FRENCH POPULATION	≤20	20-59	60 and over	75 and over
1946	40,125,000	29.5	54.5	16.0	3.4
1950	41,647,000	30.2	53.6	16.2	3.8
1960	45,465,000	32.3	51.0	16.7	4.3
1970	50,528,000	33.2	48.8	18.0	4.7
1980	53,731,000	30.6	52.4	17.0	5.7
1990	56,141,000	27.6	53.2	19.2	6.8
2000	58,226,000	25.5	53.7	20.8	7.1
2020	60,078,000	22.0	50.1	28.0	9.4

Source: INSEE.

year 2020. More than one out of three "old people" (i.e., those at least 60 years old) is at least 75 years old, as compared with one out of four in 1960. There are now about 10.7 million people over 60 years old, 7.6 million over 65 and 3.8 million over 75. This last group is the frailest and needs, therefore, to be helped with everyday activities.

But what is this group's standard of living? Since the mid-1970s, retirees' standard of living has increased continuously. Retirement pensions have increased faster than wages. Despite this overall improvement, considerable disparities still exist. The oldest are the least privileged, especially if they are women.

To have an overview of the situation, let us see how many persons are receiving minimum benefits from Social Security's Caisse Nationale d'Assurance-Vieillesse (henceforth, Old-Age Fund). Since 1975, this number has dropped significantly, even as the floor of minimum benefits has been raised (faster than retirement pensions in general). But if we look more closely at who is actually receiving minimum old-age benefits, we discover that they are mainly women. This is the poorest group among the aged. Among 70- to 74-year-olds, for instance, 8.9 percent of men receive minimum benefits as compared with 11.9 percent of women; and among 85 to 89 year-olds, these percentages are 23.1 and 32.1 percent, respectively. (These statistics and those in the following paragraphs all come from official sources–INSEE 1990).

As for living arrangements, the older one is, the more likely he or she will be living alone. This holds especially for women who, given their longer life spans, have more chances of outliving their spouses. Whereas 40 percent of women at least 65 years old live alone and only 29 percent are married, 45 percent of women who are 75 or older live alone and only 17 percent reside with a spouse. Nor do many of the elderly live with other family members (less than 10 percent of persons 65 and over), and even fewer will do so in the future. This percentage rises only very slightly with age, given the number of elderly who live in single households. Furthermore, few of the elderly live in institutions. Barely 5 percent of French people at least 60 years old live in an institution. This percentage, which has hardly changed since 1970, does, of course, increase with age: 10 percent of persons over 75 and 20 percent of those over 85 reside in such facilities. In brief, most older people have their own housing.

These population statistics and socioeconomic data help us realize the importance of the issues related to old-age policy. The needs of the growing number of aging persons who are living alone, who have meager incomes and risk becoming dependent on care, must be met.

Care for the Frail Elderly in French Old-Age Policy

In France, care for the frail elderly is provided through a complex system of measures that have been arranged without much regard for coherence. A brief history of these measures and a description of how they work will help us to assess their impact, or lack of it, on the frail elderly.

There were two major phases in the evolution of French Old-Age Policy. The first phase attempted to help the aged remain at home. This so-called "home-maintenance" policy, which was part of the Sixth National Plan (1971-1975), aimed at helping the aged avoid institutionalization or, at least, delay the time when this would occur. In this way, the consequences of such admissions (social segregation, increasing dependence, and higher costs for society) also would be curtailed.

To achieve this goal of greater community care, the state would supply services and establish new collective facilities, all of which would keep the aged integrated in society for as long as possible. Various programs were implemented in housing (renovation, group housing units, etc.), as well as in home services (Home Help and care, home delivery of meals, etc.). Moreover, facilities such as senior citizen's clubs, restaurants, and health centers were opened in neighborhoods throughout the nation.

Although national and local authorities have constantly pursued the policy of helping the aged to remain at home, problems have arisen with program implementation. In particular, the various measures have turned out to be "fragments" of a general policy, the positive effects of which have not always met expectations (Guillemard 1986). The specific programs instituted as part of the home-maintenance policy would have had to work together so that the elderly, despite their social and physical handicaps, might continue to live at home for as long as possible. The cornerstone of such a policy should have been coordination. But coordination has turned out to be very hard to achieve, given the diversity of actors, the variety of institutional rationales, and the multiplicity of budgets (and budget headings) necessary to the implementation of these myriad measures.

A major obstacle to coordination has been the extreme dualism of the health and social service sectors in France. Each of these sectors is administered under a different body of legislation. The 1970 Hospital Act has laid down the rules for organizing and financing the health sector, whereas social services are administered under a law passed in 1975. The home-maintenance policy has produced mainly social rather than health services. For example, Home Helpers' services (aides ménagères, publicly paid housekeepers) have become available, and organizations (clubs, restaurants, etc.) have been established to decrease the isolation of the aged. Home nursing services took longer to develop, practically until 1982. Furthermore, they mostly cover only practical nursing chores (help with toilet and hygiene). Today, more than half a million persons 65 and older (about 8 percent of this age group) have Home Helpers whereas only 42,000 benefit from home nurses. Of course, we should add to this the hours worked by private nurses who are reimbursed by Social Security's Health Fund.

Besides contributing to the "fragmentation" of the home-maintenance policy, this dualism also has been a factor in the dichotomy of care. Programs for helping the aged who live independently have mainly targeted the able-bodied, primarily to keep them autonomous and out of institutions. For the frail elderly, the response of old-age policy has been institutional care.

At about the time the first home-maintenance program was adopted, special hospital-type facilities were created to provide long-term care to the frail elderly. A major objective is to get this category of patients out of acute-care hospitals. Under law, these new nursing home facilities are supposed to house the elderly who have lost their autonomy and whose ill health requires constant medical supervision. As of 1990, 68,000 beds were available in this type of nursing home.

These public nursing homes are different from acute-care hospitals in two respects. First, the personnel/bed ratio is much lower. Second, these facilities receive money from two sources: a fixed sum per bed from the Health Fund; and payments from residents, their families or welfare services for accommodations, which cost about 9,000 francs a month. Since this is almost twice the minimum old-age benefit and thrice the average pension of a retiree with full career earnings, many of the elderly and their families have difficulty paying for such care.

This type of long-stay hospital accommodation is not well adapted to the needs of the frail elderly. Most of these establishments are quite large, with 120 to 240 beds. They were not designed to accommodate members of this age group who often lose their bearings. Furthermore, most of these facilities have not proven capable of creating a friendly atmosphere or maintaining a quality life for residents. In addition, they have tried to provide medical care for problems that are inseparably medical and social. Alternatively, as a result of the aforementioned dichotomy between social and health services, political leaders have developed "social" institutions which contain medical facilities; these also have been inadequate for meeting the real needs of the frail elderly.

Besides the lack of congruence between the facilities for housing the frail elderly and the requirements of this population, the aged tend to be placed in institutions as a function of costs and ability to pay, rather than on the basis of their needs and level of dependence. There is no medical reason why 40 percent of the elderly on medical or psychiatric wards are hospitalized, save that pyschiatric and acute medical care are almost fully covered by the Health Fund.

Meanwhile, attempts have been made to rationalize the costs of social services and curb Social Security expenditures. These efforts have, too often, resulted in inadequate home care at higher costs. For example, the number of hours that the Old-Age Fund reimburses for Home Helpers has been restricted, in principle, to 30 hours a month. This restriction applies despite the official priority of maintaining the elderly in their homes. As a consequence, housekeeping services cannot be provided continuously, and the slack is either taken up by families and through recourse to unspecialized personnel, such as cleaning ladies, whose services, paid by the beneficiary, cost less than that of Home Helpers, or necessary chores are left undone. There is no longer a correlation between available services and actual needs. According to one survey, 21 percent of requests for Home Helpers are not satisfied, whereas 35 percent of the beneficiaries of such services do not objectively need them.

Despite this major policy effort to help the aged remain at home, actual programs have not been sufficiently effective given the increasing number of potential beneficiaries. Moreover, since home care policy is now officially distinct from housing policy, there are no arrangements for ensuring a gradual transition from home to institutional care as individuals lose their autonomy. Due to the lack of such a transition, most admissions into institutions are made in an emergency—as a function of the availability of accommodations and their costs, instead of on the basis of the needs and wants of the recipients and their families.

Experimental programs have attempted to provide alternatives to classical institutionalization and avoid the rupture between home care and institutional custody. This is "residential care," which offers personal housing in small-scale facilities with collective services. About a dozen aged persons live in such a facility, each person occupying a single housing unit; but a professional is always present.

There are, however, few such innovations in France. Meanwhile, most of the frail elderly are receiving care from family members, though such an arrangement is difficult to maintain for a long time. No institutional support is given to family helpers, and there are still too few professional caregivers.

THE DEGREE OF DEPENDENCE

For about a decade now, dependence has been an operational concept in old-age policy. Previously, the aged population's needs were assessed on the basis of demographic trends and ratios for the number of beds in retirement and nursing homes. The concept of dependence started reaching beyond the idea of individual care when a means of measuring it was accepted in scientific circles and among practitioners. Along with this concept has come an awareness that providing care to the frail does not inevitably entail institutional custody.

A means of measuring dependence was defined in the early 1980s. Much effort was put into refining this concept, improving its measure and estimating the number of dependent elderly people. A consensus formed around the definitions of "autonomy" as the capacity to choose one's own way of life and of "dependence" as the inability to perform daily activities. Scales for measuring dependence were created, compared, and validated, in particular by a group of researchers and practitioners in gerontology headed by Alain Colvez at the National Institute of Health and Medical Research (INSERM). This work prepared the way for considerable progress in the study of aging.

The criterion of dependence gradually moved to the center of old-age policy, despite a lack of statistics about the actual size of the population concerned. Owing to a dozen studies performed between 1978 and 1988, more reliable information has become available. In fact, approximately 30 percent of persons 65 years of age or older have trouble performing at least one everyday task, but the percentage of severely dependent persons has turned out to be rather small. It has also been proven that the large majority of dependent persons (75 percent) live at home and that many of them (19 percent) do so because of professional help alone. Since most of these studies followed Colvez's methodology (1990), their results are comparable.

Let us succinctly review some of this research, which has overturned preconceived ideas about aged invalids in institutions, either abandoned by their families or unable to live at home without the latter's help. Colvez (1990) has reported the results of three regional surveys conducted between 1978 and 1988. More than 5,000 persons at least 65 years old were classified in one of four "disadvantaged groups," defined by the degree of infirmity or inability to perform daily actions. The proportion of persons confined to a bed or wheelchair was less than 3 percent, to which could be added another 3 percent who depended very much on help with elementary daily tasks (see Table 2). In addition, 12 percent did not leave home unless accompanied by someone. Extrapolating these results to all of France in 1990, these three groups would amount to about 180,000, 230,000 and 917,000 persons, respectively.

Contrary to the prevailing idea that intense dependence meant institutional custody, it was discovered that most such persons were not in an institution. Out of a hundred persons confined to a bed or wheelchair, three-quarters were living at home, and a quarter were residing in an institution. As for the other three groups, the frequency of institutional custody was inversely proportional to the degree of impairment: 12 percent, 10 percent, and 2 percent, respectively.

As for the help provided to the dependent aged, these same studies showed that the contribution from professionals was small, though perhaps significant, in comparison with all the help coming from spouses, children, friends, and neighbors. This held true even for the intensely dependent, 47 percent of whom received no professional assistance (see Table 3). Families, in particular, were actively involved in providing support to the latter. As much can be said about the three less dependent groups. In addition, professional help was supplied to all three categories in nearly the same way (except for dressing). In other words, aid was given for reasons other than dependence. This means that the policy of providing help to the aged has not been well targeted. Such a conclusion comes as

TABLE 2. Condition of frail elderly, by group (France).

Disadvantaged Group	Total (in survey)	Percent	Total Population (estimate)
Persons confined to a bed or wheelchair (group 1)	125	2.4%	180,000
Persons who need help with their toilet (group 2)	161	3.1%	230,000
Persons who do not need help with toilet but do not go out unless accompanied (group 3)	638	12.4%	917,000
Others (group 4)	4,212	82.0%	6,193,000
TOTAL	5,135	100.0%	7,520,000

Source: Table adapted from Colvez, 1990, p. 16.

no surprise, given the aforementioned fragmentation of social and health services in France. It should be noted that from 3 to 4 percent of tasks, mostly major household chores, were left undone.

The housing of the aged has its own disadvantages. Table 4 provides a glimpse of housing conditions for each of these four groups. Notice how many persons did not have hot water (12 to 18 percent), a bathroom (21 to 31 percent), or an indoor toilet (10 to 18 percent). Moreover, the most dependent were not housed very differently from the others. We can, therefore, conclude that home improvements are not targeted as a function of dependence, since all groups experience similar housing conditions.

What do these statistics imply about the future? At present, we do not know how the probabilities of impairment, and thus dependency, will evolve over time for given age groups. We might hypothesize decreases in the probabilities of death and of impairment. The number of persons to whom care will have to be provided in the coming decades depends on the relative growth of these two phenomena.

TABLE 3. Help provided to persons 65 years old and older confined to a bed or wheelchair.

Caregivers	Confined Elderly
Professional help only	19%
Family or friends/with professional help	34
Family or friends only	47
Total	100%

Source: Colvez, 1990.

COST COMPARISON OF LIVING AT HOME OR IN AN INSTITUTION

In France, no economic analysis was made of old-age policy before the late 1970s, when macroeconomic studies inquired into the financing of old-age funds. These studies focused on how to replace or supplement the usual mechanisms of redistribution with retirement plans based on capitalization. By 1990, however, such plans had not proven effective, and few had been removed.

For dependence, too, no major comparative studies were performed before the late 1970s, or even before 1982. The only exception was a short article wherein Pierre Massé (1977) showed that helping the elderly continue to live at home by providing them with up to 30 hours of work from Home Helpers cost less than housing them in institutions. This statistic has served as the basis for setting the amount of allocations for Home Help.

The arguments already reviewed account for such an absence of research. It was not thought that the same individual faced the alternative between home or institutional care. Supposedly, the "young old" (less than 75) were at home and in good health

TABLE 4. Housing conditions of the frail elderly, by condition of the frail elderly, in percentages.

Conditions in Home	Condition of Frail Elderly			
	Group 1	Group 2	Group 3	Group 4
No hot water	15%	17%	18%	12%
No bathroom	26	29	31	21
Outside toilet	10	18	13	13
Inadequate heating	8	16	13	10
Outside stairs	28	37	42	43
Inside stairs	38	48	48	49
Four rooms or more	35	39	31	37
Far from store	42	44	45	33

Source: Colvez, 1990.

whereas the "old old" (over 75) were dependent and living in institutions. As the reported data about dependence proved, this was not at all so. Preconceived ideas were widespread not just about dependence but also about the home/institutional alternatives. Lacking proof, they were grounded in common sense and backed by a few scientific notions, in particular about the economies of scale in institutions.

Starting in the mid-1980s, attention turned toward the home/ institutional alternatives. Another factor has motivated the demand for such research, namely the curbing of social expenditures. With this in mind, Social Security's Old-Age Fund asked for a preliminary methodological study (Frossard and Ennuyer 1987) and then financed further research (Frossard et al. 1990). The Sixth Plan (1971-1975) had advocated helping the elderly to remain at home not only because this is what the latter wanted, but also because it was less expensive. One hypothesis ran that, owing to economies of scale, home care costs were less below, and institutionalization costs less above, a certain threshold of dependence. As a corollary, savings would be directly proportional to an institution's size. Therefore, institutions for the aged were built with from 120 to 140 beds.

The methodology used in this research will be briefly presented, along with the results and an interpretation of them. In the original studies (Frossard 1990a; 1990b), the reader will find an analysis of "help networks" and details about the estimates of living expenses.

Methodology

To compare the costs of dependence in institutional and home care, it is necessary to do the following: compare groups with the same degree of dependence; count all expenditures on health and on help for persons in each of these groups; and estimate the actual help provided by professionals in institutions and thus modulate fixed fees for care according to the degree of dependence. Research conducted with various colleagues since 1986 has satisfied these conditions (see, for example, Frossard and Ennuyer 1987; and Frossard, Ennuyer and Jourdain 1988).

It should be pointed out that the French Social Security System pays institutions a fixed amount per elderly person regardless of either the degree of dependence or the actual help the person receives. This amount supposedly covers "normal" dependence. When costs excede it, they are covered as they would be for anyone regardless of age, namely through hospitalization or ambulatory care under Social Security's Health Fund. The originality of our three studies lay in the method used to obtain real costs: total costs were calculated by breaking this fixed amount down and then including health costs other than those covered by the State. The following calculations refer, therefore, to all the expenditures on help or care that an individual, his family, or the community pays for his dependence. Information about health expenditures came from Social Security offices, which keep individual records for a year.

The help actually provided by the personnel in institutions was estimated as a function of the time spent directly performing services for persons with the same degree of dependence. A coefficient was calculated as the ratio of this time to the average time available per resident. This coefficient was then used to modulate the fixed amount paid by Social Security to obtain an estimate of help as a function of the degree of dependence. To illustrate this, suppose that an average of 60 minutes a day is spent providing direct care to each resident. If the personnel spends 75 minutes on each intensely dependent person, the coefficient is 1.25 (75/60); and if the fixed amount from Social Security is 170 francs, the real cost of helping such a person is 212.5 francs (170 x 1.25).

To count all expenditures on help requires systematically registering assistance not only from Home Helpers and health professionals but also from unspecialized helpers (cleaning ladies as well as night-, day- or weekend-attendants). There are several ways to assess this. A valid estimate necessitates observing all help throughout a week. The differences between samples of persons who received and who did not receive free help were measured. In our initial study, such help was worth 3,500 francs a month. In the results presented hereafter, the value of a helper's time was assessed as a function of real or potential wages.

Results: The Equal Costs of Living at Home or in an Institution

The results of our 1988 survey of 2,136 persons 75 years of age or older in the French departments of Doubs and Loire-Atlantique did not confirm the hypothesis that the costs of living in an institution or at home cross at a certain degree of dependence. For the seven degrees of dependence utilized in the survey, it cost more to live at home than in an institution; and it made very little difference whether the retirement home had a medical unit or not. For the two most dependent groups, it cost as much to live at home as to undergo long-term hospitalization.

Average monthly help and health costs ranged from 1,500 to

2,000 francs for someone who was not very dependent. For the intensely dependent, this amount rose to 4,000 francs in a retirement home with a medical unit as compared with 7,000 francs at home or under long-term hospitalization. These results, which do not include housing or food costs, undermine preconceived ideas, since the costs of living at home and of long-term hospitalization are the same. The costs in nonmedical retirement homes are less, partly because the ratio of personnel to residents is lower when there is no medical unit. These results mean that the type of residence is not skewed due to global costs.

Unfortunately, this does not mean that the elderly freely choose where to live. On the one hand, the elderly, as well as their families, have an interest in keeping older individuals at home, unless their income is so low that they receive assistance from local authorities. On the other hand, Social Security has an interest in placing eldery in institutions. Given these differing financial interests, old-age policy has not been very coherent, since less is spent on housing and food at home. In effect, the fixed amounts paid by Social Security work like a cash-limit system.

Why did the common-sense hypothesis turn out false? The explanation has to do with both the economies of scale in institutions and the conditions under which the elderly who live at home are helped. Although there seems to be no reason for doubting that institutions achieve economies of scale, those made on care are probably offset by capital and overhead costs, at least in larger establishments.

What is, therefore, the optimal size for such institutions? Although this has not been thoroughly studied, the answer would seem to be less than 60 beds. Experiments are being conducted with 20 to 30 beds.

REGULATING OLD-AGE POLICY

Old-age policy developed without any regulatory mechanism. Cost containment measures have been a rather primitive means of regulation. In this respect, two factors–the growing awareness of the problem of dependence and the administrative decentralization

carried out since 1986–have raised two issues: departmental gerontological plans and the financing of the "dependence risk."

Departmental Gerontological Plans

A 1982 circular made it obligatory for local authorities in
France's departments to draw up a gerontological plan which would
help adjust supply to demand in the area. The 1986 Decentralization
Act reinforced this requirement and called for such planning for
other groups, in particular children and the handicapped. By 1990,
less than half of the departments had drawn up plans, but a few were
already working on their third.

Decentralization has led to differences in health and social services. Although the central government still controls the health
system, it has transferred to local authorities (the departments) the
responsibility for correcting the distortions wrought by the shortcomings of its interventions and the absence of regulations.

In a context of economic stagnation, criticism has been directed
at governmental involvement in the social and economic spheres;
and the Welfare State has come under question. The private sector
has adopted an offensive strategy of opening expensive old-age
establishments, often without medical facilities. This strategy is
aimed at a limited market, since monthly accommodations there
cost about 12,000 francs–more than double the average old-age
pension. Furthermore, the lack of medical facilities means that Social Security's Health Fund has to pay an uncontrollable bill.

One issue in departmental planning is whether or not to license
establishments of this sort, which are often backed by powerful
financial interests tied to the construction industry. When this decision has to be made, an important factor, apart from technical considerations (the analysis of needs, waiting lists, etc.), is locally
elected officials' political attitudes. The medical and administrative
personnel who give advice and are responsible for developing the
gerontological plans have difficulty with this component.

A second issue in these departmental gerontological plans is
whether or not to help the elderly remain at home. Although home
care has been declared a priority, it has been pursued randomly.
Several appeals for a coordinated policy have gone unheeded; and
finances as well as interventions are still fragmented. As a conse-

quence, the number of hours per month for a Home Helper's services to a very dependent person varies from 90 to 30, from three hours a day to one–obviously too little.

Why do these differences occur? It depends on the energy, tenacity and patience of the directors of Home Help services, on their bargaining abilities, since the local boards of the Old-Age Fund can decide whether to spread out help to as many people as possible, or distribute it according to the degree of dependence. Usually these boards prefer the former, rather than targeting precise groups. As a result, there are major differences from one area to another. No account is taken of whether the person can, or does, benefit from other sources of help. Frossard, Bernard, and Jordain (1988), as well as others, have shown that families are often the most important source of assistance.

A third issue raised in these plans is who should pay and how to share costs among the elderly, their families, local authorities, and Social Security–actors with varying interests. Caring for the dependent is costly; and part of the charges tends to be transferred to the beneficiaries even though they obviously cannot bear them. In each department, political forces have lined up differently around this issue. In addition, there is a variety of formulas for sharing costs between Social Security's Health Fund and local authorities.

Because of politics and conflicts of interests, only a moderate number of departmental gerontological plans has been adopted. There are, however, other important reasons for this. For one thing, there is no model methodology. For another, training in the methodology of planning is inadequate, and assistance in decision making is insufficient. The professionals involved in old-age policy have received an education in public administration. They usually have not been taught how to develop strategies and make prospective studies or economic analyses. They also have not learned organization theory, or the role that politics plays in policy making. Such topics have only recently been introduced into the curriculum at the National School of Public Health, which has a monopoly over their training. Decentralization measures have transferred the training of personnel for local administrations to the National Center of Local Government Employment, which has neither the skills nor the means to handle this responsibility.

Paying for Dependence

Awareness has grown about the costs of dependence. Although several sources help cover these expenses, such budgetary fragmentation has negative effects. Recent ministers have supported the ideas of establishing a unified system for financing dependence as well as for increasing individual purchasing power so that older people can pay for help themselves.

Critical questions confront French policymakers: Who should pay?; Should new services be paid for through income taxes, a "solidarity" payroll tax similar to Social Security, or under insurance plans taken out by individuals?; If the latter is adopted, should such plans be based on principles of redistribution, of capitalization, or, what seems more likely, should they rely on both? Despite the current strength of economic liberalism with its emphasis on personal responsibility, individual insurance plans, given the costs, obviously will not suffice alone.

Private insurance companies and the complementary retirement funds, the latter of which provide supplementary pension benefits to Social Security's Old-Age Fund, have taken the first step toward individual coverage (i.e., "dependence coverage" offered by AGIRC, a complementary fund for white collar workers–see Table 5). To cover the monthly costs of intense dependence (which, according to our calculations, range from 7,000 francs at home to 9,000 francs under long-term hospitalization), one would have to pay the most expensive premium, ranging from 102,400 to 409,600 francs, depending on the age at which the plan is taken out. Recall that the average retirement pension is between 5,000 and 6,000 francs. These figures paint the picture. Coverage under Social Security's Health Fund is also under study.

The question of how to finance costs thus remains: should it be paid for through income or Social Security taxes? and who should pay? should it be those individuals now working? retirees? persons near retirement? There are two factors that have led complementary retirement funds to offer such coverage for persons at the age of 50. First of all, the awareness of "dependence risk" arises only when the risk is looming–no one thinks about it at age 20. Secondly, a recent comparison of wages and pensions by the Center of Income

TABLE 5. Insurance coverage of the risk of dependence (under AGIRC's plan), in French francs.

AGE (at which policy is taken out)	MONTHLY PREMIUM			
50	40.40	80.80	121.20	161.60
60	59.40	118.80	178.20	237.60
65	70.60	141.20	211.80	282.40
75	102.40	204.80	307.20	409.60
MONTHLY BENEFITS	2,000	4,000	6,000	8,000

and Costs has shown that, for men, the average monthly wage is 9,233 francs, whereas a former wage-earner's average monthly pension is 8,481 francs. Given this small difference, it would not seem wise to force those still working to pay. These statistics shed light on another serious problem: the weak purchasing power of young wage-earners with children, who make up the majority of the population and whose payroll taxes go to Social Security.

A final question has to do with the sort of services to be provided to the frail elderly. Should benefits carry no restrictions? Should beneficiaries prove they have purchased certain services? Should payments be made to individuals or to a coordinating service (like the case management system in Kent, England)? At present, there seems to be a preference for payments to individuals, with no restrictions.

In France, attempts to regulate old-age policy and manage the dependence risk have led to the development of departmental gerontological plans and efforts to find a means of financing this risk. This has created a framework wherein actors adopt decentralized strategies adapted to local factors. These innovations create a local dynamics but with the risk of greater inequality. National and local authorities will have to see to it that information is made public so that all concerned can rectify these inequalities.

CONCLUSION

A policy for helping the aged remain at home seems better suited to the needs of this population. It provides services that can be adapted to the aging process, and it corresponds to what most old people want. In France, this policy emerged from an incoherent mixture of measures passed at various times. Unfortunately, it has been broken into actions and services that are essentially juxtaposed fragments. Home services and home care are on the increase; but the whole lacks coherence, thus undercutting the effectiveness of the programs. These various interventions have not helped the aged remain autonomous, but rather have made them dependent on the services and care provided. As a consequence, costs for health care and social services supplied under the home-maintenance policy have increased to a much greater extent than improvements in the well-being of beneficiaries.

Current reforms are intended to rectify this policy so as to serve the needs of the targeted population. By increasing coordination within Home Help services, as well as between such services and old-age institutions, these reforms seek to ensure a gradual transition from home to residential facilities, and eventually to institutional care, in line with the evolving needs of the elderly.

REFERENCES

Boulard, Jean-Claude. 1991. Vivre ensemble. A report on the frail elderly submitted to the National Assemble on June 20.

Colvez, Alain. 1990. Panorama de la dépendance en France. In the special issue "Personnes âgées. Le coût de la dépendance" of the *Revue Française des Affaires Sociales*, 2, pp. 15-21.

Frossard, Michel. 1990a. Maintien à domicile ou hébergement. Les coûts comparés. In *Revue française des Affaires sociales*, XLIV-1, pp.23-40.

Frossard, Michel. 1990b. Selon les lieux de vie. *Informations sociales*, 6/7, pp. 82-86.

Frossard, Michel; Bouget, Denis; Tartarin, Robert; and Tripier, Pierre, eds. 1990, *Le prix de la dépendance*. Paris: Documentation Française.

Frossard, Michel, and Ennuyer, Bernard. 1987. *Comparaison des coûts du maintien à domicile et l'hébergement collectif*. A report submitted to the Caisse Nationale d'Assurance Vieillesse at the Ecole Nationale de la Santé Publique in Rennes.

Frossard, Michel; Ennuyer, Bernard; and Jordain, Alain. 1988. Travail familial, solidarité de voisinage et maintien à domicile des personnes âgées. In *Cahiers de l'Ecole Nationale de la Santé Publique,* 3, pp. 1-130.

Guillemard, Anne-Marie. 1986. *Le déclin du social. Formation et crise des politiques de la vieillesse.* Paris: Presses Universitaires de France.

Institut National de la Statistique et des Etudes Economiques (INSEE) 1990. coll Démographic Données Sociales.

Massé, Pierre. 1977. L'adaptation des équipements des services sanitaires et sociaux aux besoins des personnes du troisième âge et du quatrième âge, étude prioritaire. *Revue RCB,* XXX, September.

Schopflin, Pierre. 1991. *Dépendance et solidarités. Mieux aider les personnes âgées.* Paris: Documentation Française.

Chapter 9

Care of the Frail Elderly in Germany

Marianne Heinemann-Knoch

SOCIO-DEMOGRAPHIC TRENDS

As in most countries of the industrialized hemisphere, the proportion of old people in Germany has been permanently increasing in the last decades, whereas the means to cope politically, socially, culturally, and economically with the consequences of this development is lagging far behind.[1]

In 1988, nearly 21 percent of the population in the Federal Republic of Germany (FRG) was 60 years and older, compared to slightly more than 18.0 percent of the population of the German Democratic Republic (GDR). The 80 and over population amounted to 3.7 percent in the FRG, and–in comparison–to 3.3 percent in the GDR (Table 1). The socio-demographic trends in the united countries are comparable,[2] although the population of the former GDR is slightly younger (KDA and ISG 1991).

The ratio of the elderly to the younger population is constantly increasing, from about 5 percent in 1880 to one-fifth currently; in the year 2030, one-third of the total population is expected to be 60 years and older. The number of the very old will probably increase even more than that of the "young old"; while the number of persons older than 70 years is expected to rise to 16.5 percent of the population in the year 2020, with 20 percent of them over the age of 80 (Tews 1990, 479).

The number of elderly who require aid is rising relatively and absolutely since chronic diseases are concentrated in old age. In

TABLE 1. Population in Germany by age and sex, 1988, in millions.

Total number of persons at given ages

	55+	60+	65+	70+	75+	80+	total population
FRG							
Male	6.5	4.8	3.2	2.1	1.4	.7	29.7
Female	9.9	8.2	6.3	4.4	3.2	1.7	32.0
Total	16.4	12.9	9.5	6.4	4.6	2.3	61.7
GDR							
Male	1.5	1.0	.7	.4	.3	.2	7.9
Female	2.4	2.0	1.5	1.0	.8	.4	8.6
Total	3.9	3.0	2.2	1.5	1.1	.5	16.4
FRG and GDR							
Male	8.0	5.8	3.9	2.5	1.7	.8	37.6
Female	12.4	10.1	7.8	5.4	3.9	2.0	40.6
Total	20.4	15.9	11.7	7.9	5.6	2.9	78.2

Source: KDA 1991a, p. 18

1989, in the Federal Republic there were 926,000 private house-holds with at least one person who needed help from others. Seventy-five percent of the elderly needed help with daily activities, and 10 percent were bedridden (Presse-und Informationsamt 1990). Most of these people were 60 years of age and more, with the highest percentage being 85 years and older: just 3 percent of the group aged 70 and over and 5 percent of those aged 75 and over needed continuous help. Thirty percent of the elderly between 80 and 90 years of age, and more than 40 percent of the elderly over the age of 90, needed help and care (Neseker and Jung 1988).

In 1980, people of 65 and more years were ill about three times as much as the group of youngsters under the age of fifteen. Until the year 2000 this ratio is expected to increase to four times, and thereafter until 2030 to eight times as much (Dissenbacher 1987). The number of impaired elderly who will need care given by relatives, in-home services, and institutional care, such as nursing homes, will probably rise proportionally.

Some of the most urgent problems are related to the increase of psychic disorders, especially dementia, in later life. An estimated 25 percent of the 65 and over population suffers from psychic diseases, including dementia (Grond 1984; Häfner 1986; Häfner and Weyerer 1986; Cooper and Bickel 1989; Häfner 1990). In 1991, there were between 790,000 and 1.1 million elderly with dementia in the "old states"[3] of the FRG; more than 500,000 of these suffered from Alzheimer's disease.

Again, dementia is a problem of advanced age since only 5 percent of the 65- to 69-year-old population, but more than 30 percent of those above the age of 90 years, suffers from it (Clade 1991). Hence, dementia has developed as one of the most critical problems of old age. It requires special efforts and enormous engagement of caregivers since they are not only confronted with impairment of their elderly kin but also with behavioral problems and changes in character (Heinemann-Knoch, Kardorff, and Klein-Lange 1991).

Moreover, old age is increasingly female due to the fact that life expectancy of women is higher than that of men. In 1989 the average female life expectancy in the Federal Republic was 79.2 years and that of males was 72.7 years; in the German Democratic Republic the figures were 76.3 and 70.2 years, respectively (KDA and ISG 1991).

In addition, single households have been rising steadily, with females overrepresented among them. Whereas most men aged 60 to 75 years are still married, one-third of the women between 60 and 70 years, and two-thirds of the women between 70 and 75 years are widows (Bojanovski 1986). In 1988, 60 percent of the 6.6 million households of the 65 and over population consisted of single people–the majority of them (namely 86 percent or 3.2 million) was women (Statistisches Bundesamt 1988).

Although the older generations have never been as well off as presently, poverty still exists. Because of lower wages for females in the labor force and because of their fewer working years, women's income in old age is lower than that of men: old age poverty is female poverty.[4] For example, 78 percent of those impaired elderly who received social assistance in 1987 were women (Behrmann 1990; Beyer, Dill, and Heinemann-Knoch 1990).

Quite a high percentage of elderly in the FRG lives in owner-occupied homes. In 1978, 36 percent of elderly households lived in such housing (BMJFFG 1986; Steinack 1987; KDA and ISG 1991). On the other hand, the percentage of old people living in substandard housing is fairly high.[5] Some communities offer special counselling and financial support for the elderly in order to renew substandard housing or to reconstruct their dwellings to meet the special needs of old age and impairment. A high proportion of elderly also receives a housing allowance (*Wohngeld*) since there is a shortage of low cost housing in Germany.

Poor older women, in particular, tend to live in substandard circumstances (Steinack 1987). Sheltered housing with domiciliary services in the vicinity is lacking for this sector of society. In fact, their housing needs are neglected in general in Germany.

FAMILY CARE

Until very recently, about 80 to 90 percent of the frail, chronically ill and impaired German elderly has been dependent on family care, primarily by daughters and spouses (Thiede 1988). Whereas most of the frail and functionally impaired old men get help from their spouses, most of the women are single, and therefore dependent on help given by their children or others (Thiede 1988). Even the elderly who live in single-person households tend to rely on the help of their relatives if they live in the vicinity. When there is a significant distance between the households of caregivers and dependents, the potential for family caregiving falls to about 30 percent.

Many of the caregivers provide support until they are emotionally and physically exhausted. Above all, their work remains unpaid and is not covered by social security (Bracker, Dallinger, and Middeke 1987; Grunow 1982; Thiede 1988). About 50 percent of the caregivers themselves are beyond their midlife (Thiede 1988). Moreover, their caregiving often negatively effects their health, financial status, and housing situation (Beyer, Dill, and Heinemann-Knoch 1990).

Changes in generative behavior, the rising percentage of divorces, more single households, greater quantity and quality of female employment, job mobility, women's emancipation and striving for self-fulfillment and self-esteem, and the breakdown of the extended family all have already diminished the potential for family care. These will have even greater effects on caregiving in the future as well as increase the demand for better quality formal services (BMJFFG 1986; Bracker, Dallinger, and Middeke 1987).

The number of potential caregivers in society (i.e., the population between the ages of 15 and 65 years) also has decreased continuously with the falling of the birth rate. This is true both for family and professional caregivers (Lehr 1984).

It is possible that the changing life styles of the "young olds" will have an impact on caregiving, as well, since that age group may be less willing to care for the "old olds" in the future; they are increasingly more healthy, vital, educated, and financially secure than previous generations. Moreover, the current "young olds" will spend a longer period as pensioners than any previous generation. Most of these older people want to be active during retirement and seek new social networks rather than enter into family or other obligations that would tie them down (Karl and Tokarski 1989; Tews 1989).

It should be noted that there was a remarkable difference in family care between the FRG and the GDR; in the latter, females who cared for their relatives were covered by a pension. In addition, many women were employed by *Volkssolidarität*, the caregiver organization for domestic help and mobil meals. These and other disparities in long-term care have had to be reconciled, although many problems remain unresolved.

AMBULATORY CARE

Until the early 1970s, long-term care for the elderly belonged to the duties of the family. Institutional care, mostly provided in substandard facilities, was available for a small percentage of old people who tended to be poor and without any informal source of help. To an even lesser degree, a third possibility of getting help was in-home care, delivered by parish nurses (*Gemeindeschwestern*) of the Protestant and Catholic Churches. Formal long-term care was a branch of the voluntary welfare sector, organized mainly by the church communities and welfare organizations (Dahme and Hegner 1982).

The autonomous organization of long-term care by the voluntary welfare sector has not changed over the years, although the parish nurse has largely disappeared (Hüssler 1982). In the early 1970s, the voluntary sector was responsible for reorganizing long-term service delivery while political authorities (the German federal states) set the framework for institutionalized conditions. Heiner Geißler, then social minister of Rhineland-Palatinate, and later Secretary General of the Christian Democratic Party, was one of the first to point out the necessity of reorganizing long-term care. Future socio-demographic projections, as well as incipient threats to health care insurance funding, were among the primary reasons for reform. Since that time, in-home care has been viewed as more humane and less expensive than institutional care (Heinemann-Knoch, de Rijke, and Schachtner 1985).

The reorganization of the 1970s aimed at providing more effective and professional domiciliary services. "Catchment areas" were defined, which meant that one organizational unit (*Sozialstation*, or social service station), administered by a social welfare organization, delivered in-home services both to old or sick people and families with small children (whose mother was hospitalized). In general, these agencies consist of office rooms with telephones. Here, administrative work is done, clients call in, some medical equipment such as beds, crutches, and wheelchairs is borrowed, and the otherwise mobile staff of nurses, caregivers for old people (*AltenpflegerInnen*), Home Helpers, social workers, semi-skilled helpers, volunteers, and those who refuse military service (*Zivildienst-*

leistende) hold their staff meetings. The available services include: family welfare; nursing, care, and treatment of old and ill persons; Home Help; meals-on-wheels; neighborhood activities; and several other social services. There is no standardized catalog of services or personnel requirements; however, service stations are subsidized by state and local community funds only when they offer a minimum of defined services and employ a minimum number of trained staff (Heinemann-Knoch, de Rijke, and Schachtner 1985;, Steinack 1987).[6]

The funding of in-home services is an admixture of state and local subsidies, health insurance payments, social assistance, client fees, and agencies that run the service stations and balance the deficits. Both funding levels and deficits differ considerably among the social service units (Wohlleber, Frank-Winter, and Kellmayer 1991).

Most of the clients (about three-fourths) are old and impaired or chronically ill. The clients themselves have to apply for help; in order to be eligible for any refunds from the health insurance system they must have physician authorization, as well. In addition, clients must bargain with the leader of the unit as to the amount and time of service provision (Heinemann-Knoch, de Rijke, and Schachtner 1985).

A network of social service stations currently exists throughout the old federal states of the FRG, and since politicians as well as social welfare authorities and consumers all seem to agree, they have precedence in the chain of care. The structure of social service stations has been exported to the five new states of the FRG, where they replaced the ambulatory facilities of the former GDR. In the latter structures, community nurses and physicians had worked together to secure home care and treatment.[7]

In recent years, there has been a slight decline in the ratios of family help to formal aid: domiciliary services appear to be replacing family care to a limited extent (Presse- und Informationsamt 1990). Care by in-home services has been increasing since about 1985; in 1990 there were about 4000 social service stations (*Sozialstationen*) in the FRG, plus about 400 in the new states of the FRG (KDA and ISG 1991). In Northrhine-Westfalia (NRW), the number of these stations increased steadily from 382 to 424 during 1983 to 1984, and reached a total of 477 by the end of 1987 (MAGS 1989). However, the growth of domiciliary care has now come to an end in the old parts of the FRG.

Importantly, not all of those who need domiciliary care get help from these services: in 1989, about 30 percent of the frail and impaired who required such care received it (Presse–und Informationsamt 1990). This figure, however, overestimates the aid provided specifically to older people: the available data for 1987 indicate that about 2 to 6 percent of those elderly living at home and needing care received professional domestic help (MAGS 1989). This raises the question of whether older people receive sufficient formal support. In particular, the most needy families still do not seem to request or receive the domiciliary help they need (Rückert 1990; Steinack 1987, 88).

In addition, although the net of care is spread all over the country, it is too wide-meshed and has systematic holes (Heinemann-Knoch, de Rijke, and Schachtner 1985). For example, while medical care for somatic illness is adequate, there is a lack of supportive services for homemaking, social stimulation, rehabilitation, gerontopsychiatric problems and dementia, day care, and short-term care.

Domiciliary services also tend to be fragmented. The mobile social services mainly work together with unskilled staff, voluntary helpers (*Ehrentamtlichen*), and those who refuse military service (*Zivildienstleistenden*). Culturally oriented services (*Altenclubs* and *Altentagesstätten*) are mainly operated by voluntary helpers. Moreover, social service stations, meals-on-wheels, mobile social services and domiciliary psychiatric services (*Sozialpsychiatrische Dienste*) are only beginning to work cooperatively.

Other urgent issues relate to staffing (Deutscher Verein 1987; MAGS 1989; LDS 1988; MAGS 1991; and Heinemann-Knoch 1989). Most personnel working in domiciliary services are highly oriented toward somatic medical care. In fact, about one-third of its staff has been trained as nurses. Approximately another 40 percent is semi-skilled. While the professional staff works full-time and gives treatments (*Behandlungspflege*), the semi-skilled staff mainly works part-time and provides personal care (*Grundpflege*) and other services.

In addition, the standards of care are oriented to professional rather than consumer needs. Not only should there be more planning of care, but it also should include input from clients and their families.

The growing shortage of personnel, low wages for professionals, and burn-out effects have to be confronted, as well. Measures aimed at better recruitment and improved training are urgently needed. Although there have been initiatives to raise pay rates, efforts to standardize professional training for the nonmedical staff have been delayed. Yet, there is a lack of professional training by the state, and welfare organizations are unwilling to support the costs of on-the-job training (Heinmann-Knoch and Kardorff 1989).

Ambulatory care in the new countries of the FRG, the former GDR, has developed in diametrically different directions, as this author discovered in Chemnitz. It should be noted that it is difficult to compare the conditions of domiciliary help in the FRG and GDR, especially because of large differences in statistical material, quality of service delivery, and standards of housing (KDA and ISG 1991). In the GDR, domestic help and cultural work with the elderly (by employees of the *Volkssolidarität*) developed to a higher quantitative level than in the FRG. Thus, in Chemnitz there was one domestic help for every 97 pensioners (September 1990) in comparison to one caregiver of a domiciliary service for every 200 persons above the age of 60 years in NRW (1987) (MAGS 1989 and Heinemann-Knoch 1989). On the other hand, there is much less medical in-home care for the elderly by community nurses in the GDR. For example, in Chemnitz there was one community nurse for every 1,342 pensioners (Heinemann-Knoch 1989).[8]

INSTITUTIONAL CARE

It was not until 1961 that care for the elderly became a sociopolitical target. As we pointed out earlier, the previous decades had been characterized by institutionalization of the ill and poor elderly who could not rely on family help. Institutional care was provided by voluntary welfare organizations in poor quality nursing homes. Aid for the elderly was just a "muddling through."

With the passage of the Social Welfare Act of 1961, the issue of the aged emerged as a focus for social concern. At that time, communities and political leaders of the federal states started to plan for the elderly and to fund more institutional facilities. While the newly constructed nursing homes of the 1960s merely fulfilled quantitative goals, new funding guidelines since 1970 have been aimed at improving conditions. For example, they require single-bed apartments in residential homes, and double-bed rooms in nursing homes (Brandt, Dennebaum, and Rückert 1987).

Both investment and administrative costs of residential homes and nursing homes are funded by the provider, normally a welfare organization; local and state authorities, along with voluntary agencies, provide subsidies under certain conditions. Residents pay for the remaining costs, which are decided upon through bargaining among statutory funders (Pflegesatzverhandlungen) (Rückert 1990; Wohlleber, Frank-Winter, and Kellmayer 1991).

Health insurance covers only the cost of medical treatment and necessary hospitalization for nursing home residents; ordinary living expenses and supportive services are excluded (Rückert 1990). These latter costs tend to be higher than the pensions received by the vast majority of residents. In fact, the ratio of those economically dependent on relatives or social assistance has risen continuously over the last three decades, currently reaching two-thirds of all nursing home inhabitants. Such financial dependency, along with the character of these facilities–which tend to be custodial, "total institutions" (as Goffman has analyzed)–compels frail and impaired older people to remain at home as long as possible (IGF 1991; Brandt, Dennebaum, and Rückert 1987; Knobling 1983; Goffman 1972).[9]

Consequently, the average age of new residents has reached more than 80 years. Most of them come directly from the hospital where they have been discharged as no longer treatable. Because of cuts in health insurance payments, hospitals are obliged to dismiss their patients as early as possible (Rückert 1990). Between 1983 and 1989, the average stay of patients over 65 years of age was cut from 21.2 to 16.9 days (Völlink 1992; KDA and ISG 1991). The staff of nursing and residential homes (as well as of domiciliary services) point out that residents who are released from hospitals enter their facilities with more serious health conditions than in the past. Many of them are highly disabled.[10]

Between 1960 and 1990, the percentage of people aged 65 and over living in homes for the aged rose from about 4.6 percent to 5.5 percent[11] (Rückert 1990); this ratio rises to about 15 percent of the elderly between 85 and 90 years and to more than 20 percent of those aged 90 and over (KDA 1988, 25). Nearly 18 percent of the elderly aged 65 and over in Germany die in an institution (Rückert

1987; Bickel and Jaeger 1986). Although most of the residents are women, the primary reason for institutionalization is their single status rather than their gender (Rückert 1990).

The available statistics show evidence that there has been a shift from the nursing home to the family care system, with the exception of those who are single females older than 85 years. One reason for this, according to Rückert, is that the elderly population has grown faster than available institutional facilities. He writes:

> Though in Bavaria during the 1974 to 1986 period, the number of places in homes for the aged has risen from 63,000 to 82,000, they would have had to build an additional 7,700 places in order to keep up the 1974 level. (Rückert 1990, 9)

In 1990, there were about 6,600 residential and nursing homes in the FRG with slightly more than 500,000 places; 300,000 of the latter were in nursing homes (Rückert 1990).[12] The evidence suggests that the need for institutional places will rise in the coming decades.

Semi-institutional or short-term care in Germany recently emerged as an alternative to full-time institutionalization. Since 1990, funding for such services by health insurance has been regulated by The Health Reform Act. However, this type of aid is considered too expensive to be publicly supported on a regular basis (Heinemann-Knoch 1989; Claussen 1990). Nevertheless, there is a rising tendency to provide short-term care.

Both short-term care and day care must be paid for, in most cases, by the consumers themselves, unless they are eligible for social assistance. Day care tends to be financially unattractive both to consumers and suppliers. In 1990, there were only 70 day-care centers with 1,000 places in Germany (Rückert 1990).

THE POLITICAL, ECONOMIC, AND SOCIAL CONTEXT

Private, Voluntary, and Statutory Sources of Care

One of the outstanding German welfare principles is the subsidiary principle: individuals and the family system have to solve their own problems; if they fail, the public sector is obliged to provide aid. Consequently, an admixture of private, voluntary and statutory sources of help has been established: family; social security; welfare and church organizations (voluntary welfare); and communal and state authorities (public welfare).

Social security is based on the solidarity of the labor force which pays for the triple insurance system against the risk of becoming ill (health insurance), unemployed (unemployment insurance), and retired (old-age insurance). Health insurance covers only medical treatment and prescriptions by physicians as well as hospitalization; it excludes the risks associated with impairment and dependency in old age. Caregiving is viewed as within the private rather than the public domain. Therefore, the frail elderly are forced to pay for their own care, or depend on privately organized help from families and voluntary welfare organizations (Asam and Heck 1985; Heinemann-Knoch, de Rijke, and Schachtner 1985; Holz 1990; Steinack 1987).

In-home care and household help through domiciliary services are financed by the health insurance system only up to four weeks, and only if they are necessary to prevent hospitalization or involve medical treatment by a physician. Otherwise, these services–as well as institutional care in nursing homes–are paid by the consumers or, if they are economically needy, by social assistance.

For those highly disabled elderly whose family caregivers need a temporary rest from their obligations, the Health Reform Act of 1989 (*Gesundheitsstrukturreform*) mandates coverage of short-term care for up to four weeks. However, the fixed annual limit of 1,800 DM for this service generally is not adequate to pay for the maximum allotted time (Claussen 1990). Day care, another potential aid to family caregivers, is not funded by health insurance at all.

The purpose of the Health Reform Act is to bring relief to highly disabled persons (*Schwerpflegebedürftige*) who need intensive care and help with activities of daily living. Beginning in 1991, such individuals can claim either 25 hours of care and domestic help per month, which is paid for by health insurance up to 750 DM or 400 DM in cash. However, this benefit has not substantially aided highly disabled persons who are dependent on social assistance; many communities (the local bodies of social assistance) have reduced the amount of social assistance commensurate with any gains from health insurance. Overall, long-term care is still within the private domain of the family.

Roots of Caring: Christian Charity and Female Role Ascription

The historical and cultural roots of caring for the aged have fostered, in part, some of the exclusion of care from medical treatment. Caring and politics for the aged have developed as part of christian charity and welfare for those poor and ill people who could not afford to take care of themselves nor had any kin to aid them. Over the centuries, caring also was viewed as the "natural" task of women. Moreover, as an integral role of the female in the family, it was assumed that such efforts did not require training. The concepts of christian charity and female role ascription contributed to the rise of the denominational nurse as well.

Along with the professionalization of familial tasks, secularization of christian charity, and demographic changes, care for the aged and the assessment of their needs were legalized for the first time in Germany in 1961 with the passage of the Federal Social Welfare Act (*Bundessozialhilfegesetz*). At the same time, courses were instituted for care of the elderly, aimed at housewives whose children had grown up. Since then, the profession of caregiving for the elderly (*Altenpflegerin*) has been developing, although there is still no formalized state job training requirements (Lohmann 1984; Voges and Koneberg 1984; Balluseck 1980; Ostner and Beck-Gernsheim 1979; Garms-Homolova 1977).[13]

THE GERMAN HEALTH CARE SYSTEM AND LONG-TERM CARE FOR THE ELDERLY

The basis for the present German health care system was laid in 1883, when the German parliament (*Reichstag*) passed the first Act of health care for workers (*Gesetz betreffend die Krankenversicherung der Arbeiter*). This act was followed in 1884 by legislation for social security against the risks of accident at work, and in 1889 against worker disability and retirement. Such social security legislation was enacted to appease and control the working class and its representatives, the labor unions and the Social Democrats (*Sozialistengesetze*, whose party had been forbidden in 1878) (Holz 1990; Ploetz 1956).

The principles of health care have not changed fundamentally since that time, despite several reform acts (Holz 1990; Steinack 1987; Heinemann-Knoch, de Rijke, and Schachtner 1985). German health care is an insurance system with a primary purpose to finance medical treatment for the labor class so as to enhance worker employability. It is a solidarity-based, statutory system which is funded by workers and their employers. Health insurance pays for medical prescriptions as well as treatment of and hospitalization for curable illnesses. Although since 1956 there also has been statutory health care for pensioners, the group of secured risks is still confined to potentially treatable illnesses. Thus, health insurance tends to exclude the special health needs of old age (Holz 1990) by restrictively interpreting its financial obligations toward the elderly.

Geriatric knowledge and special treatment of the elderly in Germany is seriously deficient and rehabilitation is seldom provided (in contrast to rehabilitation of the employed members of the society). All of these factors contribute to increases in the need for long-term care.

Long-term care was–and with some exceptions still is–explicitly excluded from health care insurance. Those people who need long-term care, whether at home or in an institution, have to rely on informal and unpaid family help or in many cases have to pay for formally delivered services themselves. Only those who live below the legally defined minimum income level are eligible for social welfare and social assistance for long-term care.

In the last decades there also has been a shift from the hospital sector to the nonhospital sector in caring for elderly people in the FRG. In the past, "social indicators" were utilized when deciding whether or not to hospitalize an older person. This was done to prevent the breakdown of family help or to compensate for lack of it. However, legislation and the health insurance system forced the hospitals to disregard social indicators and to dismiss elderly patients as early as possible. On the other hand, until the unification, impaired older people in the GDR could stay in the hospital as long as there was no appropriate alternative. (Rückert 1990; KDA and ISG 1991).

SEPARATION OF TREATMENT AND CARE

Due to the types of problems experienced by frail older people, both medical intervention and supportive services should be integrated.

Caring cannot be confined to the medical aspects of treatment. It must be humane and comprehensive (*ganzheitlich*), and as such include the social context within which the elderly person lives. This is particularly important for those with mental conditions such as dementia.

Effective caring also implies geriatric knowledge, including the study of special groups of chronic diseases and impairment which are both severe and progressively debilitating. Heart conditions and circular disturbances, rheumatism, pneumonal diseases, neurological and urological conditions tend to worsen and, because of their severity and disabling potential, are among those chronic diseases which demand a considerable amount of care (Schlierf 1988). These illnesses require specific types of services in order to meet the needs of the frail elderly and their caretakers.

The separation of care and treatment in the German health system (Holz 1990) has had serious consequences, including the belief that impairment is not treatable in old age. Although the restructuring of health insurance in 1988 (Health Reform Act) provided for some geriatric rehabilitation, there have been only limited efforts to carry this out. Few frail or impaired older people receive such rehabilitation services. There also is a lack of standards for rehabilitation of the elderly. Consequently, the impaired elderly are more dependent on help as well as more often bedridden than their physical condition would warrant.

Economically and socially, most old people suffer when they retire; old age too often is labelled as a period of incompetence and impairment. Indeed, the 30-year-old discussion over whether to establish an insurance program against the risk of getting old and impaired reflects the poor social and political status of care for the elderly and the ineffectiveness of political lobbying on their behalf.

Three positions have been taken in this issue: the first aims at instituting a solidarity-financed insurance system. This model is preferred by Social Democrats and the labor force oriented wing of the Christian Democrats and their representative in the Federal Government, and the Minister for Labor and Social Affairs. The second stance (which is no longer discussed) favors a model financed by general taxes. The third position is based on funding by private insurance (this model presently is preferred by the Liberal

Democratic Party and by the employer-oriented wing of the Christian Democrats).

CONCLUSION

This chapter suggests that families in Germany have been forced to take on increasing burdens of care. These caregivers, most of them women, are not paid,[14] nor is their social insurance for old age covered. This means that they risk their economic stability and diminish their own income in old age. Although formal, community-based services are growing, they are unable to meet the needs of the increasing number of elderly, especially those who are poor.

At the same time, institutional care is overburdened and characterized by long waiting lists, unskilled and poorly paid staff, rising age levels of residents, an increase of highly impaired old people, limited planning for care, and lack of rehabilitation (Brandt, Dennebaum, and Rückert 1987; Heinemann-Knoch and Kardorff 1989). Institutional care statistics in the new countries of the FRG are comparable, although the quality of care and especially housing standards are lower (KDA and ISG 1991).

Moreover, the costs of the German health care system are permanently rising. This holds for the medical care system as well as for the institutional care system and in-home care, although these three systems are funded differently and the costs are differently structured.[15]

The cost explosion may be illustrated by the rising proportions of the total social budget allocated to health insurance: from 1970 until 1983, state expenditures for health insurance grew by 500 percent; while in 1963 less than 20 percent of these outlays were for the health insurance of pensioners, this rose to about 27 percent in 1973 and to nearly 30 percent by 1984 (Diessenbacher 1987; Heinemann-Knoch and Kardorff 1989).

Despite rising expenditures for the health and care system and the growing rates of health expenses for the elderly—which are not only due to the growth of the elderly—the quality of geriatric treatment, care, and rehabilitation remains inadequate. There continues to be wide gaps between the costs of the health care system and the quality of geriatric treatment and rehabilitation (Bundesarbeitsgemeinschaft für Rehabilitation 1984; Holz 1990). In addition, gerontological knowledge and training of professionals continues to be extremely limited. The German Health system does not even have geriatric nurses or medical specialists in geriatrics.

Further, the risk of becoming frail and impaired in old age is not covered by the social security system in Germany. Consequently, most of the costs of care have to be paid privately, unless social assistance covers those costs for the needy. Since in-home care–and even more so, institutional care in nursing homes–is very expensive and surmounts the average income of pensioners, older people who are in need of care often become dependent on social assistance.

An additional issue confronting Germany is the threat to the old age pension system. Because of the rise of older generations and the falling rate of the productive labor force, adequate future funding for the German pension system is in jeopardy. In reaction to this, the Rent Reform Act of 1989 increased the age of pension eligibility from 65 to 67 years beginning in the twenty-first century. However, two problems are unresolved: female poverty in old age, which has become a critical issue with the unification of the two German states; and the inability of a large percentage of frail and impaired elderly to pay for care services.

The risk of becoming frail and impaired has been dramatically postponed to advanced years during the last century. The elderly are, overall, more competent, healthier, and live longer than ever before. Yet, chronic illness and impairment in high age call for action, especially since demographic and structural changes indicate a rising gap between those who need care and those who can provide it.

The current system of long-term care in Germany not only has structural holes but it also appears increasingly unstable; the German unification will probably intensify these tendencies. Clearly, creative public and private alternatives are lacking for meeting the requirements, expectations, and hopes of growing numbers of frail older people.

EXPLANATORY NOTES

1. The availability of nationwide statistics in the FRG is quite poor. Among other reasons this is due to extensive legal protection of personal statistics; nationwide protest against census taking; and the splitting of responsibilities between medical and social care.

2. Since October 1990.

3. Since the unification of FRG and GDR in 1990, the united countries form the FRG. To mark the difference, the federal states of the former FRG are called "old states," while the territory of the former GDR has been restructured into five "new states."

4. "The average contributory pension in 1985 amounted to: wage earner's contributory pension: 1,240 DM for men and 454 DM for women; salary earner's contributory pension: 1,710 DM for men, 810 DM for women; the average amount for a widow's pension in the care of a wage earner's contributory pension was 699 DM, in the case of a salary earner's contribution pension 982 DM." (Steinack 1987, 55).

5. For example, during 1978 in the FRG nearly 50 percent of elderly households, as compared to only about 40 percent of all households, lived in buildings built before 1948. At that time about 6.2 percent of elderly households lived in dwellings that did not have toilet facilities within them. The problem of substandard housing of the elderly is very severe in the five new states: in 1990, 25 percent of elderly households did not have toilet facilities inside their dwellings. Additionally, more than 50 percent of elderly households did not have central heating (KDA and ISG 1991; Steinack 1987).

6. The standards for funding by state and local communities differ between the federal states and local communities.

7. A report issued by the German Gerontological Association in September 1990 indicated that the number of ambulatory facilities in the former GDR was more than 5,700, with about 6,700 community nurses.

8. In 1989, in the GDR 4 percent of pensioners received household help and 8 percent of them received meals either in their homes or in a meals service unit (Schwitzer 1990).

9. There exists, however, a slightly growing small minority of old, well-off people who move to a comfortable residential home where they may remain in case of impairment and chronic disease (IGF 1991).

10. One of our studies in the city of Munich showed that in 1988 between 50 to 80 percent of the newcomers in nursing homes had been dismissed directly from hospitals. Their average was 84 years old; about 30 percent was highly impaired (IGF 1991).

11. This percentage holds also for the former GDR, although the age structure and gender of the residents in the GDR were different; they consisted of younger residents, fewer residents of advanced age, and more males than in the former FRG (KDA and ISG 1991).

12. At the same time, there were only two hospices in Germany (Rückert 1990).

13. There have been several initiatives to bring about a federal law for the professional training of caregivers; although the last one failed in 1990, it may be renewed during the current session by both the Ministers of Health and of Families and Seniors (Mrs. Hasselfeldt and Mrs. Rönsch).

14. Since 1991, the health insurance system has been reformed so that caregivers–also family caregivers–can be paid for 25 hours of care per month up to a limit of 750 DM. If the family is poor, and lives on social welfare, there is the possibility of receiving some of the costs of caring refunded by social assistance.

15. The cost structure of the German health and care system and its financing methods are extremely complicated and will not be explained in this chapter.

REFERENCES

Asam, W., and Heck, M., eds. 1985. *Subsidiarität and Selbsthilfe*. München.

Balluseck, H. v. 1980. *Die Pflege alter Menschen*. Institutionen, Arbeitsfelder und Berufe. Berlin.

Behrmann, G. 1990. Armut im Alter. In *Lehrbuch der Psychologischen und Sozialen Alternswissenschaft*, edited by J. Howe. Vol. 2: 141-161. Heidelberg.

Beyer, J.; Dill, H.; and Heinemann-Knoch, M. 1990. Golden oldies? In *Psychologie Heute, Frauenleben heute*. Weinheim, Basel, 51-62.

Bickel, H., and Jaeger, J. 1986. Die Inanspruchnahme von Heimen im Alter. *Zeitschrift für Gerontologie*, 30-39.

Bojanovski, J. 1986. *Verwitwete-Ihre Gesundheitlichen und Sozialen Probleme*. Weinheim, München.

Bracker, M.; Dallinger, U.; and Middeke, M. 1987. Altweibersommer (Beiträge zu den späten Jahren der Frau).

Brandt, H.; Dennebaum, E.; and Rückert, W., eds. 1987. Stationäre Altenhilfe. Problemfelder–Rahmenbedingungen–Perspektiven. Freiburg.

Bundesarbeitsgemeinschaft für Rehabilitation e.V. 1984. *Die Rehabilitation Behinderter*. Köln.

Bundesminister für Jugend, Familie, Frauen und Gesundheit (BMJFFG), ed. 1986. Vierter Familienbericht: Die Situation der älteren Menschen in der Familie.

Clade, H. 1991. Gerontopsychiatrische Erkrankungen: Differenzierte, gestufte Versorgung notwendig. *Deutsches Ärzteblatt*, 88 (Heft 4), C116-C117.

Claussen, F. 1990. Kurzzeitpflege in Völklingen-Ludweiler. Abschlußbericht der wissenschaftlichen Begleitung (Arbeitsbericht des Instituts für Gerontologische Forschung). München.

Cooper, B., and Bickel, H. 1989. Prävalenz und Inzidenz von Demenzerkrankungen in der Altenbevölkerung. Ergebnisse einer populationsbezogenen Längsschnittstudie in Mannheim. *Nervenarzt*, 60, 472-482.

Dahme, H.-J. and Hegner, F. 1982. Wie autonom ist der autonome Sektor? *Zeitschrift für Soziologie*, 11.

Deutscher Verein für öffentl. und private Fürsorge, E. 1987. Bestandsaufnahme der ambulanten sozialpflegerischen Dienste (Kranken- und Altenpflege, Haus- und Familienpflege) im Bundesgebiet (bearbeitet von Höft-Dzemski). Stuttgart, Berlin, Köln, Mainz. (Schriftenreihe des BMJFFG, Bd. 195).

Diessenbacher, H. 1987. Recht auf Leben–Pflicht zum Sterben. Universitas, Heft 9, 905-912.

Garms-Homolova, V. *Situation und Tendenzens in der Altenpflegeavsbildung.* Berlin: Deutsches zentrum für Altersfragen.

Goffmann, E. 1972. *Asyle.* Frankfurt.

Grond, E. 1984. *Die Pflege verwirrter alter Menschen.* Freiburg.

Grunow, D. 1982. Hilfe zwischen den Generationen als Bezugspunkt der Sozialpolitik. In F.-X. Kaufmann, *Staatliche Sozialpolitik und Familie.* München, Wien, 213-242.

Häfner, H. 1986. Psychische Gesundheit im Alter. Stuttgart, New York.

Häfner, H. 1990. Epidemiology of Alzheimer's disease. In *Key Topics in Brain Research,* edited by K. Maurer, P. Riederer, and H. Beckmann. Heidelberg, New York, Tokyo, 23-39.

Häfner, H., and Weyerer, S. 1986. Psychische Gesundheit im Alter. *Wiener klinische Wochenschrift,* 98. Heft 19, Sonderdruck.

Heinemann-Knoch, M. 1989. Modelleinrichtungen der Kurzzeitpflege. Abschlußbericht des Instituts für Gerontologische Forschung. München.

Heinemann-Knoch, M., and v. Kardorff, E. 1989. Sozialpolitische Aspekte der Pflegebedürftigkeit. In *Wie sicher ist die soziale Sicherung?* edited by B. Riedmüller and M. Rodenstein. Frankfurt, 182-209.

Heinemann-Knoch, M.; v. Kardorff, E.; and Klein-Lange, M. 1991. Verwirrte alte Menschen, Empirische Studien zur Versorgungslage und zur alltäglichen Problembewältigung. Arbeitsbericht des Instituts für Gerontologische Forschung. München.

Heinemann-Knoch, M.; de Rijke, J.; and Schachtner, C. 1985. *Alltag im Alter: Über Hilfsbedürftigkeit und Sozialstationen.* Frankfurt, New York.

Holz, G. 1990. Die Alterslast–in Gewinn für andere? Bd. I und II. Berlin.

Hüssler, G. 1982. Grundfragen der Caritas. Schwerpunkte und Perspektiven in der Gegenwart. Caritas, 83, Heft 2.

Institut für Gerontologische Forschung (IGF). 1991. *Fachliche Standards in der Altenhilfe–Bestandsaufnahme und Empfehlungen zur Qualitätsverbesserung und Qualitätssicherung.* München.

Karl, F., and Tokarski, W., eds. 1989. Die "neuen" Alten. Beiträge der XVII. *Jahrestagung der Deutschen Gesellschaft für Gerontologie.* Kasseler Gerontologische Schriften 6. Kassel.

Knobling, C. 1983. *Konfliktsituationen im Altenheim.* Freiburg.

Kuratorium Deutsche Altershilfe (KDA) 1988. 25 Jahre Kuratorium Deutsche Altershilfe. Köln.

Kuratorium Deutsche Altershilfe (KDA). 1991. Im Gesamtgebiet der heutigen Bundesrepublik hatte am 31.12.1988 jeder zehnte Einwohner das siebzigste Lebensjahr überschritten. Presse- und Informationsdienst, (Heft 4), p. 18.

Kuratorium Deutsche Altershilfe (KDA), and Otto-Blume-Institut für Sozialforschung (ISG). 1991. Analyse der Situation älterer Menschen und der Altenhilfe in den fünf neuen Bundesländern. Ein Werkstattbericht. Köln.

Landesamt für Datenverarbeitung und Statistik NRW (LDS), ed. 1988. Statistik der ambulanten sozialen Diesnte am 31.12. 1987. Düsseldorf.

Lehr, U. 1984. *Perspektiven zukünftiger Altenarbeit.* Caritas, 256-262.

Lohmann, S. 1984. Altenhilfe. In *Gerontologie*, edited by Oswald, W. D.; Herrmann, W. M.; Kanowski, S.; Lehr, U., and Thomae, H. Stuttgart. 11-18.

Ministerium für Arbeit, Gesundheit und Soziales (MAGS), ed. 1989. Ältere Menschen in Nordrhein-Westfalen (Wissenschaftliches Gutachten von Bäcker, G. Dieck, M. Naegele, and G. Tews, H. P.). Düsseldorf.

Ministerium für Arbeit, Gesundheit und Soziales (MAGS), ed. 1991. Gesundheitsreport Nordrhein-Westfalen 1990. Düsseldorf.

Neseker, H., and Jung, C. 1988. Ist der Pflegenotstand beseitigt? Nachrichtendiesnt des Deutschen Vereins, 314-322.

Ostner, I., and Beck-Gernsheim, E. 1979. Mitmenschlichkeit als Beruf. Frankfurt.

Presse- und Informationsamt der Bundesregierung. 1990. Familiäre Pflegebereitschaft sinkt. Sozialpolitische Umschau, Nr. 386.

Ploetz, K. 1956. *Auszug aus der Geschichte*. Wiesbaden.

Rückert, W. 1987. Demographische Grundlagen zur Altenhilfeplanung. In *Stationäre Altenhilfe*, edited by H. Brandt, Dennebaum, E., and W. Rückert. Problemfelder–Rahmenbedingungen–Perspektiven, Freiburg, 59-98.

Rückert, W. 1990. Nursing homes and hospices in Germany (MS in preparation for publishing).

Schlierf, G. 1988. Die gesundheitliche Situation älterer Menschen. In StaatsministeriumBaden-Württemberg, Altern als Chance und Herausforderung (Kommissionsbericht im Auftrag der Landesregierung, 41-51). Stuttgart.

Schwitzer, K. 1990. Zur sozialen Lage von AltersrentnerInnen in der DDR vor der Währungs-, Wirtschafts- und Sozialunion. WSI- Mitteilungen, 43 (Heft 8), 492-498.

Statistisches Bundesamt. 1988. Statistisches Jahrbuch der Bundesrepublik Deutschland. Wiesbaden.

Steinack, R. 1987. The elderly in the Federal Republic of Germany: Basic data, life situations, requirements, provision of services. In Social Integration, Social Interaction, Material and Non-Material Resources, edited by M. Dieck and Steinack, R. Berlin, Dublin, 3-139.

Tews, H. P. 1989. Die "neuen" Alten–Ergebnis des Strukturwandels des Alters. In *Die "neuen" Alten*, edited by F. Karl and W. Tokarski. (Beiträge der XVII. Jahrestagung der Deutschen Gesellschaft für Gerontologie, 126-143). Kassel.

Tews, H. P. 1990. Neue und alte Aspekte des Strukturwandels des Alters. WSI-Mitteilungen, 43 (Heft 8), 478-491.

Thiede, R. 1988. Die besondere Lage der älteren Pflegebedürftigen. Sozialer Fortschritt, 37 (Heft 11), 250-255.

Voges, W., and Koneberg, L. 1984. Berufsbild Altenpfleger and Altenpflegerin. Augsburg.

Völlink, J. 1992. Patienten in Akutkranken häusern 1990. *Das Krankenhaus*, (Heft 2): 66-69.

Wohlleber, C.; Frank-Winter, A.; and Kellmayer, M. 1991. Leistungen und Kosten von Sozialstationen. Stuttgart.

Chapter 10

Japan's Welfare Vision: Dealing with a Rapidly Increasing Elderly Population

Harry Kaneharu Nishio

Galbraith's *Affluent Society* witnessed the beginning of postwar economic and technological growth and advancement in North America, western Europe, and Japan. The ramifications of this development included an extensive demographic restructuring which was accompanied by other changes such as a postwar decline in fertility rates, nuclearization of the family, and an extension of life expectancy. In this chapter, I shall attempt to elucidate the rapidly changing Japanese age structure with particular reference to the emergence of the need for providing social, medical, and health care for those aged 65 and older. With this objective in mind, I shall make a brief but broad explanation regarding past and current Japanese demographic trends. This analysis will reveal some of the special characteristics of the aging process which are unique to Japan.

THE CHANGING JAPANESE AGE STRUCTURE

Since the beginning of Japan's modernization in 1868, it has maintained a relatively young age structure, with an elderly population (65 and older) of less than 5 to 6 percent. Because of this, the need for old-age welfare support and assistance was limited. However, the percentage of young people began to decrease due to a change in Japan's fertility rate which declined rather rapidly; in 1990 there were only 1.57 children per married female. This trend, coupled with advancing life expectancy (in 1989 this was 75.54 years for males and 81.3 years for females) (MHW 1990c), has significantly affected Japan's age structure.

The United Nations states that to be classified as an "aged" society, a country must have a minimum of 7 percent of its population consisting of individuals aged 65 or older. The Japanese population reached this landmark in 1970 when Japan joined the group of industrialized nations considered to have "aging societies." But, as Table 1 shows, the percentage of elderly in Japan is expected to reach 14 percent as early as 1995, attaining this level in just 25 years.

The U.S. attained the 7 percent level in 1945, but is not expected to reach the 14 percent level until 2015–70 years later. It took Sweden 85 years to reach the 14 percent level from 7 percent. It is predicted that France will take 130 years to reach the 14 percent level, with this probably occurring in 1995; it attained the 7 percent level as early as 1890. For any phenomenon, it is socially and economically easier to accommodate forces of change if these changes occur gradually over a long period of time. Conversely, it would be extremely pressing and stressful for any society to adjust to the rapid demographic transition of the type that Japan is now experiencing. Japan will have *the* oldest age structure on earth by 2020 if current predictions hold (Table 2). Not only will it have the oldest society in terms of people over the age of 65 years, but it will also have an alarming proportion of the society in the *very old* age group, aged 75 and older.

In October 1989, the proportion of those older than 75 years of age was 4.7 percent of Japan's total population; this is expected to increase to the 11.3 percent level by 2020, the latter figure also representing the 1989 percentage for Japanese people already aged 65 and older. Further, those aged 75 and older are expected to compose approximately one-half of the total elderly population (MHW 1991).

TABLE 1. International comparison of the speed of aging.

Country	Year in which given percentage of population is aged 65 and over		Number of years taken
	7 percent	14 percent	
Japan	1970	1995	25 years
U.S.A.	1945	2015	70
Britain	1930	1975	45
W. Germany	1930	1975	45
France	1865	1995	130
Sweden	1890	1975	85

Source: MHW, Population Research Center, *World Population Prospects,* Tokyo, Koseisho, 1988c.

If current trends can be relied upon for prediction, this proportional increase suggests that there will be an alarming rise in the number of bedridden or senile elderly who will require care and assistance. When we examine statistics for the elderly aged 65 to 74, and for those aged 75 and older, we find that the probability of the latter age group becoming bedridden or senile is far greater than for those in the former age category. In the period of 25 years from 1985 until 2010, the population of bedridden elderly potentially will rise from about 600,000 to 1.4 million. The number of senile elderly is expected to rise from 600,000 to 1.6 million. For the age group 64 to 74, 6.9 elderly persons per 1,000 are likely to become bedridden while the rate for those 75 and older is predicted to be 35.1 per 1,000 (General Affairs Bureau 1991, 26). There will certainly be a

TABLE 2. International comparison of 65 and over populations (1950-2020), in percentages.

Country	1950	1985	2000	2020
Japan	4.9%	10.3%	16.3%	23.8%
U.S.A.	8.1	11.9	12.8	17.3
England	10.7	15.1	15.4	18.7
W. Germany	9.4	14.7	16.8	22.3
France	11.4	13.0	15.3	19.1
Sweden	10.3	17.9	17.6	22.8

Source: MHW, Population Research Center, *World Population Prospects,* Tokyo, Koseisho, 1988c.

need for a much larger number of caregivers, as it is a well-known fact that the very elderly are far more vulnerable to debilitating illnesses due to the decline of their physiological strength. After becoming ill, they tend to lose the ability to care for themselves and eventually may become totally dependent upon others.

There is one additional demographic phenomenon which is likely to increase the difficulty of Japan's adjustment to the social process of aging; there is a severe regional variation in the distribution of the aged population. For example, rural areas such as Shimane (where the proportion of the aged population over 65 is 16.8 percent), Kochi (15.9 percent), Kagoshima (15.4 percent), Tottori (15.0 percent), and Nagano (14.9 percent) surpass the national average by 3 percent to as much as 5 percent. On the other hand, the highly industrialized regions such as Saitama (7.8 percent), Kanagawa (8.3 percent), Chiba (8.6 percent), Osaka (9.0 percent), and Aichi (9.1 percent) are below the national average by 2 to 3 percent. Unlike the already aged rural regions, these populated, industrial areas will grow old very rapidly until the national average reaches the predicted 22 to 23 percent by 2020 (MHW 1990c, 186-187). Consequently, the problems and adjustments of an aged population will be acutely concentrated in and around the industrial centers of Japan. Moreover, any solutions will need to be undertaken not only by the central government, but also by particular cities in which the elderly are concentrated, particularly during the first two decades of the twenty-first century.

What are the social implications of this increased number of very old, frail, and dependent people; particularly, what are the ramifications of the rapidity with which the aging process has occurred in Japan? We need to take special note of the dramatic rise which is expected to occur in the number of very elderly people in industrial areas who will become frail, bedridden, or senile within the next twenty to thirty years. If we consider together these various demographic indicators, we cannot help but realize the enormity of the social and economic pressures which will come to bear on Japan to resolve the problems of care and support of an aging, physically dependent population. Judging from the various predictions, Japan has no time to lose.

In the following section, I shall assess the existing traditional care institution in Japan which has, for many years, borne the main responsibility for looking after the elderly–the family. The question we must keep in mind is: Can the institution of the Japanese family continue to bear the major responsibility for caring for elderly individuals? If not, what are the other alternatives?

THE FAMILY AS A CARE-GIVING INSTITUTION

Japanese modernization and Japan's traditional familism, though seemingly incompatible (at least as seen from the Western vantage point), have maintained their dynamic harmony and cooperation for many years; indeed, the latter has been very instrumental in promoting and directing the former. Erdman Palmore's work, *Honorable Japanese Elders* (1975), stresses, perhaps somewhat strongly, that familism is a way of Japanese life. By comparison with the individualistic West, the Japanese family is far more integrative in relating the older generation to the young, a practice which evolved from the centuries-old Confucian concept of filial piety. According to this doctrine, the younger generation "owes" the older generation because since their birth, everything has been done for the children by the parents. The expected way of repayment is to give care and assistance to their aging parents under the same roof until their death. Ostensibly then, many, if not all, aged Japanese expect to be looked after by their own children, preferably by the family of the eldest son.

In Japan as well as elsewhere in East Asia, where Confucianism originated, the aging parents and the supporting adult (often married) children form the so-called three-generational living arrangement which functions, in many ways, to protect the aging generation emotionally, socially, and financially. "Dependency" is culturally and customarily condoned for the elderly even though, in actuality, dependency relationships are often delayed until the aged have developed some physical impairment or have grown too frail to care for themselves.

Table 3 below shows the postwar trends with regard to multigenerational living arrangements. In 1989, according to a study conducted by the Ministry of Health and Welfare (1991), those aged 65 and older have developed the following living arrangements: 61.9 percent live with their adult children; 24.2 percent live independently as married couples; and 10.4 percent live alone. One thing we must remember is that those elderly living as married couples probably will join the group of those living with their adult children as they grow older or develop physical ailments. Though there has been some decline in the frequency of multigenerational living arrangements, this pattern still appears to be preferred by the Japanese elderly. The pattern becomes even stronger as the parents age–among those aged 65 to 75 years, the frequency of multigenerational living arrangements is just over 50 percent, but among those older than 80 years of age, the frequency increases to as much as 76.1 percent (Table 4).

One final account which will help to explain the prevalence of the Japanese preference for multigenerational living as opposed to "individualistic" living as in the West is the longitudinal study conducted by the Aging Division of the General Affairs Bureau in 1988 (GAB 1991). This survey asked the opinion of the elderly

TABLE 3. Changes in bi/multi-generational living arrangements of males and females in Japan, by year (rounded to the nearest percentage).

Year	60	63	68	73	78	81	82	83	86	87	88
Total	82%	80	79	74	73	69	68	67	64	63	62
Males	80%	77	77	69	69	63	62	61	59	58	56
Females	83%	82	81	78	77	73	72	71	68	67	66

Source: Office of the Director of General Affairs, *The Third Follow-up Report on Measures for Japan's Aging Trends,* Tokyo, Koseisho, June 1990.

concerning their wishes and expectations regarding their preferred living arrangements. It also questioned younger individuals on their own predicted future preferences. Although a few changes have occurred among the younger people, with some preferring "separate residence" to "sharing" with their aging parents, the extent of the change is not significant. In contrast to the Japanese preference for multigenerational living, a much lower percentage of elderly in the West live under the same roof as their married child; even fewer would choose such an arrangement if they could manage independently. Moreover, in the West, multigenerational living usually involves a married daughter rather than a married son, as is the case in Japan (Nishio 1974). These differences and preferences are, generally speaking, culturally patterned and therefore likely to endure, even though in some cases spatial limitation may be the overwhelming reason for living together in the first place.

To recapitulate, the Japanese family institution continues to function in its traditional caregiving role and provide protective welfare service to the growing number of elderly individuals. Older people's life satisfaction is, to a large extent, tied to the younger generations and their family members. This connection provides the Japanese aged population with a positive self-image, because they are still an integral part of society and their families. Of course, this

TABLE 4. Percentages of bi/multi-generational living arrangements by age.

Age	Total 65 and over	65 to 69	70 to 74	75 to 79	80 and over
Percent	61.9	53.7	59.9	65.7	76.1

Source: Ministry of Health and Welfare (MHW), *The Basic Survey of the Japanese Life Style* (1989 – nen Seikatsu fukushi kiso chousa), Tokyo, Koseisho, 1990a.

generalization must be made with caution because of the socially significant incident of elderly suicide, deprivation, and social isolation among those detached from their family relations. In general, though, the statistical data and descriptive information appear to indicate a rather contented, socially active, and generally healthy elderly population in Japan.

Contrary to generalized expectations drawn from the "Modernization Hypothesis," there has not occurred–at least not so far–a shift from the private sector (the family) to the public sector (welfare agencies) in providing care and support for elderly individuals in Japan. The Western individualistic approach to the care of the elderly does not prove to be adequate in explaining Japanese welfare practices. This is probably one of the reasons why a public sector approach to social welfare in Japan has tended to lag behind the Western welfare states. In the next section, this chapter shall look at the governmental mechanisms which have been developed to address welfare issues. I will note some of the flaws and limitations inherent in these programs, most of which are expected to be rapidly modified as a result of a ten year strategy designated by political officials as "The Basic Measures toward Japan's Becoming a Super-Senior Society."

THE JAPANESE WELFARE SYSTEM

Elsewhere (Nishio 1982), I have discussed the Japanese welfare system as consisting of the state welfare system, the family, and the enterprise welfare system. Each plays its particular role and performs a limited function; together, in a largely unsystematic way, they manage to more or less fulfill Japan's welfare needs. Unlike the European system which is characterized by bureaucratic uniformity, using the phraseology of Professor Tadashi Fukutake, the Japanese welfare programs are "patched together" (1983), are institutionally diffused, and attempt to solve rapidly arising problems with no consistent national policy. Instead, they create new policies as they go. As Ian Gough comments, the system of welfare in Japan is "in a class of its own" (1979).

The institutions providing welfare seem to have appeared rather haphazardly in Japan with no clear definition of objectives and rules, at least until the early 1970s when Japan began to feel strong demographic pressure to develop a more coherent and systematic welfare structure. However, even during the 1980s, many Japanese welfare specialists complained about the government's approach which was viewed as lacking systematic planning and methods of implementation. It was argued that under existing conditions, Japan could not provide solutions to the mounting gerontological problems or a means of dealing with the approaching "tidal waves" of elderly and their demands.

When Japan joined the "Club of Aged Countries" in 1970, it clearly had a pressing need to develop a coherent welfare policy. Consequently, many government leaders and welfare specialists visited Sweden and other European welfare states. Sweden, in particular, was viewed as the model for future programs. During this period, however, demographic shifts and the establishment of a welfare state were eclipsed by the oil crisis of the early 1970s; the government was instead forced to put its efforts into finding a solution to Japan's energy needs. Large scale government measures aimed at social welfare were tabled temporarily.

Many Japanese analysts interpreted the period of 1960 to 1975 as the heyday of the developing European welfare states. Because of their extensive income redistribution schemes, the latter nations were seen as an alternative, more humanistic capitalist model. However, social scientists in Japan became somewhat disenchanted with the European and Swedish prototypes as they began to observe the many social ills spreading through some of these countries. In particular, they pointed out the following five negative economic and social consequences: (1) because of generous welfare payments, which often surpassed average wages, the motivation to work was greatly weakened; (2) heavy taxes and social insurance payments fostered the development of an "employment black market" damaging the practice of fair and regulated employment; (3) "Tax-flation" occurred due to a spiral path of anticipatory wage hikes and the payment of high taxes; (4) individual savings declined; and (5) the cost per unit of production tended to increase, resulting in the weakening of these countries' competitive advantage in the international market (Marumi 1989, 124-130).

Japanese analysts were also concerned with what they called "pathological symptoms" arising in European welfare states. These included: a high frequency of absenteeism; alcoholism and drug addiction among the youth; fatalism among the elderly; old age suicide; excessive reliance upon the public sector for the care of the aged; the social isolation of older people; a growing trend toward the impersonalization of welfare agencies; and an increasing dominance of treatment-oriented medical practices which were both more costly and less family oriented (Marumi 1989, 131-132).

Whether these criticisms are warranted or not, many Japanese policymakers chose to develop a different model which became known as "Japanese style welfarism." It is a model which caters to traditional Japanese values and orientations and, according to its designers, would not contain the seeds of "welfare pathology." The underlying theme of the Japanese model is to accentuate the importance of developing a viable, energetic, and forward-looking "welfarism" capable of being supported by Japan's expanding economy. It attempts to duplicate the successful Japanese-style management model which is based on such ideas as life-long employment, mutual support and cooperation, dedication to community needs, and promotion of health. Thus, instead of individualism or individual rights along the line of universal rules and principles, the foundation of Japanese-style welfarism is mutual dependency, obligations, and responsibilities. It also emphasizes harmonious cooperation between central and local government agencies, between the public sector and the private sector, and between enterprise and the state. The end product is a "gemeinschaft" welfarism within the system of "gesselschaft." (Fukutake 1983, 187-206).

Within this framework of a Japanese-style welfarism, the Prime Minister's Cabinet outlined the government's position vis-a-vis the long-term welfare policy of Japan as a rapidly aging society. In June 1986, the Cabinet adopted a basic guideline entitled "The Basic Political Measures Toward Japan's Becoming a Super-Senior Society." Pursuant to this guideline, a number of specific policies and regulations have been put into practice, with an annual increment in government spending for social welfare purposes over the past several years. Indeed, the annual spending for welfare items far exceeded those of other budgetary items belonging to the General Accounts category (MHW 1990d, 27). "Basic Political Measures" represents the government's step-by-step approach to the solution of many pending welfare problems which are expected to increase both in complexity and enormity as the 21st century draws near. This political "manifesto" appears to be the most significant indication of the Japanese government's position regarding present and future welfare matters.

The document contains four objectives, each articulating specific policies: employment, income security, health, and welfare. Importantly, it urges a systemization and unification of three distinct, independent pensions (National [*Kokumin*] Pension, Welfare [*Kosei*] Pension, and Cooperative [*Kyosai*] Pension) so as to avoid the continued development of inequity and confusion.[1] The systemization and unification of the existing pension systems will become more and more pressing with the growing number of pension recipients who will be able to withdraw their full pension payments. In 1988, only 17 percent of national pension recipients and 14.7 percent of Welfare Pension recipients received fully matured pensions.

A more dramatic rise will occur in 2020 when the "baby boomers" will have "grayed." At this time, as much as 48.4 percent (nearly one-half of the total pension recipients) of the National (*Kokumin*) Pension and 39.9 percent of the Welfare (*Kosei*) Pension

---

1. Cooperative (*Kyosai*) Pension is by far the smallest of the three major pension funds, with eight smaller groups within this category. In this study, National (*Kokumin*) and Welfare (*Kosei*) Pension programs are the two principal pension programs analyzed.

subscribers will be fully pensioned. In 1990, each Welfare Pension recipient, if fully pensioned, received 132,308 yen per month. This amount is considerably more than in the U.S. (99,931 yen per couple per month), Sweden (70,582 yen per couple per month), and in West Germany (99,801 yen per month for an ex-office employee). Further, the ratio of the amount of annuity over the average wage is comparable to that of the countries cited above (MHW 1990d, 44-45).

The government data show that the total social expenditure calculated according to the International Labor Organization (ILO) amounted to 406,536 oku (oku = 100 million yen), or 332,500 yen per person (1.06 million yen per family unit). This is a substantial increase when compared with a meager 1,261 oku in 1945 (MHW 1990d, 19).

Until recently, the ratio of social security spending to Japan's GNP was significantly lower than any other welfare nation. This was probably due to two factors: the relatively smaller size of the aged population in Japan and also to the government's deliberate policy of restricting social spending in favor of economic growth. Comparing the ratio of social security spending to GNP of various countries, we find that in 1987 Japan had a ratio of 14.8 percent; the U.S., 16.2 percent (1986); England, 25.5 percent (1986); West Germany, 29.1 percent (1983); France, 36.9 percent (1983); and Sweden, 40.7 percent (1986).

Although Japan currently lags behind the rest of the welfare countries in the amount of money allocated to social security spending, this trend will disappear within the next ten years; ever-increasing demands will be placed on the budget due to the rise in the number of the elderly, as well as an increase in their life spans. It is estimated that the ratio of social security expenditure over GNP will rise to the 22 to 23 percent level by the year 2000, and possibly even to nearly 45 percent by the year 2010. In the latter year, the percentage of the elderly in Japan will reach 24 percent of the total population.

Equally important is a progressive change which will occur in the dependency ratio. In the year 2000, the dependency ratio (the number of those 65 and older versus the population between 20 and 64) will be .25 (four people supporting one elderly person). In 2020, it will rise to 0.4, or 2.5 persons supporting one elderly person (Fuku-take 1983, 78). Such a change has enormous monetary implications. The Japanese government has little time left to waste in planning coherent and workable policies which will cope with the mounting demands that will be made on the national budget.

The aims of the government (as set down in "Basic Political Measures" for dealing with the fiscal problems caused by the coming increase in the amount of social security payments appear to be twofold: to make it possible for the elderly to continue to work beyond the retirement age, and to institute a four day work week system which is intended to decrease the national work hour average; this is currently 2,162 hours per week, 520 hours longer than Germany's average of 1,642 (Asahi Shimbun 1991). The Japanese government hopes to improve the quality of life for the Japanese worker by reducing the work commitment and at the same time to provide an opportunity for aging individuals to continue working.

It is not clear whether this policy alone will have an impact of any significance on government spending and government monetary policy in the future. As of January 1989, 61.9 percent of Japanese enterprises had adopted age 60 as the age of retirement; this percentage will rise to 79.3 percent in the near future. At the moment, however, nearly 30 percent of Japanese workers are obliged to retire before commencement of the National Pension which occurs at age 60 (MHW 1990d, 28). Moreover, "Basic Political Measures" argues for an extension of the retirement age to 65.

HEALTH WELFARE AND THE ELDERLY

It is a given that any aged individual is more vulnerable to illness. Physiological decline due to aging is inevitable and unavoidable although this process can be slowed by means of effective health management which includes attention to diet, exercise, and life style.

According to a survey conducted in 1987, 85.5 percent of people aged 60 to 69 reported that they were most concerned about health-related issues (MHW 1988a). Age differences in the type of health complaints and in the frequency of medical treatment were clearly evident in the study. In fact, in the 1989 *Basic Survey of the Japa-*

nese Life Style it was found that 64.4 percent of those aged 65 and older had some illness. This figure is about four times the 15.3 percent illness rate of those between the ages of 15 and 24. However, when the elderly (excluding those hospitalized or regularly bedridden) were asked about their health condition in general, as many as 74.2 percent (three out of four) reported feeling "good," "pretty good," or "normal." This suggests that most elderly people, even though they have some sort of illness, continue to maintain their daily life as actively as possible (MHW 1990a).

Improvements in living standards and in sanitary conditions, plus the introduction and wide use of penicillin and other antibiotic medications, have dramatically reduced the frequency of communicative diseases. In contrast, there has been an increase in the rate of occurrence of malignant tumors, cardiovascular ailments, and strokes.

A brief comparison of mortality statistics for 1945 and 1989 will serve to illustrate this point: in 1945, tuberculosis accounted for 13.4 percent of all deaths, pneumonia and bronchitis for 8.6 percent, cancer for 7.1 percent, cerebral hemorrhage for 11.7 percent, and heart disease for 5.9 percent. In 1989, cancer accounted for 25.9 percent, strokes for 16.2 percent, heart disease for 19.9 percent and tuberculosis for 0.5 percent. Cerebral hemorrhage is said to have declined due to widespread reduction in the amount of salt intake. However, heart ailments are more prevalent due to a significant increase in the consumption of animal fat. Also on the rise are mental disturbances, and as can be seen from the above data, cancer, and strokes. In recent years, there has been a growing number of outpatients receiving periodic follow-up for hypertension (MHW 1989).

A 1988 patient survey showed that of those hospitalized patients who are 65 years and older (225.3 million), 60.5 percent had circulatory ailments. The rest of the patients in that age group suffered from cerebral arterial illnesses (41.8 percent), muscular bone disease (7.3 percent), bronchial/digestive disorders (4.6 percent), injuries and illness due to poison (4.3 percent), and other problems (18.5 percent) (MHW 1989). Moreover, of those Japanese who are older than 70 years of age, 17.5 percent spent more than 31 days in bed during the year, although another 50 percent remained free from any illness and were able to enjoy healthy and active lives (MHW 1989).

Generally speaking, after prolonged convalescence, very old, frail, elderly individuals experience a significantly decreased ability to use their arms and legs, and in many cases they can become semipermanently bedridden. Such individuals have special needs, as do the elderly who develop symptoms of senility, for daily care and assistance. The 1989 Welfare White Paper reports that the rate of bedridden patients per 1,000 between the ages of 65 to 74 was 6.9 percent; the rate for those aged 75 and older was considerably higher at 35.1 percent (MHW 1990b). Senility appears at the rate of 1.9 percent for those aged 65 to 74 and 9.5 percent for those older than 75.

Earlier, it was noted that the proportion of the total Japanese population older than age 75 will increase from 4.7 percent in 1989 to 11.3 percent, or two and a half times higher, by the year 2020. This sudden growth in the number of citizens aged 75 and over will most certainly lead to a greater number of bedridden and senile people in Japan. It has been predicted that the number of bedridden patients requiring care and assistance will double by the year 2000 and triple by the year 2025. Likewise, the number of senile patients is expected to more than double by the year 2000 and almost quadruple by 2025 (Table 5).

Within the next three decades, Japan will be compelled to fulfill social and medical demands made on the welfare system which may be two to three times greater than those which the Japanese currently face. This increase in welfare assistance will require a dramatic growth both in allocated funds and in the number of personnel and institutions necessary to handle the large number of elderly patients.

The financial implications of caring for a significantly increased aged population with a much longer life expectancy than ever before will be considerable. Japan's bill for medical care is expected to leap sixfold from 20.9 trillion yen in 1990 to 119 trillion yen in 2025, at about the time Japan's aging population is expected to reach its peak. This medical bill is expected to be financed by various sources. According to the Japan Medical Association, taxes and social insurance premiums paid by the Japanese as a whole are

TABLE 5. Increase in the number of Japanese bedridden and senile elderly (1981 to 2025).

	1981	1990	2000	2025
Bed-ridden	520,000	730,000	1,020,000	1,650,000
Senile	540,000	790,000	1,130,000	1,920,000

Source: Economic Planning Bureau, *Plans for Japan's Aging Process,* Tokyo, Ministry of Finance, August 1988.

expected to cover 58.9 percent of the cost of medical care by 2025 (*Japan Times* 1990).

Overall outlays for social welfare programs are expected to inflate to 484 trillion yen from 49 trillion yen; this is expected to consume 36.8 percent of the national income, representing an almost twofold increase over the present rate of 16.5 percent.

Further, projections made at the request of the Japan Medical Association by Nihon University's research institute on population predicted that, by 2025, bills generated at clinics and hospitals nationwide by people aged 65 and older will account for 58.7 percent of the medical costs incurred by the entire population; this represents a substantial rise from the current 38.7 percent (*Japan Times* 1990).

Data published by the Welfare Ministry show that for 1989 the medical costs per elderly person older than age 70 was approximately 550,000 yen, which is 4.23 times as much as the national average. Other studies show that the medical cost of caring for bedridden elderly patients was 26.7 percent of the entire national medical expenditure in 1989 (MHW 1989).

Japan's medical costs are not only rising due to changes in demographic trends, but also because the medical profession is relying more and more on technologically advanced and costly medical equipment on a daily basis. The old age medical insurance system can certainly not be reduced–it can only be expanded. This expansion will occur in different ways and in different directions.

HOME AND COMMUNITY-BASED CARE

At this point, let us turn back to the 1986 political manifesto which reviewed the specific strategies the government had implemented prior to that time in providing health and medical care for elderly Japanese. "Basic Political Measures" stresses various optimistic and forward-looking attitudes toward health. For example, it emphasizes the creation of appropriate social environments and conditions in which many elderly Japanese, with their extended life expectancies, can continue to enjoy life in good health. One government measure resulting from this goal has been to develop and promote many different kinds of health-preserving programs which include such facilities as fitness clubs or physiotherapeutic establishments for physically impaired people. The latter allow the elderly to pursue either preventive or corrective health care in their own familiar environment, with the intention of reducing the probability of serious illness. Another aim of the government is to enhance and improve the elderly's quality of life. In sum, the government's basic approach is to develop a meaningful and workable linkage between the traditional medical treatment in hospitals and clinics and preventive medicine and welfare services available to the aging population, particularly to those aged 75 and older. The strategy, therefore, is to broaden the concept of "home care" so as to reduce the need for hospitalization, and to encourage the elderly to remain at home if at all possible.

Along with the general objectives embodied in "Basic Political Measures," specific goals are identified in the "Ten-Year Welfare Strategy (1990-2000)." With the expected increase in the need for home care for those older than 75 who have become semipermanently bedridden or senile, the Japanese government enacted legislation to create two new social work related positions: social workers and care specialists. To qualify for these official titles, candidates must take and pass government tests. This official recognition of social work and care provision as distinct professions will help to attract qualified individuals who will become involved in welfare-type work in the future (Editorial Committee for the Promotion of Welfare Worker Education 1990, 25).

As part of the ten year welfare strategy, the Japanese policy is to rapidly increase the number of professional helpers and the number of nursing homes to accommodate more elderly people in the future. The "home care service ten year plan" provides for the creation of 100,000 jobs for Home Helpers. Fifty-thousand beds will be created for short stays by the elderly in hospitals, and 10,000 Day Service Centers and 10,000 Home Care Support Centers will be built to aid the elderly and their caretakers.

In order to reduce the number of bedridden elderly, buses will be provided to transport them to physiotherapy centers. A fund of 70 billion yen is to be established for Senior Social Welfare Activities. In the ten year plan for new institutions, 240,000 beds will be available in special nursing homes. An additional 280,000 beds will be created in Senior Health Centers. Another 100,000 people will be accommodated in care houses and 400 Remote Senior Welfare Centers (see #4 in Table 6). Gerontological Research is to be encouraged through the development of National Gerontological Research Institutes. Six hundred billion yen will be allocated for the Improvement of Comprehensive Welfare Facilities for the Elderly.

In addition to the increase in the number of caregiving personnel and institutions (see Tables 6 and 7), periodic medical tests will be available to provide early detection of such illnesses as stomach cancer and cervical cancer (for these, mortality rates can be reduced by as much as 30 percent); lung cancer and breast cancer (the aim is to reduce the incidence of these diseases by as much as 50 percent); cardiovascular illnesses (the goal is to reduce these by 60 percent through periodic monitoring of high risk individuals); and strokes (to be reduced by 50 percent) (MHW 1990d, 120). Medical personnel (doctors, technicians, nurses, and social workers) can expect cooperation from community leaders in posting notices as to when these tests are to be available. The Japanese community social networks seem to work extremely efficiently in encouraging community members to take advantage of these preventive medical screening tests. No one, of course, can estimate with any accuracy just how much of a reduction in the number of critical illnesses has been or will be attained through these preventive measures.

Because of the rapid growth of Japan's aged population requiring care and assistance, the availability of caregiving personnel has been lagging behind the demand for such service. The gap between

TABLE 6. 10-year plan for developing the Japanese home-care welfare program.

Type of Service	Number of Helpers		
	1989	1990	1999
Home Helpers	31,405	35,905	100,000
Short Stay	4,270	7,674	50,000
Day Service	*1,080	*1,780	*10,000
Home Care Assisting Centers	*0	*300	*10,000

Source: MHW, Secretariat, *Social Welfare*, Tokyo, Koseisho, 1988b.
*Number of centers

the availability of trained personnel and the demand for care services has narrowed somewhat over the past few years, but will still not be eliminated until 1994 or 1995 (see Table 8).

To supplement this lack of caregiving personnel, many individual volunteers and groups of volunteers offer services to assist the elderly bedridden at home. In fact, there has been a sharp increase in both the number of volunteer groups as well as in the number of volunteers since 1988.

These volunteers are, no doubt, significantly reducing the need for personnel to care for the elderly, but, at the same time, more entrepreneurial input may very well help to stimulate both private and public participation in solving the need for care and assistance of the elderly. For example, the government has decided to give a substantial tax deduction to enterprises which generate facilities for the elderly such as physiotherapeutic gyms, sports arenas, convalescent homes, etc. (General Affairs Bureau 1991, 124). This type of collaboration between the state and enterprise may prove to be a workable and beneficial means of increasing facilities for the elderly.

TABLE 7. 10-year plan for the development of Japanese elderly care institutions.

Type of Institution	Numbers		
	1989	1990	1999
Nursing Homes (a)	162,019	172,019	240,000
Infirmaries (b)	27,811	47,811	280,000
Care Houses (c)	200	1,700	100,000
Welfare Centers (remote areas) (d)	0	40	400

Source: MHW, Secretariat, *Social Welfare,* Tokyo, Koseisho, 1988b.
a) Number of persons
b) Number of beds
c) Number of houses
d) Number of centers

What are the main characteristics of the so-called Japanese style care systems which make them different from the Swedish or the British systems of care and assistance? There have been debates about the shift of care institutions from the private to the public sector as it is held by some analysts that the public sector care system is more bureaucratic and therefore more impersonal.

The Japanese-style care system depends a great deal on the family institution, and more specifically upon the caregiving role provided by the wives of the aging parents' sons. Because of the gradual increase in the nuclearization of the Japanese family and the decline in multigenerational living arrangements, the Japan of the future must devise a comprehensive and compromise plan for care and support of the elderly. This means that the Japanese style of

TABLE 8. Increasing Japanese Demand for Geriatric Care Workers

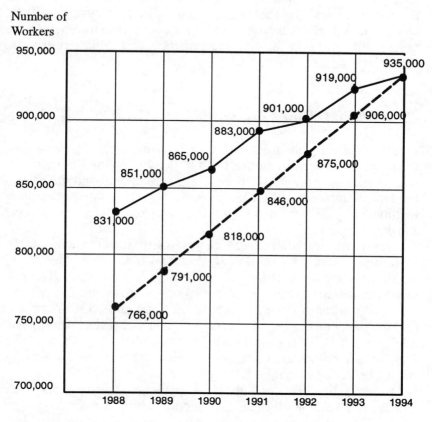

Source: MHW, *White Paper*, 1990b.

_____ (required)

- - - - - - - - - (in service)

caregiving will continue to play a role but to a lesser extent. It will be necessary to supplement the decreasing role of the Japanese family by perhaps adopting particular aspects of the American and European models. In the end, the Japanese care system will be broadly identified as a community-based care system, open to the family institution, to the state bureaucracy, and to entrepreneurial efforts.

THE PHYSICALLY IMPAIRED ELDERLY IN JAPAN

Let us now, as our final and most critical problem for analysis, focus on the increasing number of physically impaired individuals, with particular reference to the present care system and the role of the family. In so doing, we shall begin to explore some alternative methods of care which will have to supplement the role of the Japanese family.

According to a 1980 survey of physically impaired individuals, there were about 1.07 million aged 60 and older, or 54 percent of the entire population of the physically impaired in Japan. The rate of physical impairment for all ages was found to be 23.8 persons per 1,000, while for the age groups 60 to 64 and 65 to 69, it was 55.8 and 68.7 per 1,000, respectively. There was a sharp increase to 87.6 per 1,000 for the age group 70 and older (Yamashita 1988). Clearly, individuals are more likely to develop physical impairment or sustain injury with age.

We normally define an individual as having a physical disability if there is a notable physical malfunction which has a a long-term effect on the functioning of the person concerned. Aging individuals who experience a decline in their physical functioning often develop multiple impairments and associated illnesses. Earlier, we briefly analyzed the sociological implications concerning the increase in those aged 65 years and older who are bedridden on a more or less semipermanent basis. As noted, a 1982 government survey disclosed that there were about 520,000 such patients in Japan in that year with differing rates of incidence, depending on age (see Table 5). For the age group 65 to 69, the rate was 19 per 1,000 people; for 70 to 74, it was 34; for 75 to 79, it was 57; and for those 80 years and over, the rate was 126 per 1,000. Clearly, there is an increase with advancing age.

When one examines the various causes of physical impairment which occur with aging, it is clear that there is a tendency for bones to become brittle, and consequently they can easily crack or break. Other changes may occur in muscles, the brain, nerves, glands, and joints; these changes result in slower movement. The aging process also affects the heart, arteries, lungs, and digestive system. All of these changes increase the vulnerability to illness, often fostering chronic and/or multiple conditions. Further, because of prolonged convalescence in bed, many aged people develop secondary impairments such as contraction of joints, shrinkage of glands, and hardening of bones. These secondary symptoms often lead to the person becoming permanently bedridden.

According to a 1980 Tokyo Metropolitan survey, 26 percent of the bedridden elderly had become impaired due to accidents while 63.8 percent had become impaired because of illness (Tokyo Metropolitan Office 1981). If we limit our analysis to those aged 65 and older who are physically impaired, we discover that the major causes for the elderly becoming bedridden include strokes, hypertension, rheumatism, and arthritis. The survey indicated that 34.6 percent of those bedridden had become so due to strokes, a finding supported by a number of other studies (MHW 1982a).

Of those people older than 65 who are bedridden, 76.5 percent are not capable of bathing themselves, 69.2 percent are unable to dress by themselves, 59.8 percent require someone to change their diapers, 55.6 percent is not at all mobile, even with the use of canes or walking support equipment, and 46.3 percent are unable to feed themselves (MHW 1982b). These bedridden elderly individuals are often totally dependent on others for their daily care and fulfillment of their basic needs. The caregivers who provide continuous services to these bedridden people must maintain close contact for many hours.

In Sweden, and in Europe generally, thousands of trained helpers and social workers are employed to assist those who are permanently bedridden. Earlier it was noted that there has been a significant rise in the number of trained social workers, care specialists, and volunteers in Japan. At present, however, the majority of bedridden patients in Japan are being cared for within the family, with little outside help or trained assistance.

I have noted that three-generational living arrangements, though experiencing a decline over the past few decades, are still very much intact. Those families with bedridden aged people are far more likely to observe the traditional custom of the three generations living together. While 71.7 percent of Japanese families with an aging member maintain the three-generational living arrangements, as many as 82.0 percent of those families with an elderly, bedridden family member follow this custom. Moreover, when one member of an elderly couple living independently becomes bedridden, there is a tendency for the couple to move into the home of their married son's family. This tendency represents a most intriguing social consequence of having a bedridden aged person in one's family. It tends to restructure the Japanese unit, to increase the size of the family membership, and to provide support for the physically impaired individual. Thus, even today, caregiving in Japan is a family responsibility.

Aging males who have become bedridden are likely to be cared for by their wives (61 percent), by daughters-in-law (21.7 percent), and by their children (10.8 percent). For female elderly bedridden people, daughters-in-law will become the caregivers in 50.4 percent of the cases, an adult child in 27.7 percent, and husbands in 11.4 percent (Table 9). Gender is clearly a significant factor in determining who will perform the role of caregiver.

Of the three major groups giving care (spouses, children, and daughters-in-law), the most frequent complaints are that they cannot go out when they want to, or when they need to, and that their sleep is often disrupted at night. Often the role of caregiver necessitates a change in the person's job. Among caregivers, 37.5 percent are forced to quit work; 5.9 percent to take a leave of absence; and 6.7 percent to change jobs; about one-third continue to work while providing care.

When one considers the situation regarding work as outlined above, it is clear that there are often significant economic ramifications that caregiving families have to face. Income may be lost as one of the family members is forced to quit work or take a leave of absence.

TABLE 9. The relationship of the bedridden Japanese elderly to their primary caregiver, by gender.

Caregiver	Bedridden Elderly		
	Total	Male	Female
Spouse	31.6%	61.0%	11.4%
Child	20.9	10.8	27.7
Daughter-in-law	38.1	21.7	50.4
Grandchild	2.0	0.8	2.7
Other relative	1.7	1.0	2.3
Non-relative	2.8	1.5	2.8

Source: Japanese Social Welfare Association, "The Conditions of Caring for the Elderly," 1990.

CONCLUSION

As outlined earlier in this paper in the discussion of the "Basic Political Measures," the government hopes in the future to increase the number of professional Home Helpers. However, current care-giving practices are heavily dependent upon the Japanese family. This can be dramatically demonstrated if one compares the situation in Japan with that of Sweden and England. The Social and Economic National Congress compared the types of welfare services available and the costs incurred in Sweden, England, and Japan. Two comparable cities, Malmo in Sweden and Kamakura in Japan, were compared with reference to the public expenditure allocated for the employment of Home Helpers. In Malmo, over 100,000 yen (for a family of four) was allocated for Home Helpers annually, while the expenditure for this in Kamakura was no more than 267 yen (Marumi 1989).

There are two factors which should be kept in mind when one considers these data. First, Sweden currently has the world's highest proportion of elderly in its population. Secondly, Sweden has a much higher proportion of elderly living alone. Only 10 percent of those aged 65 and older in Japan live alone, whereas in Sweden about 30 percent live alone. Consequently, considerably more elderly are living with their families in Japan than is the case in Sweden.

Within the next twenty-five years, this situation will change dramatically and, by the year 2008, the proportion of the old age population in Japan will come to equal that of Sweden. If Japan is to adopt the Swedish style of Home Helpers, it is estimated that approximately 1 million Home Helpers will be needed in Japan as a whole. For Tokyo alone, 100,000 Helpers will be required (Marumi 1989).

In Sweden, 4.1 percent of those aged 65 and older live in homes for the aged with an additional 2 to 3 percent living in service housing. Currently in Japan, only 1.5 percent of the elderly aged 65 and older live in these types of institutions. By the year 2008, there will be twice as many old people in Japan, and the country will likely need 8 to 10 times as many public institutions such as homes for the aged and nursing homes. Can Japan afford to increase the number of Home Helpers by 10 times or more? Many would agree that Japan's resources will not be able to keep up with the extremely rapid rate of aging in Japan, and that adoption of the Swedish model seems rather unrealistic (Marumi 1989).

The British model appears to fall somewhere in between the Swedish and the Japanese welfare models. In Britain, neighborhood volunteer activities are extremely advanced in terms of effectiveness and reliability, and these fulfill a very large portion of the Home Help need. By comparison, the number of volunteers working in Japan is rather minute. As we have seen, the Japanese model exploits family members, particularly the females who fulfill the caregiving role in the majority (86.9 percent) of cases. While the Japanese welfare model continues to utilize the institution of the family (this has, of course, many important merits as far as those being cared for are concerned), this will continue to decrease due to the falling fertility rate on one hand and to the expanding number of the elderly on the other.

Are there any measures which can reinforce this caregiving role of the family? One suggestion is to develop compensatory measures such as providing substantial allowances to those families supporting elderly individuals or paying the caregivers for their work and service to the elderly. Another alternative is for the young elderly (those aged 65 to 70) to act as caregivers. This is a viable alternative as, in the future, some Japanese families may consist of four and even five generations. Effective training and education of this group of young elderly may help provide significant manpower for the expanding need for home assistance.

Various holistic ideas and approaches have been presented for making the Japanese-style welfare system more adaptive to demographic and gerontological needs. The road to the solution for the needs of Japan's increasing elderly population appears quite rugged, twisting, hazardous, and most of all, costly. As emphasized in the "Basic Political Measures," the Japanese-style welfare state must preserve a dynamic, expansive economy which supports future-looking, active, and participatory members, regardless of age, sex, or occupation.

REFERENCES

Asahi Shimbun. "Salaried Men's Affluent Life Style Still Out of Reach." January 13, 1991.

Economic Planning Bureau, *Plans for Japan's Aging Process,* Tokyo, Ministry of Finance, August 1988.

Editorial Committee for the Promotion of Welfare Worker Education (*Fukushi yousei kouza kenkyuu iin-kai*). *The Old Age Welfare* (*Roujin fukushi-ron*). Tokyo: Chuo Houki Shuppan, 1990.

Fukutake, T. *Some Aspects of the Social Welfare Debates.* Tokyo University Press, 1983.

General Affairs Bureau (GAB), Old Age Division (*Soumu-chou, roujin-ka*). *Trends and Prospects Regarding the Measures Towards an Aging Society* (*Chouju shakai taisaku no taisaku no doko to tenbou*). p. 26, 1991.

Gough, Ian. *The Political Economy of the Welfare States.* London: The Macmillan Press, 1979.

Japan Times. "Medical Costs to Soar with Aging of Society." October 10, 1990.

Japanese Social Welfare Association. "The Conditions of Caring for the Elderly," Tokyo, Japan.

Marumi, N. *Japanese Style Welfare System (Nihon-gata fukushi shakai)*. Tokyo: Nihon Housou Shuppan-kai, 1989.

Ministry of Health and Welfare (MHW) *(Kousei-shou)*, Welfare Secretariat. *Introduction to Social Welfare*. 1982a.

Ministry of Health and Welfare (MHW) *(Kousei-shou)*. *1981 Health Survey* (1981-nen Kenkou Chousa). 1982b.

Ministry of Health and Welfare (MHW) *(Kousei-shou)*. *1987 Basic Survey of the Japanese Life Style (1987-nen Seikatsu fukushi kiso chousa)*. 1988a.

Ministry of Health and Welfare (MHW), Secretariat, *Social Welfare*, Tokyo, Ko-seisho, 1988b.

Ministry of Health and Welfare (MHW), Population Research Center, *World Population Prospects*, Tokyo, Koseishu, 1988c.

Ministry of Health and Welfare (MHW) *(Kousei-shou)*. *Patients Survey 1988* (Byounin chousa 1988). 1989.

Ministry of Health and Welfare (MHW) *(Kousei-shou)*. *1989 Basic Survey of the Japanese Life Style (1989-nen Seikatsu fukushi kiso chousa)*, Tokyo, Koseisho, 1990a.

Ministry of Health and Welfare (MHW), *(Kousei-shou, Jouhou-bu)*. *Welfare White Paper 1989 (Kousei hakusho)*. 1990b.

Ministry of Health and Welfare (MHW), Division of Information *(Kousei- shou, Jouhou-bu)*. *Actuarial Chart (Shibou zuhyou)*. 1990c.

Ministry of Health and Welfare (MHW), Policy Making Division *(Kousei-shou, Seisaku-ka)*, *Introduction to Social Welfare (Shakai hoshou nyuumon)*. 1990d.

Ministry of Health and Welfare (MHW), *(Kousei-shou, Jouhou-bu)*. *Welfare White Paper 1990 (Kousei hakusho)*. 1991.

Nishio, H. K. "Aging and the Aged in the Japanese Social Structure." *Asian Profile*, Vol. II, No. 5, Nov. 1974.

Nishio, H. K. "Can Japan be Called a Welfare State?" Unpublished Manuscript, 1982.

Office of the Director of General Affairs, *The Third Follow-up Report on Measures for Japan's Aging Trends*. Toyko, Koseisho, June 1990.

Palmore, Erdman. *Honorable Japanese Elders*. Duke University Press, Durham, NC, 1975.

Tokyo Metropolitan Office *(Tokyo-to)*. *Survey on the Bed-Ridden Elderly (Neta-kiri roujin no chousa)*, 1981.

Yamashita, S. *The Old Age Welfare (Roujin fukushi)*. Tokyo: Kawashima, 1988.

Chapter 11

The Changing Role of the Elderly in the People's Republic of China

Philip G. Olson

INTRODUCTION

China, like other Eastern civilizations, has long been considered a society which revered its elderly citizens. The tradition of reverence has been an integral part of its value system and was undergirded by the teachings of Confucianism. China has been portrayed as the paramount example of obedience to the word of the elder and even of basic political and social rule by the elderly segment of the population. However, the ideals of a society and the realities of daily life may be quite different. The actual treatment and regard for elders in any society can be influenced by many factors. In China, elders are not always given the respect and reverence that tradition dictates. Evidence exists of elder abuse, inadequate housing conditions for some childless elders, and insufficient retirement programs. Examination of various historical periods reveals that elders were sometimes discriminated against by political regimes or by the day-to-day activities of other age groups. In fact, the most well-known period in China's history, the Cultural Revolution (1966-1975), was a period in which all those, including the elderly, who represented the traditional values of the past were persecuted.

Social theory, in attempting to explain the factors that affect how elders are regarded in society, points to an interplay of social, economic, and political structures. These structures interact so that, for example, changes in the economic conditions of a society can be associated with changes in the form or functioning of social structures, such as the family. Changes in the family may correspond to changes in people's attitudes and behaviors, influencing not only the private family, but also the public sphere of life (Whyte and Parish 1984). This interplay is also true of changes in a political system's priorities and strategies, which in centrally controlled States, like the People's Republic of China, have more power and are more immediately influential (Wolf 1986) than in a market-based society.

The purpose of this chapter is to examine the relationship of this constellation of social, economic, and political factors to the care and treatment of elders in China during the period following the Cultural Revolution. This period coincides with the death of Mao Zedong and the emergence of major reforms within the society and Community Party, which control the economic and political structures of China. This chapter will first provide a background by tracing the historical role of aging in China as it moved from an agrarian society into a communist-dominated political economy. Next, modernization policies in post-Mao China, the period following the Cultural revolution, will be examined as a means for understanding current policies and practices toward elders. Empirical evidence from this same period following the Cultural Revolution will then be examined in an effort to trace the relationship between the political agenda of the state and care of elders. One particular segment of the elderly population, the frail elderly, will be the focus of this last discussion. Concentrating on the frail elderly, those needing health care and assistance with daily living due to physical and mental disabilities, will serve to highlight a number of vital issues when examining the treatment of the elderly in a society.

THE ROLE OF THE ELDERLY IN CHINA

Traditional Agrarian China

Agrarian China was characterized by centrality of the family and reverence for the elderly. Indeed, the two are related and form an essential base upon which the social structure of China was built. China as an agrarian society, in the period before the Republic was founded in 1911, was rooted in a tradition of ancestor worship and filial piety. The society was patrilineal and dependent on the land. One's future resided in the male offspring, for he inherited property, carried on the family name, cared for parents in their old age, and produced offspring who carried on the family lineage, ensuring continuity with both the past and future. The male was seen as a link in an unending chain of kin stretching back as far as ancestors could be traced, and forward into the future through his descendants. To break the chain by not having a male child was a failure to honor one's obligations to both past and future generations (Baker 1979; Chai and Chai 1969).

Confucianism built on this premise of ancestor worship and provided a moral and intellectual foundation for revering the elderly. Older persons, by virtue of their years of accumulated experience, were the moral and ethical models of their society. They were to be respected, honored, and followed. Because this idea was so central to Confucian philosophy and because this philosophy was so central to Chinese society during the two millennia preceding its entry into Western industrialization, it is understandable that the elderly have played an important role in the history and development of the Chinese social structure (Ganshaw 1978). This veneration of both age and the past served to preserve the importance of the family over the single person, the dominance of male over female, and the power of age over youth.

However, it should be noted that Confucianism was not as widespread among the Chinese as popularly believed (Freedman 1961; Ikels 1975; Leslie 1979). It was limited to perhaps the upper 20 percent of society, and, for the vast majority of Chinese, the Confucian practice of venerating the elderly was an ideal rather than daily practice (Yin and Lai 1983). However, children were still important, if not for veneration, at least for security in one's old age.

Also underpinning the importance of the family and reverence for the elderly was Chinese folk religion, which forebode the dangers of Hungry Ghosts wandering alone in the Underworld. One became a Hungry Ghost by failing to leave descendants. Descendants were vital in the role of worshipping the ancestor after his demise. To face old age and death without natural or adopted descendants was indeed a grim prospect (Sankar 1981). To avoid this prospect, unmarried persons or childless couples went to great lengths to ensure that they had some descendants who could care for them after death. As Sankar points out, there were thousands who found themselves in this position, and they coped with their dilemma through a variety of cultural solutions, including adopting nephews. The two most common means for unmarried women to avoid this outcome were to either become servants within a home where they established family-like relationships or to enter a secular sisterhood (Sankar 1981, 32).

The Role of the Elderly After Liberation

The era of Mao Zedong, which began on October 1, 1949, marked the beginning of the Chinese Communist Party era and a historic redistribution of wealth, property, and power in China. The economic upheavals of the years during which Mao had power impacted the elderly, whose well-being depended on the overall prosperity of the society. However, among those who have observed the role and status of the elderly during these years, there is little consensus over whether the elderly fared better or worse under Maoism. Some argue that the status of the elderly declined under Communism (Ganshaw 1978; Woon 1981; Cherry and Magnuson-Martinson 1981), and some believe there is considerable evidence for the equal or increased status of the aged under Mao (Tien 1977; Kinoy 1979; Treas 1979; Yin and Lai 1983; Davis-Friedmann 1981, 1983).

The enactment of the new marriage laws in 1950, and their revision in 1981, marked efforts by the political system to institutionalize new attitudes toward elderly parents and women. Under the new laws, the following changes occurred: men and women were considered equal under the new law; monogamy became the only recognized marriage form; parents were responsible for proper care of their children; and children became responsible for the proper care of their parents in old age. Though it is certain that the passage of this new law did not instantly transform millions of relationships within existing families across China and did not compel all young people to obey the spirit of the new law, it did establish a public ideology and expectations for the new generations of Chinese. In the forty-one years since its enactment, there have been many changes in family relationships, especially in urban areas: children marry later and have more freedom in choosing partners, and women have greater rights and freedoms, as well as greater economic independence. This contrasts to traditional family life, in which the wife had no property rights and remained unskilled except in domestic work. She is now more likely to have a skill, an income, and a participatory role in the society, especially in the urban neighborhood, where she is likely to serve on a neighborhood council, the Resident's Committee. Also, in her work role she is more likely to have responsibility and authority. The younger women, in their positions of greater autonomy, are now becoming especially visible, and possibly even enviable, to the older women (Yue 1986).

Mao's personal attitudes concerning elders and youth were unquestionably a factor in the state policies toward the elderly following liberation. Those who have closely examined his writings and his political career conclude that he was not Confucian in his outlook. He looked not so much to the elderly for leadership or wisdom, but to the vigor and enthusiasm of youth for the success of the economic and political revolution he had mounted (Ganshaw 1978, 307-309). Though there is debate over the precise role Mao played in launching the Cultural Revolution, there is little doubt that he believed in purging the system of traditional values such as the sacredness of age, the importance of the old, and the inviolateness of tradition, and replacing them with continued new revolutions (Mao 1969).

Yet it seems quite certain that Mao never intended that the old should undergo as much vilification as they did; as the Cultural Revolution unfolded, efforts were initiated to redirect the attack against tradition away from the elderly. Old people themselves were no longer defined as evil, but only as having lived through periods of an evil political economy. Thus the elderly were called upon to join publicly with the young and form a "three-in-one" alliance: "The old cadres and the young cadres must acquire each others' strong points, unite as one and do their work still better together" (quoted by Ganshaw 1978). In addition, the old were called upon to bear witness to how bad the "old" China actually had been (Ganshaw 1978, 318; Davis-Friedmann 1983, 8; Woon 1981, 253). These activities were undertaken by bringing old people to schools to tell children stories of the evil practices of the past eras in which old people especially were poorly treated and where general conditions were miserable.

In rural China, despite the economic gains made through collectivization, the primary responsibility for the aged during Mao's era remained with the family. Parish, in his analysis of rural family life, notes, "The welfare system is still based on the family" (1975, 616). This process has been largely accomplished "through the ability of the elderly to share the rewards earned by younger family members, and not through increases in direct state intervention" (Davis-Friedmann 1981, 53). Rural care of the elderly depended upon the economic successes of the communes, and although there were almost no pension systems for older farm workers during this period, the wealthier the collective, the better were medical care and other benefits to retired persons. However, the masses of rural elderly had no major programs or policies directed toward their needs. This condition, tagged by Lipton (1977) "urban bias," typifies developing societies, which direct resources first toward urban areas. Szelenyi (1983) notes this bias under State socialism in Eastern Europe, and Davis (1989), examining Chinese data, documents the same bias there.

For the childless elderly, those who bore only daughters (daughters usually moved to the household of their husband and took little or no responsibility for care of their own parents), and the frail and disabled, the rural communes developed a system of relief. In 1956, during the era of expansion of the collectives, the system of "Five Guarantees" (*wu bao*) was developed, providing food, clothing, shelter, medical care, and for the young, education, or for the elderly, a burial. Although it was far from uniform in its formative period (Dixon 1981, 191-195), this system did provide the childless elderly with a degree of security in their old age.

In addition, by the end of 1958, a massive campaign to build old age homes began. One hundred thousand homes were opened in the countryside, with a resident population of two million elderly (Dixon 1981, 198-199). These homes were short-lived, and after the failure of the "Great Leap Forward" in 1958-59, there was no comprehensive welfare program for the rural elderly, except the "Five Guarantees" and a few homes for the childless and disabled. For those elderly with children, the family remained the principal welfare unit.

In urban areas the care of the elderly under Mao was quite different than in the countryside. The development of retirement programs and pensions for workers began on a small scale in the mid-1950s and grew rapidly during the 1970s (Davis-Friedmann 1981). By the mid-1970s nearly 75 percent of all urban workers were covered by a pension plan. The development of pensions for retired workers removed the burden of care from the children, and the retirement of workers at ages 55 and 60 opened the way for younger, more vigorous workers to fill the factory jobs of the often less skilled and less efficient older workers. Medical care and other benefits to the aged were also better in urban areas than in the countryside. Davis-Friedmann concludes, "The overall security of the aged has markedly improved since 1949" (1981, 52), and "the Communist revolution has thus strengthened rather than weakened traditional views of old age and the elderly have benefitted from government support" (1983, 13).

MODERNIZATION POLICIES IN POST-MAO CHINA

The death of Mao Zedong in 1976 brought an end to one era in Chinese history and the beginning of another. In the new era, full-scale modernization accelerated. In January 1975, Premier Zhou En-lai announced the Four Modernizations Program and set the year 2000 as a target date for its achievement. The program centered on the development of agriculture, the military, industry, and science and technology. The adoption of the program in 1978, together with the downfall of the "gang of four" following the death of Mao, promoted China's development through technological growth rather than through class struggle, as the "cultural revolution" had promoted.

Three major reform policies form the core of the modernization policy in the 1980s and 1990s: (1) population reform, (2) economic reform, and (3) party reform.

Population Reform

Among the first policies reformulated in the period following Mao's death was population reform; the new policy was aimed at further reduction in the growth of population as a necessary step in economic reform (Saith 1981). Unless population growth could be stopped, economic development could never be realized because the increasing population would erode gains in economic development. Although population control began as early as 1962, its impact was not substantial until the "one child" policy became fully operational in the early 1980s (Wolf 1986; Kallgren 1985). In the decade since its inception, it has shown dramatic signs of success, largely in urban areas and in those rural counties closely linked to urban centers along the eastern coast of China (Bianco 1981; Poston and Gu 1984; Chen 1985).

Economic Reform

The political successor to Mao, Deng Xiaoping, "encouraged unity through increased economic interdependence, through reliance on effective, planned allocation of material goods and capital, and through a regularized promotion and personnel management system" (Oksenberg 1982, 170). The decade of the 1980s witnessed a remarkable reform of the entire economy, including the abolition of the farm commune, the opening of "free markets" for many goods and services, the institutionalization of a work incentive policy, greater decentralization of enterprise management, implementation of a mixed controlled and market economy, and greater reliance on Western technology, capital, and markets. Most of the economic indicators available suggest that the economic reform efforts have resulted in growth in nearly all parts of the system, large-scale improvements in the standard of living, inflation, and greater "Westernization" of the lifestyles of the Chinese peoples, especially those living in urban areas. It has been suggested, however, that there continue to be inequities between rural and urban elders, and the principal reason for those inequities is the unwillingness of the central government leaders to break from the policy "that defines most social welfare goods as rewards to job statuses and thereby allocates the best quality services to the most highly ranked employees," who live in cities (Davis 1989, 581).

Party Reform

Begun in the early 1980s, the major political reforms included abolishing life tenure for cadres, encouraging retirement of veteran cadres, and promoting younger cadres to leading posts (An 1982). In a speech delivered in 1981 on the occasion of the sixtieth anniversary of the founding of the Chinese Communist Party, Party Chairman Hu Yaobang said, "It is now a pressing strategic task facing the whole party to build up a large contingent of revolutionary, well-educated, professionally competent and younger cadres . . . and they [old, veteran cadres] should free themselves from the onerous pressure of day-to-day work . . . . " (Liu 1986, 355). A major thrust of party reform has been to streamline the bulging bureaucracy, often cited as a cause of the sluggishness of the reform, the major impediment to efficiency, and a drain on the economy. This policy was launched in 1982 when the Party Central Committee passed a resolution establishing a veteran cadre retirement system (Zhao 1987). In the words of Deng, the goals are "to make the ranks of cadres more revolutionary, younger in average age, better educated, and more professionally competent" (1983). In 1983, over 800,000 veteran cadres retired, signaling the new retirement policy was underway (Ding 1984).

THE STATE AND THE FRAIL ELDERLY

The three policies outlined above, though aimed at economic and political reform, have had and will continue to have significant consequences for today's elderly population, and specifically for the frail elderly. China currently faces the dilemma of dealing with a growing proportion of frail elders while at the same time undergoing modernization and struggling to meet the needs of its enormously large population, including its massive peasant population.

The Frail Elderly in China

The modernization of China contributes to the increase in the proportion and number of older persons in that society. Modernization theory attributes this growth in the elderly population to improved hygiene, health care, diets, and other sociomedical changes (Cowgill 1986). In 1985, China's age 65 and over population constituted 5 percent of the total population. Within 30 years, by 2015, it will double to 10 percent (Banister 1988, 75). The very old, those over 80, constituted 11 percent of the over 65 population in 1985 and by 2015 will grow to 19 percent (Banister 1988, 75), nearly a fifth of all elders. The group of elderly over age 80 is most likely to include those who need health care and other assistance as their frailty increases.

An emphasis on the frail elderly in the discussion to follow is important because frail elders highlight the issue of competing interests on the systems of support. The dilemma presented by this constituency involves defining, through social policy, how resources should be allocated among the nonproductive sectors of the domestic public. It raises the question: How does the political system allocate resources among the needs of the youth, the needs for stability of the family, the need for continued economic growth, and the need to care for elders? Frail elders, who can offer little or no return on the investment in their long-term care, are in an especially unusual and important position in a society that is struggling with its economic development.

Theoretical Perspectives of Political Economy

In attempting to understand the issues surrounding social and economic change and their influence on a population such as frail elders, it has been argued that sociologists have long overlooked the State as a variable (Skocpol 1985). However, this appears to be changing. Myles (1984) does factor in the role of the State when he points out that it is primarily capitalistic societies that provide welfare for their elderly population in the form of retirement pensions. Estes et al. (1984) focus on the political economy and identify it as the overriding factor in determining how elder care is addressed.

"Political economy" refers to the economic system as it is supported and promoted by the political system that has garnered the power to operate the government and thus regulate or control the economic system. The question of how economic growth gets transformed into expenditures is a central issue of the political economy perspective (Estes et al. 1984). This perspective highlights the fact that, in the U.S., health care is a part of the market economy, and the management of illness is a business. Furthermore, elder care is an integral part of that market economy. Since the ethos of the U.S. political economy is profit and growth, the system is benefitted when the aging population is defined in terms of its illness.

In China, however, the health care system is not a central part of the economy, and illness is not defined as an element of economic growth. While the health care system in China is a necessary system and is being modernized along with other sectors, health care technology and training are costly investments for a society, and in China it is no advantage for there to be a large "sick" population. Developing societies, like China, first address problems of communicable diseases. Only when these diseases have been controlled does attention turn to dealing with chronic diseases, which are not only costly to the society but focus largely on the older population. In China, this issue is now before the government. "Success in the control of communicable disease has transferred the burden of China's health problems to the older age groups. . . . Prevention is relatively difficult for most chronic diseases, and development of effective, yet low-cost, strategies for dealing with these disorders is a priority. The major pitfall is the temptation to emulate high-cost curative approaches that have proved relatively inefficacious and that, even in high-income countries, have resulted in a massive drain on national economic resources" (Jamison, Evans, and King 1984, xvii). How China deals with its frail elder population is then a reflection of the political decisions on how that "problem" is defined.

Treas and Logue (1986) suggest that policies of development are in part influenced by how the aged population is defined relative to economic development. They identify four perspectives in defining the aged: (1) as a low priority; (2) as an impediment; (3) as a resource; or (4) as victims of the development process. However, they argue, these four categories are not mutually exclusive. Most developing societies define the older population in a combination of ways. The evidence from China suggests that it publicly defines the old as resources who can play an important role in the development of the society (China News Analysis 1983; Ikels 1990b). However, examining the programs currently underway suggests the old are a low priority in the allocation of public resources.

The Role of the State and the Family in Elder Care

Consistent with their ideology of minimizing illness and maximizing self-sufficiency, the government and the Communist Party promote local initiatives that foster a minimum role for the government and a maximum role for the family and community in care of its elders, especially for the old-old, the frail, and the dependent (Ikels 1990a; Henderson 1990). The development of modernization in China under communism, together with the political intervention of the Chinese Communist Party, have reinforced the role of the family and have clarified a balance of responsibility between the State and the family for elder care, especially within the decade of the 1980s (Whyte and Parish 1984; Wolf 1986).

In traditional China, both rural and urban, the extended family was the primary unit that provided for elders. In the current period, while the family remains a central element in care of elders, other factors influence the role of the family. One such factor, the rural-urban distinction, influences all of Chinese life. In 1982, 80 percent of China's population was rural. Although, according to the 1990 Chinese census, the rural population dropped to 73.8 percent, China remains predominantly rural and agricultural. In addition to a predominantly rural population, China's economy is bifurcated. This dual economy has endured through the 30 years of Communism, with the urban sector becoming semi-modernized and receiving about 70 percent of the state investment, while the rural sector continues to depend on local surpluses. More comprehensive social and health care services accrue to urban elders due to subsidization from the state; in rural areas social and health services are primarily the result of "regeneration through one's own efforts" (*zi li geng sheng*) (Davis-Friedmann 1984, 207). Such a dual economy has led to very different programming for rural and urban frail elders and alters the role of the family in long-term care.

In rural areas, parents expect to guarantee their care in old age through a married son who will provide for them in the absence of a pension system and other social services. Family reciprocity is the basic system that ensures elder care in rural areas. Living with a married son offers both economic and social security for the elder, and, in exchange, the elder contributes to the household economy through child care, gardening, and household work.

In urban areas, where 75 percent of all adults are state employees, parents look to the state to provide for them through a retirement pension and social services, and children are seen as dependents rather than as supports. Because of seniority, older workers receive more pay than younger workers, and the additional household income earned by elders is often used to subsidize expenses of children through household purchases, gifts for grandchildren, vacations, and medical expenses (Sankar 1989; Davis-Friedmann 1985a). However, despite the fact that the state in urban areas plays a major role in providing economic support for the aged, the family still provides the majority of elder care. Studies in two of the largest cities in China, Tianjin and Beijing, reported that when elders became ill, 96 and 87 percent, respectively, were cared for directly by family members (Yuan 1987).

Health Care of the Frail Elders

One particularly important issue in a discussion of elder care is the specific question of how the society addresses the health and long-term care needs of the chronically ill and frail elders who are unable to care for themselves on a daily basis due to mental or physical disability. Long-term care as defined here includes the continuum of activities directed toward the physical, medical, and social care of persons unable to provide for themselves. It includes institutional care as well as in-home family care, and is provided by both skilled personnel as well as family members, friends, or neighbors.

Though the principal support for elders, including frail elders, is the family unit, there are health care supports in place to supplement the family. These supports are, however, much less extensive than one would expect given the long tradition of respect toward elders. As early as 1983, observers of social welfare policies in China noted that it was the overall intention of China "to avoid the creation of large welfare agencies which have drained the capacity of richer governments" (China News Analysis 1983, 8). Instead, the evidence is quite clear that the family and local communal organizations are expected to provide much of the long-term care for frail elders to prevent otherwise costly institutionalization. This policy is evident in both rural and urban areas, although the higher standard of living and the generally better medical care in urban areas conceals the extent to which urban areas rely on these informal support systems. The visible exception to this policy in both rural and urban areas is the childless elderly population, who receive special benefits.

In rural China, health care for both acute and chronically ill frail elders is available through primary health care stations, rural hospitals, "barefoot" doctors, nurse aides, and some nursemaids (*bao mu*) (Davis-Friedmann 1984; Liang and Gu 1989; Jamison, Evans, and King 1984).

Primary health care stations are clinics operated in small quarters of existing public buildings or sometimes in separate structures. These stations are in small villages, and there are also larger clinics in the township (*xiang*). The village stations contain basic medical examination features, but provide little privacy to the patient. Medical treatment includes traditional (herbal) medicine and acupuncture, depending on the diagnosis and preference of the attending doctor and the patient. Minor illnesses and injuries are treated; immunizations and birth control are also administered (Hu 1984). A typical staff includes two or three doctors and one or more nurses. The stations keep regular hours, but are also available on an emergency basis. There is great variance in the size and equipment of these stations: in wealthier areas, particularly in agricultural areas along the eastern coastal region, facilities are substantial and include equipment such as X-ray machines; in the poorer counties, there may be little more than a sparsely furnished room with no equipment. In the mid-1980s over half of these rural stations were privately operated by village doctors and only 4 percent were supported by the state (Ministry of Public Health 1986). In 1986, among the 7.38 million villages in China, there were approximately 6.48 million primary health stations (Liang and Gu 1989, 277).

The village doctor, sometimes referred to as a "barefoot" doctor, is typically a peasant with a primary school education, receiving three to six months of medical training and qualified to treat minor diseases and injuries. He also oversees local public health workers.

The term "barefoot" doctor derives from the fact that many of them are peasants who dress and live much like the rural peasants. In 1986, there were estimated to be 12.8 million village doctors (Liang and Gu 1989, 277). Herbal medicine and traditional measures like acupuncture are widespread and low cost measures are administered by these barefoot doctors as well as by the primary health care stations. However, the decollectivization of agriculture has been accompanied by a decline in the number of village health clinics and barefoot doctors–now called "countryside doctors." Between 1975, the year with the highest number of barefoot doctors, and 1986, the number of barefoot doctors declined by 18 percent and the total number of brigade health personnel declined by more than 50 percent (Henderson 1990, 271).

Nursemaids (*bao mu*) are semiskilled workers in health care who are hired by families to take care of a bedridden person either in the hospital or at home. To keep hospital costs low, nursing staffing is limited, and it is expected that family members will be present at the bedside of the sick relative most of the time. To relieve the family burden, the family may hire nursemaids to perform this task; and they are also hired for in-home care of the bedridden.

Some rural areas have adopted the *bao hu zu* (voluntary nursing service) in which supervised in-home care is done by neighbor volunteers who are sometimes paid minimally for their services. In many small villages, a local committee signs a "guaranteed community service agreement with nearby neighbors, schools, or other service units to provide certain services such as delivery of groceries, medicines, or coal, and regular monitoring of the health status of frail childless elders" (Zhu 1990, 2-3).

As a reflection of the dual economy, health services in rural areas are not as advanced as in urban areas. In 1986, the number of hospital beds per 1,000 persons in rural areas was 1.54, compared to 4.48 in urban areas, nearly three times as many (Henderson 1990, 270). Hospitals are generally a unit of the county, and care is primarily for short-term and acute illnesses. Patients who cannot be adequately treated at the primary health care stations in the *xiang* (township) are sent to the county hospital.

The services described here are designed primarily to supplement family care for the frail and chronically ill elderly. This situation is changing under the economic reforms brought about in the early 1980s; the change, however, is toward reduced health services in rural areas, increased costs, and fragmented programs of health insurance from one rural area to another (Henderson 1990). Retrenchment places more responsibility on the family unit.

The major exception to these trends in health care for frail elders in rural areas is the policy toward the childless elderly. The policy has two parts: the *wu bao hu,* five guarantee households (described earlier), and *jing lao yuan,* homes for the aged (Zhang 1986). During the last ten years, thousands of homes for the aged have been built. The government reported an increase from 7825 homes in 1978 to 33,295 in 1986 (*Shehui Baozhang Bao* 1987). These homes serve as a symbol to rural families that, should they have no one to care for them in old age, the community will provide that care. As others have noted, these homes also function to reinforce the one-child policy by reassuring young families who fear that having only one child will increase their risk of having no one to provide for them in their old age (Olson 1987; Ikels 1990a; Davis-Friedmann 1985a; Zhang 1986).

Criteria for admission to a home are that the person (1) has no living children near enough to provide care; (2) is not bedridden or requiring constant medical care; (3) is willing to enter the home; and (4) qualifies for local welfare assistance (*wu bao*). Typically, a local committee monitors the status of older childless persons and determines when "the time has come" for them to be admitted to the local *jing lao yuan.* A committee member who knows the person visits with them and suggests the idea; typically it takes a few visits to get them to "come around" to seeing that it is best to be in the home. Once in the home, should long-term hospitalization or medical care be needed, the person is sent to a county hospital.

The China National Committee on Aging, a governmental unit, has been engaged in a campaign to promote the establishment of *jing lao yuan* in every rural township throughout China (Olson 1988, 253-254). Yet even though it is national government policy to develop supports for childless elders, the financing of these measures is left largely to the local governmental unit. Each township is expected to design, build, administer, and maintain a *jing lao yuan.* The typical *jing lao yuan* contains 15 to 25 living units usually arranged in a motel-like configuration, L- or U-shaped, is single storied, and, depending on climate, includes covered or enclosed walkways. Each unit consists of one room furnished with a bed, nightstand, wash stand, chair, and dresser. The dwelling is occupied by one person, except in cases of married couples. Toilet and bathing facilities are communal, segregated by sex. A common room functions as both dining center and recreation center. Many facilities have vegetable and flower gardens and interested residents garden for pleasure; but vegetable gardens are also operated to provide food for the residents. In many cases light industry, such as the raising of rabbits or the production of commercial products, results in income for the home and serves as a reminder of the "regeneration through one's own efforts" policy that characterizes the rural social service system. A doctor and one or more nurses are on duty to tend to illnesses or accidents that may occur, and a clinic facility is available, in which are practiced Western medicine, acupuncture, and herbal medicine. Round-the-clock staff provide minor nursing care, personal grooming such as haircuts, laundry service, meals, cleaning, and recreation programming. Some homes have a reading room supplied with local newspapers, magazines, and some books. Periodic trips are planned to nearby towns for personal shopping and recreation such as a movie.

In terms of urban areas, fragmentary data from a number of small-scale surveys performed in different cities in China give some hint of the magnitude of long-term care issues for the urban aged. A study done in Shanghai in 1985 indicates that the proportion of those needing long-term care increases with age (Yu et al. 1989). For those over age 75, 10.5 percent can engage in activities only with help, and 10.3 percent of all women over age 65 have severe cognitive impairment (Table 1).

Some researchers believe that perceived health status is yet another measure of the degree to which a population may be described as needing long-term care. From the Shanghai study, the proportion of those who perceived themselves to be in poor health was nearly one-fifth of the total population aged 75 and over. A 1987 study done in Guangzhou shows that of those with self-reported impairments, half or more of those over age 85 indicated

TABLE 1. Health status in Shanghai, 1985.

CATEGORY	55-64	65-74	75 & OVER
PHYSICAL HEALTH: PERCEIVED AS POOR	11.4%	16.0%	19.5%
CAN DO PERSONAL CARE W/OUT HELP	98.7%	96.0%	85.0%
CAN DO MOBILE ACTIVITIES ONLY WITH HELP	.7%	1.8%	10.5%
SEVERE COGNITIVE IMPAIRMENT:			
MEN	4.1%	6.9% (65 AND OVER)	
WOMEN	N.A.	10.3% (65 AND OVER)	

Source: Yu et al. 1989

moderate or major impairments in vision, mobility, and mental functioning (Table 2).

Although there are special provisions of welfare and health assistance from the State to certain groups of those urban elders needing long-term care, including the childless, nonstate employees, and others who are a small proportion of the population, the majority of assistance to urban elders comes through direct assistance plans from an individual's work unit (*dan wei*), or community unit, the Street Station (*jia dao*). All employees of the state, which includes those persons in most work units in the cities in addition to government office employees, are covered by health insurance, which continues into retirement. Though this insurance covers most medical care, it does not provide for long-term care. In 1986, this program was changed through the addition of a copayment, ranging from 5 to 10 percent, for medication and hospitalization; several expensive procedures were no longer covered (Ikels 1990a, 280). This policy has led to a shift of a greater share of medical costs to the users. Disabilities that force workers to retire prior to retirement

TABLE 2. Impairment of Urban Elderly, Guangzhou

THOSE REPORTING MODERATE OR MAJOR IMPAIRMENT

AGE	VISUAL	MOBILITY	MENTAL
70-74	9%	15%	2%
75-79	25	25	0
80-84	22	64	40
85 & OVER	50	92	62

Source: Ikels 1990a; adapted from a survey of 100 elders in Guangzhou in 1987.

age are compensated for by both a retirement pension and a stipend to employ a *bao mu*. The amount of money depends on the length of employment by the disabled worker, but it is a lifetime guarantee (Davis-Friedmann 1985b, 306). Except for the addition of a copayment, recent analyses indicate that there have been only minor changes in medical care benefits for retired workers during the 1980s (Liu 1990, 20).

Yet economic reforms during the 1980s that have led to a reduction of health care services for rural elders have resulted in increased services to urban elders. Greater growth in hospital construction, in high-tech equipment such as CT scanners, and in the number of health care personnel have occurred during the late 1980s (Henderson 1990, 269-271).

Long-term care in urban areas for the childless has basically two components: (1) social welfare institutes (operated by the Bureau of Civil Affairs) where frail, bedridden elders needing total care live permanently; and (2) community-based in-home care (*bao hu zhu*) (Liang and Gu 1989; Sankar 1989; Zhu 1990).

Social welfare institutes vary in size, function, and financing depending on the city. As shown in Table 3, Shanghai has a well-developed set of facilities compared to Beijing and Tianjin. The overall rate of growth of these facilities has not been significant; in 1978 there were 577 homes and in 1985 the number had risen to 752. However, the expenditure per capita did rise significantly from 553 yuan in 1978 to 1782 yuan by 1985 (Liu 1989, 113), but much of this increase may be accounted for by inflation.

Urban welfare institutes, the counterpart of the rural *jing lao yuan,* provide the same kind of services although their physical plants are very different. The urban facilities are often multistoried, and also function as long-term care centers for totally bedridden elders and for those requiring continuous physical care. Usually residents who are bedridden and require continuous care live on the upper floors, are served meals in their rooms, and seldom leave their floor. Residents on the lower floor are fully ambulatory, well, and reside there permanently. Normally they live three or four to a room. The same services found in rural homes are also available in these facilities; but the average number of residents is greater. Some urban facilities resemble their rural counterparts in other ways. For example, some are single storied, and some operate money making enterprises, the income from which is used to offset expenses of operating the facility.

Community-based in-home care in urban areas is developing rapidly. Under this program, the Street Station (*jia dao*) has responsibility for administering the funds it receives from the municipal government and dispersing them to the Resident's Committees that serve local neighborhoods. These local Resident's Committees identify childless elders and others needing in-home care and train and supervise a person who is assigned to regularly visit, prepare meals, run errands, notify the doctor, and in other ways attend to the needs of the homebound elder. This system, called *bao-hu zu,* has been operating since the early 1980s (Olson 1987, 291-292; Liang and Gu 1989, 274), but has grown dramatically during the late 1980s. According to one set of data, there were 36,000 persons in 1986 looking after 66,000 persons; by 1988 these had grown to 54,000 caring for 88,000 older persons (Zhu 1990, 1). The kinds of services vary from short-term volunteer in-home care to exchanges between household units in which the elder provides household

TABLE 3. Social welfare institutes in three cities, 1985.

City	No. of Institutes	Funds (1000 Y)	Number of Elderly
Beijing	6	2169	416
Tianjin	7	1987	416
Shanghai	15	4031	1598

Source: Liu, W. 1989b:114

services to a younger working family in return for which the elder receives care during times of illness (Zhu 1990, 2; Liang and Gu 1989, 274).

In addition to the welfare institutes and the *bao-hu zu,* frail elders are cared for through a variety of other means. There are organized efforts of students, military personnel, factory employees, and local government employees to provide such assistance as home repair, carrying of heavy supplies, and home decorating (Olson 1987, 287-288; Liang and Gu 1989, 274). Another approach, one that is relatively new, is the "home-based sick bed" (Henderson 1990, 290). A medical care organization, such as a hospital, designates the sick bed. The designation of sick bed means that services, under the management of a doctor, are provided to the elder in his or her own home. Elders seeking medical care at a neighborhood clinic or hospital will be designated, after having been examined, as eligible for a home sick bed if they are not sick enough for in-hospital care, but too sick to be sent home with only medicine. The practice is designed primarily for persons with chronic illnesses, those who are convalescing, or those who need rehabilitation. Services offered in the sick bed system include drug therapy, physical therapy, nutrition, exams, mental health counseling, and traditional Chinese treatments (Liang and Gu 1989, 277). The number of sick beds in operation rose from 490,000 in 1984 to 831,000 in 1986 (Liang and Gu 1989, 277). Of major significance is the cost savings; reports of savings of 37 to 57 percent over hospital beds have been reported.

Other newly emerging strategies for addressing issues of frail elders are the *bao mu,* elder-care centers, and additional family-oriented policies. The *bao mu,* or nursemaid discussed earlier, offers a low-cost approach to in-home care in urban areas (Ikels 1990b, 234). Elder-care centers are another new approach being developed in Guangzhou and Linghai (Ikels 1990b, 240). They are residential facilities for ambulatory elders not needing medical care. In terms of policies oriented specifically toward the family as a source of care, a study cited by Sankar (1989, 213-214) describes a new policy directed toward family caregiving of elders: college graduates who are only-children are placed in jobs in the same city, physically near their parents so they will be available as caregivers when needed. Recent evidence points to one other alternative to long-term care that places emphasis on the family rather than on the state, and that is encouragement to widows and widowers to remarry. Begun in the mid-1980s, this approach, though not universally accepted, is growing in urban areas (Ikels 1990a, 238).

CONCLUSION

Policies of elder care in the People's Republic of China have undergone significant changes during the regime of the Chinese Communist Party. Undergirding these changes are the traditional strength of the family unit and its function of providing social, economic, and emotional supports to its members. The modernization now underway and the attendant policies toward population containment, bureaucratic and party reform, and economic reform appear to be having a significant impact on the role and care of the elderly population (Olson 1988). These reforms, together with the growth in the proportion of elderly, have an impact on how the society addresses the issues of long-term care and other issues surrounding an increasing frail population.

The evidence available from China suggests that the dominant policy addressing the growing proportion of frail elders centers on minimizing the role of the state and constraining the growth of costly medical treatment programs. However, there continue to be policy suggestions that focus on the centrality of the family in elder care in partnership with the state. In a recent symposium on aging it was proposed that "while giving full play to the functions of family care for the aged, we should. . . perfect such care . . . by combining the state, collective, and family . . . " (Wei and Hu 1989). There is a hint in this proposal that the state will have to assume a larger role in the future of elder care.

Nonetheless, as long as the major responsibility for elder care is placed on the family, the community and the work unit, the political system defines the responsibility for frail elders primarily as residing in the social system and secondarily as a responsibility of the state-operated medical care system. In so doing, economic resources are directed toward economic growth and increases in the standard of living, especially in urban areas. The policy of reducing the burden to the state in elder care is reflected in several initiatives now underway: (1) adopting a copayment plan in medical benefit programs; (2) targeting only special elders (the rural childless and urban influentials) for benefits; (3) encouraging family obligations; and (4) encouraging elders to be resources to their families and communities (Ikels 1990b, 221-222).

Other analysts have made similar observations which indicate the emphasis on local or community initiatives to address the issue of elder care. Jia (1988) gives an example of rural initiatives now underway in China which relieve the State of the economic burden of care for elders. She reports efforts in one village to establish a local pension system for its retirees based on voluntary contributions from workers. Zhang (1986) identifies efforts in rural communities to expand local retirement systems for elders, to institute old-age insurance programs, and to promote bank savings for older workers. To the degree that the state does play a role in elder-care, and this is almost entirely in urban areas, it is done largely through increases in the number of hospitals, training of more doctors, a stabilized pension system, and a cost-effective medical insurance program.

The direction of these initiatives remains to be seen, and the decade of the 1990s will reveal more clearly how far the state will shift its policy away from local care of frail elders to a centralized program and whether the differences in rural and urban long-term care practices will grow or disappear. In addition, the question of the future of state policy is complicated by recent, mounting evidence from research during the last decade suggesting that although elders still live predominantly with other family members, that proportion is declining (Goldstein, Ku, and Ikels 1990). Several studies performed in both rural and urban settings point to more elders living alone, including one study, done in Lanzhou (Yue 1986), which found that nearly half of the women over age 65 preferred to live separately from their married children. The question raised is to what degree, if at all, the increase in independent living will contribute to erosion of the family as the principal long-term care unit.

It seems clear, to the degree changes such as that noted above occur in the structure of the family, that there will have to be changes in the long-term care practices for frail elders. This does not mean, of course, that there are simple cause-effect relations between family systems and elder care, but rather that there are complex interrelated social systems that change in some discernible pattern. However, the complex interrelations among (1) the traditional values of the family, (2) the economic reform programs, (3) the thrust of the political agenda, and (4) the differences between the rural and urban social and economic systems make predictions difficult. An increased understanding of future elder care practices will require a careful watch on the family, economy, and political system.

REFERENCES

An, Z. 1982. "Reforming the Cadre System." *Beijing Review* 25 (9):3-4.

Baker, H. 1979. *Chinese Family and Kinship*. New York: Columbia University Press.

Banister, J. 1988. "The Aging of China's Population." *Problems of Communism* 37:(6) 62-77.

Bianco, L. 1981. "Birth Control in China: Local Data and Their Reliability." *China Quarterly* 85:119-37.

Chai, C., and Chai W. 1969. *The Changing Society of China*. New York: Mentor.

Chen, X. 1985. "The One-Child Population Policy, Modernization, and the Extended Chinese Family." *Journal of Marriage and the Family* 47:193-202.

Cherry, R., and Magnuson-Martinson, S. 1981. "Modernization and the Status of the Aged in China: Decline or Equalization?" *Sociological Quarterly* 22: 253-61.

China News Analysis. 1983. "Socialist China, Social Policy and the Elderly." 1257 (March 26):1-8.

Cowgill, D. O. 1986. *Aging Around the World.* Belmont, CA: Wadsworth.

Davis, D. 1989. "Chinese Social Welfare: Policies and Outcomes." *China Quarterly* 119 (September): 577-597.

Davis-Friedmann, D. 1981. "Retirement and Social Welfare Programs for Chinese Elderly: A Minimal Role for the State." In *The Situation of the Asian/Pacific Elderly,* edited by Nusberg, C. and Osako, M. Washington: International Federation on Aging, 52-65.

_____. 1983. *Long Lives.* Cambridge: Harvard University Press.

_____. 1984. "The Provision of Essential Services in Rural China." In *Rural Public Services,* edited by Lonsdale, R. Boulder: Westview Press, 205-224.

_____. 1985a. "Old Age Security and the One-child Campaign." In *China's One Child Family Policy,* edited by Croll, E., Davin, D., and Kane, P. London: Macmillan, 149-161.

_____. 1985b. "Chinese Retirement: Policy and Practice." *Current Perspectives on Aging and the Life Cycle.* 1:295-313.

Deng, X. 1983. "On the Reform of the System of Party and State Leadership." *Beijing Review* 25 (9):3-4.

Ding, H. 1984. "Glorious Retirement of 813,000 Veteran Cadres Throughout the Country." *Chinese Elderly* 11:9.

Dixon, J. 1981. *The Chinese Welfare System.* New York: Praeger.

Estes, C.; Gerard, L.; Zones, J.; and Swan, J. 1984. *Political Economy, Health, and Aging.* Boston: Little, Brown.

Freedman, M. 1961. "The Family in China, Past and Present." *Pacific Affairs* 34:326-36.

Ganshaw, T. 1978. "The Aged in A Revolutionary Milieu: China." In *Aging and the Elderly: Humanistic Perspectives in Gerontology,* edited by S. Spicker, K. Woodward, and D. Van Tasel. Atlantic Highlands, NJ: Humanities.

Goldstein, M., Ku, Y.; and Ikels, C. 1990. "Household Composition of the Elderly in Two Rural Villages in the People's Republic of China." *Journal of Cross-Cultural Gerontology* 5.

Henderson, G. 1990. "Increased Inequality in Health Care." In *Chinese Society on the Eve of Tiananmen,* edited by Davis, D. and Vogel, E. Cambridge: The Council on East Asian Studies/Harvard University, 263-282.

Hu, T. 1984. "Health Services in the People's Republic of China." In *Comparative Health Systems,* edited by Raffel, M. University Park, PA: Pennsylvania State University Press, 141-152.

Ikels, C. 1975. "Old Age in Hong Kong." *The Gerontologist* 15:230-35.

_____. 1990a. "Family Caregivers and the Elderly in China." In *Aging and Caregiving,* edited by Biegel, D. and Blum, A. Beverly Hills: Sage Publications, 270-284.

_____. 1990b. "New Options for the Urban Elderly." In *Chinese Society on the Eve of Tiananmen,* edited by Davis, D. and Vogel, E. Cambridge: The Council on East Asian Studies/Harvard University, 215-242.

Jamison, D.; Evans, J.; and King, T. 1984. *China: The Health Sector.* A World Bank Country Study. Washington, DC: The World Bank.

Jia, A. 1988. "New Experiments with Elderly Care in Rural China." *Journal of Cross Cultural Gerontology* 3 (2):139-148.

Kallgren, D. 1985. "Politics, Welfare, and Change: The Single-Child Family in China." In *The Political Economy of Reform in Post-Mao China,* edited by Perry, E. and Wong, C. Cambridge: Harvard University Press, 131-156.

Kinoy, S. 1979. "Services to the Aging in the People's Republic of China." In *Reaching the Aged, Social Services in Forty-four Countries,* edited by Teicher, M., Thursz, D. and Vigilante, J. Beverly Hills: Sage, 69-83.

Leslie, G. 1979. *The Family in Social Context,* 4th ed. New York: Oxford University Press.

Liang, J., and Gu, S. 1989. "Long-Term Care for the Elderly in China." In *Caring for an Aging World: International Models for Long-Term Care, Financing, and Delivery,* edited by Schwab, T. NY: McGraw-Hill, 265-287.

Lipton, M. 1977. *Why Poor People Stay Poor.* London: Temple Smith.

Liu, A. 1986. *How China is Ruled.* Englewood Cliffs, NJ: Prentice Hall.

_____. 1990. "Social Security for State-Sector Workers in the People's Republic of China: The Reform Decade and Beyond." Unpublished paper.

Liu, W., ed. 1989. *China Social Statistics 1986.* Compiled by the State Statistical Bureau of the People's Republic of China. The China Statistics Series. New York: Praeger.

Mao, Z. 1969. "The Dead Still Rule Today." In *The Political Thought of Mao Tse-Tung,* edited by S. Schram. New York: Praeger, 368.

Ministry of Public Health. 1986. *1985 Chinese Health Yearbook.* Beijing: Chinese Health Press.

Myles, J. 1984. *Old Age in the Welfare State.* Boston: Little, Brown.

Oksenberg, M. 1982. "Economic Policy-making in China: Summer 1981." *China Quarterly* 90:165-94.

Olson, P. 1987. "A Model of Eldercare in the People's Republic of China." *International Journal of Aging and Human Development* 24:279-300.

_____. 1988. "Modernization in the People's Republic of China: The Politicization of the Elderly." *Sociological Quarterly* 29:241-62.

Parish, W. 1975. "Socialism and the Chinese Peasant Family." *Journal of Asian Studies* 34:613-30.

Poston, D., and Gu, B. 1984. "Socioeconomic Differentials and Fertility in the Provinces, Municipalities and Autonomous Regions of the People's Republic of China, Circa-1982." *Texas Population Research Center Papers.* Series 6: Paper No. 6.011. Austin: University of Texas.

Sankar, A. 1981. "The Conquest of Solitude: Singlehood and Old Age in Traditional Chinese Society." In *Dimensions: Aging, Culture, and Health,* edited by Fry, C. New York: Praeger, 65-83.

_____. 1989. "Gerontological Research in China: The Role of Anthropological Inquiry." *Journal of Cross Cultural Gerontology* 4:199-224.

Saith, A. 1981. "Economic Incentives for the One-child Family in Rural China." *China Quarterly* 87:492-500.

Shehui Baozhang Bao (Social Security News). Untitled News Release. April 10, 1987 (No. 54), 1.

Skocpol, T. 1985. "Bringing the State Back In: Strategies of Analysis in Current Research." In *Bringing the State Back In,* edited by Evans, P., Rueschemeyer, D. and Skocpol, T. New York: Cambridge University Press, 3-37.

Szelenyi, I. 1983. *Urban Inequalities Under State Socialism.* NY: Oxford University Press.

Tien, Y. 1977. "How China Treats its Old People." *Asian Profile* 5:1-7.

Treas, J. 1979. "Socialist Organization and Economic Development in China: Latent Consequences for the Aged." *The Gerontologist* 19:34-42.

Treas, J., and Logue, B. 1986. "Economic Development and the Older Population." *Population and Development Review* 12 (4): 645-673.

Wei, H., and Hu, R. 1989. *International Symposium on Aging: Policy Issues and Future Challenges.* Proceedings. Beijing: China National Committee on Aging.

Whyte, M., and Parish, W. 1984. *Urban Life in Contemporary China.* Chicago: University of Chicago Press.

Wolf, A. 1986. "The Preeminent Role of Government Intervention in China's Family Revolution." *Population and Development Review* 12 (1): 101-116.

Woon, Y. 1981. "Growing Old in a Modernizing China." *Journal of Comparative Family Studies* 12:245-55.

Yin, P., and Lai, K. 1983. "A Reconceptualization of Age Stratification in China." *Journal of Gerontology* 38:608-13.

Yu, E.; Liu, W.; Levy, P.; and Zhang, M. 1989. "Cognitive Impairment Among Elderly Adults in Shanghai, China." *Journal of Gerontology: Social Sciences* 44 (3):S97-106.

Yuan F. 1987. "The Status and Roles of the Elderly Chinese in The Families and Society." *Journal of Beijing University* (Philosophy and Social Sciences) No. 3: 1-8.

Yue, Qing. 1986. "Family Changes and Trends in Lanzhou." *Xibei Renkou* [*Northwest Population*] 3:8-12.

Zhang, C. 1986. "Welfare Provisions for the Aged in Rural China." *Australian Journal of Chinese Affairs.* No. 15:113-124.

Zhao, S. 1987. "The Retirement of Veteran Cadres in China: Its Causes and Impact on Elderly Chinese." M.A. thesis. Kansas City: University of Missouri-Kansas City.

Zhu, C. 1990. "Community Service with Chinese Characteristics–Guaranteed Community Service." Unpublished paper.

Chapter 12

The Elderly in Yugoslavia:
A Forgotten Group in Time of Crisis

James H. Seroka

INTRODUCTION

In the period from 1988-90 there have been epochal changes in the political, economic, and social systems of Eastern Europe. In each East European state, with the exception of Albania, there have been dramatic changes in the structure and composition of the decision-making apparatus. Single-party dictatorships of the proletariat have been replaced by multi-party parliamentary democracies. Planned economies have been abandoned for the creativity and apparent chaos of the free market. Overall, the entire network of social institutions has been abandoned or transformed.

Nevertheless, through all these revolutionary changes, the new governments and movements have kept faith with the major underpinnings of socialist social policy, including policy toward children, the aged, and the infirm. These policies have remained virtually intact, despite the huge economic and social burdens they incur. In addition, no significant political movement in any of these emerging regimes has advocated dismantlement, abandonment, or even drastic retrenchment of such programs for the elderly, young, or infirm.

Yugoslavia, like its neighboring socialist republics, formulated and implemented a program for the material well-being of the elderly population. This program, however, had been decentralized among Yugoslavia's six republics and two provinces since the early 1970s. Decentralization, although contributing to inequalities in services and protection, did permit experimentation and programmatic flexibility. Thus, social policy for the elderly in Yugoslavia could be adapted to local situations.

We must remember that Yugoslavia is a poor nation and that its per capita income ranks among the lowest in Europe. Significantly, however, Yugoslavia is a nation with large income and productivity inequalities among the republics and provinces. A worker in the primarily Albanian-speaking province of Kosovo, for example, earns on average only 40 percent of the income of a worker in the republic of Slovenia; and if one were to compare per capita income between the two regions, the ratio would be at least five to one in favor of the Slovenian resident (Savezni Zavod za Statistiku 1989).[1] To make matters worse, during the last decade, income inequalities among the republic and provinces have been growing, as illustrated in Table 1.

In addition to growing income inequalities, Yugoslavia, like the other nations in East Central Europe, has been experiencing a marked deterioration in the living standards of the population and gross domestic product of the nation. Until 1989, the national hard currency debt for Yugoslavia hovered around $1,000 (U.S.) per capita, an enormous sum considering that this debt nearly equalled the annual gross personal income of the nation. In 1988, real personal income per worker was only 70 percent of the income of 1978; and in 1989, it is estimated that the real income per worker had fallen to the level reached in 1965 (Savezni Zavod za Statistiku 1989, 161). The immense hardships imposed by the decline in income and production, as well as real living standards were even greater than those experienced in Western Europe and the United States during the Great Depression of the 1930s. Moreover, the active population (i.e., the proportion of the population employed) had dropped from 49 percent in 1948 to 44 percent in 1981; this decline represents the overall aging of the population, increased unemployment, and the extension of the duration of education for the young.

The strain that the economic crisis placed on the maintenance of

TABLE 1. Index level of net personal income per worker 1983-1988 by republic and province (Yugoslavia = 100).

YEAR						
REPUBLIC/ PROVINCE	1983	1984	1985	1986	1987	1988
Bosnia-Hercegovina	95	93	91	87	84	84
Montenegro	84	81	79	81	74	73
Croatia	109	108	107	107	107	109
Macedonia	83	79	73	70	69	68
Slovenia	115	122	135	145	156	152
Serbia (Proper)	95	94	93	93	90	91
Kosovo	81	78	77	73	69	66
Vojvodina	102	102	97	92	91	96
Yugoslavia (Total)	100	100	100	100	100	100

Source: Savezni Zavod za Statistiku. *Statisticki Godisnjak Jugoslavije 1989.* (Belgrade: Savezni zavod za statistiku), 1989, p. 475.

social welfare programs fell disproportionately across the republics and provinces. In the poorest regions, such as Kosovo and Montenegro, a single actively employed person supports 2 to 3 non-employed individuals, and the disparity among republics and provinces also has been growing over time (Table 2). In Kosovo, less than 24 percent of the population in the 1981 census was actively

TABLE 2. Percent of population actively engaged in the economy, 1948-1981, by republic and province.

YEAR					
REPUBLIC/ PROVINCE	1948	1953	1961	1971	1981
Bosnia- Hercegovina	42.9	42.5	39.2	36.7	38.7
Montenegro	36.9	36.4	34.3	32.7	34.3
Croatia	51.6	47.7	47.0	45.5	45.6
Macedonia	43.4	40.8	39.4	38.3	41.8
Slovenia	52.9	48.0	48.3	48.4	50.3
Serbia (Proper)	54.2	52.4	51.1	51.5	51.8
Kosovo	35.3	33.2	34.8	26.0	23.8
Vojvodina	49.4	45.4	44.0	42.7	44.3
Yugoslavia (Total)	49.1	46.3	45.0	43.3	44.0

Source: Savezni Zavod za Statistiku. *Statisticki Godisnjak Jugoslavije 1989.* (Belgrade: Savezni Zavod za Statistiku), 1989, p. 453.

participating in the economy, compared to slightly over 50 percent in Slovenia.

Among the former socialist states, Yugoslavia is characterized by a unique theoretical approach to social policy making; namely, self-management. The intended purpose of self-management is to transfer responsibility and power from the state to the work community. Ideally, the system intended to put power to make decisions— ranging from the distribution of income to the selection of leaders—in the hands of the workers at each work unit. Theoretically, the workers, through an institution called the "self-managed interest of the community" (i.e., SIZ) decided where to place their social welfare funds.

For general social policy decision making, self-management meant a limited public choice model through which various social services would compete among themselves for resources from the work units. Most social policy institutions were guaranteed a minimum contribution from the firm, but it was still necessary to solicit additional support to fulfill one's social welfare responsibilities. In the 1980s, as the economy worsened and as inflation picked up in tempo, the competition intensified among the social welfare providers for the increasingly scarce and diminishing resources. In practice, the health, education, rehabilitation, elderly, and other social welfare interests competed with one another for the distribution of an increasingly smaller income.

As could be expected, the process was frustrating both to the social welfare interests and to the work-place providers. Over time the system became increasingly politicized, and those groups with a strong constituency in the work place generally triumphed over others with weaker constituencies. Needless to say, inequalities in levels of service among the republics and provinces become more pronounced with time. With the 1000 percent annual inflation of the late 1980s, however, the competitive system collapsed and a more responsible framework may be emerging. Beyond doubt, the unrestrained, quasi-free market, competitive environment for social welfare funds contributed to the rejection of the socialist self-management model in Yugoslavia and the rejection of a one-party communist state.

PROFILE OF THE ELDERLY IN YUGOSLAVIA

The demographic structure and relative position of the aged in Yugoslavia have changed remarkably in the period since the end of the second World War.[2] In 1948, the population age structure of Yugoslavia resembled the classical pyramid. Only 5.58 percent of the population was 65 years of age or older, and only 1.66 was age 75 or older. This is contrasted to 32.6 percent of the population which was under 15 years of age. By 1981, the percentage of the 65 and over age cohort increased by 63 percent to constitute 9.1 percent of the population, and the proportion of those aged 75 or more nearly doubled to 3.1 percent of the total population. Meanwhile, the percentage of those under 15 years of age had dropped 25 percent to 24.47 percent of the total (Savezni Zavod za Statistiku 1989, 129).

Over the long-term, the situation will become more acute. The expectations for the 1991 census project an increase in the proportion of the elderly population (i.e., age 60 or more) to 14 percent of the national total in 1990 and over 16 percent in the year 2000 (Socialist Federal Republic of Yugoslavia 1987). In addition, the fall in the birth rate and rise in life expectancy for Yugoslavs (68 years for males and 73 for females) should alter the demographic pyramid even more radically into the twenty-first century.

Considerable variation in population structure exists among the republics as well. Kosovo, for example, still maintains the traditional pyramidical population structure of an underdeveloped region. In the 1981 census, only 4.6 percent of the Kosovan population was aged 65 or more. This contrasts with the republic of Croatia, which had recorded 11.6 percent of the population in the age 65 or higher cohort. By the year 2000, republics such as Croatia and Serbia are expected to have 20 percent or more of their population in the elderly cohort (aged 60 or more), compared to only 7 percent in Kosovo (Table 3).

The implications for macro-social policy among the Yugoslav republics are clear and ominous. Those republics with an expanding aged cohort are also the more economically advanced regions. As these governments devote proportionately more of their surplus income to care for the elderly, there will be much less available to redistribute to the poorer republics and provinces. Thus, regional income inequality is perpetuated and potential social conflicts among the regions are exacerbated. Inequality, even among the population structure, inevitably becomes a source of political conflict in a plural society such as Yugoslavia.

The elderly in Yugoslavia differ from the general population in a number of significant ways. This cohort tends to be poorer, less educated and disproportionately rural, with a significant number

TABLE 3. Share of aged population (in percent) over 60 years of age in total population, 1921-2000, by republic and province.

REPUBLIC/ PROVINCE	YEAR					
	1921	1953	1971	1981	1990	2000
Bosnia-Hercegovina	5.6	5.2	7.7	8.3	9.6	12.8
Montenegro	9.8	10.4	11.0	10.7	11.6	14.4
Croatia	8.8	10.2	14.9	14.9	16.8	19.6
Macedonia	11.1	8.2	8.8	9.2	10.6	12.3
Slovenia	14.4	11.1	14.8	14.6	15.2	17.1
Serbia (Proper)	8.5	8.9	13.6	13.2	17.3	20.8
Kosovo	9.7	7.6	7.1	6.4	6.3	7.1
Vojvodina	9.7	10.7	14.8	14.8	18.1	21.3

Source: Dusan Breznik, "Demographic process of aging with special reference to the situation in Yugoslavia." First Gerontological Congress of Yugoslavia, Belgrade, 1977, pp. 138-139.

involved in agriculture. The elderly literally represent a rural peasant Yugoslavia that is gradually disappearing from view. Of the 9 percent of the population that is aged 65 or older, 33 percent live in agricultural areas, compared to 20 percent of the population as a whole. According to the 1981 census, the aged (i.e., 65 or older) constitute 15.8 percent of the total population in rural communities, and their relative share of the rural population is growing (Table 4). In Croatia, the aged represent less than 12 percent of the population, but constitute more than 20 percent of the agricultural population. In Slovenia, where the agricultural population is only 9 percent, the elderly constitute 17 percent of that group. In Macedonia, 33 percent of the aged are in agriculture, compared to 22 percent of the population as a whole.

The decade of the 1980s saw an intensification of the rural isolation of the elderly. Many villages in Dalmatia, for example, appear to be inhabited solely by the elderly. As the productivity of those communities decline with an increase in the average age of their population, these communities become increasingly isolated and unattractive to younger, more energetic age cohorts. Thus, the traditional system whereby the children would support the elderly has collapsed as the younger cohorts have abandoned the villages for an urbanized life style. In Yugoslavia, the rate of urbanization has been precipitous. In 1948, 67.2 percent of the population lived in villages. By 1981, the percentage had dropped to 19.9 percent. Increasingly, the elderly have been left behind in communities where the death rate exceeds the birth rate by as much as 50 percent.

Aged citizens in these rural areas are often involved in subsistence agriculture. They generally lack most basic social services such as health care and sewage, and they have little or no access to public transportation or to urban services.

Yugoslavia's self-management institutions have been very slow to respond to the problems of the rural elderly. Before 1986, for example, Serbian peasants were not included in the system of social security (Markovic 1985). Medical care in many areas is nonexistent and the delivery of social services for the elderly are very dispersed and not readily available. In the rural commune of Donji Lapac, Croatia, an area of 606 square kilometers with 33 settlements and 8,447 people, there were only four doctors and no hospital facilities in 1981. Sadly, the situation in Donji Lapac is typical for much of rural Yugoslavia where the needs of the rural elderly have been neglected.

The republics of Yugoslavia have a well-developed system of pension and income supplements for the retired. While the specifics vary by republic, a retired individual is guaranteed a pension based on household size and the average monthly income of a worker in the commune (i.e., county) in which the individual resides. A large

TABLE 4. Comparative share of aged and rural populations (in percent), 1981, by republic and province.

REPUBLIC/ PROVINCE	MEASURE (IN PERCENT)			
	RURAL TOTAL	AGED TOTAL	AGED % IN RURAL TOTAL	% OF AGED IN RURAL AREAS
Bosnia-Hercegovina	17.3	6.1	11.3	30.8
Montenegro	13.5	8.3	13.4	21.3
Croatia	15.2	11.5	20.4	25.9
Macedonia	21.7	6.7	10.9	33.3
Slovenia	9.4	11.6	17.1	14.2
Serbia (Proper)	27.6	10.0	18.7	49.4
Kosovo	24.6	4.6	6.6	34.7
Vojvodina	19.9	11.3	18.9	32.2

Source: Savezni Zavod za Statistiku. *Statisticki Godisnjak Jugoslavije 1989.* (Belgrade: Savezni zavod za statistiku), 1989, pp. 452-456.

number of firms and institutions supplement this basic pension, thereby permitting retirees to live more comfortably. In Serbia, for example, a pensioner is guaranteed an income according to a formula which is based on the average family income in the commune computed in the previous month.[3] In those circumstances when the pensioner's firm cannot pay, the republic makes a direct contribution and utilizes those statutory provisions which require working children of the elderly to provide assistance. Retired peasants receive remuneration depending upon the market price of the commodities they would have produced, if able.

Approximately half of the aged population is covered under the Serbian social security system, and only a small fraction of those

who receive benefits derive a significant share of their
the social assistance (i.e., public welfare) provisions. O...
Yugoslavia in 1988, 66.3 percent of pension income we from
from savings or the personal income of the pension ho. in
percent was derived from the work organization, and only 5 p...
from the federation or republic (i.e., social assistance) (Posrk
1989).

Again, there is dramatic variation among the republics in their
level of support and in their legal requirements and accounting
procedures (Table 5). In Montenegro, for example, 14.7 percent of
all pension income is derived from the republics or federation,
reflecting its weak economic and industrial structure. Sixty-two
percent of pension income in Serbia is contributed by the work unit,
while only a negligible 1 percent is contributed by the work unit in
Macedonia and Slovenia.

The pension and compensation system in Yugoslavia is rapidly
approaching a crisis point. The contributing base of active workers
has increased by only 8 percent during the 1984-88 period, and the
worker base may have shrunk dramatically with the 1990 depression in the Yugoslav economy. Nevertheless, total pension holders
increased 27 percent during the 1984-88 period, which suggests that
the pension system is under increasing strain (Posrkaca 1989). In
some republics, such as Slovenia, the ratio of pension recipients to
participants in the social security fund approaches two pension
holders per five contributors (Table 6). The high pensioner/worker
ratio can have a significant negative impact on future productivity,
economic growth, and social peace.

As the current economic depression deepens in Yugoslavia, the
financial base of the pension funds becomes seriously endangered.
The work unit and state pension contributions are paid out of current revenues; and as these revenues decline, there will be mounting
pressure to avoid responsibility and to erode the level of pension
benefits. In the 1984-88 period, the typical Yugoslav firm increased
its pension burden from 15.7 percent of total firm revenue in 1984
to 19.3 percent of total firm revenue in 1988. The five year increase
in pension payments was 43 percent in Bosnia, which had 17.4

TABLE 5. Distribution of pension and worker's compensation income by source, 1988.

REPUBLIC/ PROVINCE	INCOME SOURCE			
	PERSONAL INCOME	ENTERPRISE INCOME	FEDERATION OR REPUBLIC	OTHER
Yugoslavia (Total)	66.3	28.0	5.0	0.7
Bosnia-Hercegovina	80.2	12.7	7.0	0.1
Montenegro	82.7	2.6	14.7	—
Croatia	51.6	42.9	5.4	0.1
Macedonia	91.3	1.3	4.6	2.3
Slovenia	95.4	1.3	3.0	0.3
Serbia (Proper)	33.4	62.2	3.9	0.5
Kosovo	78.0	14.0	6.4	1.6
Vojvodina	83.3	7.2	6.0	3.5

Source: Dragan Posrkaca, "Penzijsko i invalidsko osiguranje, 1984-1988," *Jugoslovenski Pregled* (July-August, 1989), p. 311.

percent of firm revenue earmarked for pensions in 1988, and 39 percent increase in Macedonia, which had 14.9 percent of firm revenue allotted to pension payments. Croatia was the republic which was most heavily burdened, with pension expenditures accounting for 23.9 percent of total enterprise revenue (Posrkaca 1989).

As is the case for nearly every aspect of Yugoslav life, the quality of one's old-age pension heavily depends upon the republic or province of origin. In 1988, old-age pensions throughout Yugoslavia equalled 86.3 percent of the average personal income (Posrkaca 1989). The low end of the range was held by Slovenia at 68.6 percent, and the high end was captured by Montenegro, whose pensioners received on average 106.2 percent of the average income for a worker in that area.[4] In 1989, a Slovenian old-age pensioner generally received a pension that was two-thirds larger than the average Yugoslav payment, while the Kosovan counterpart received a sum that was only two-thirds the size of the Yugoslav average. In Kosovo in 1989, 24 percent of the pension payments totalled 500,000 dinars or less, while fewer than 1 percent of Slovenian beneficiaries received such limited benefits (Stojakovic 1990).

There also has been a marked, narrowing gap between pension payments and worker income during the 1984-88 period. In 1984, elderly pensioners received approximately 70 percent of the average personal income of a worker, and by 1988 that figure climbed to 86.3 percent (Posrkaca 1989, 310). Throughout the 1984-88 period, the annual increase in the level of pension payments exceeded the annual increase in the cost of living and in the personal income of workers. This trend occurred in each republic and province.

The above data do not let us conclude that Yugoslav old-age pensioners live well and comfortably. Prior to 1984, pension payments were a national scandal (Zenenovic 1986). Also, the increases during the past decade have not yet given a level of assured dignity to the pension holders. It should also be noted that the narrowing of the worker-pensioner income gap actually reflects the sharp and catastrophic erosion in the standard of living of workers during the runaway inflation of the 1980s. In reality, pensioners did not improve their objective situations, but rather the living standards of the workers had worsened. Finally, the mega-inflation of 1989 had completely erased all the gains which the elderly had made during the past decade. By June 30, 1989, average pension payments in Yugoslavia dropped from 86.3 percent of average worker income to 62 percent of average worker income (*Bilten za Pitanja Zdravstenog* 1989).

To summarize, the social and economic positions of the elderly in Yugoslavia are endangered. A substantial proportion of the aged lives in rural areas and is deprived of essential health services and social amenities. In addition, the projected explosion in the numbers

TABLE 4. Comparative share of aged and rural populations (in percent), 1981, by republic and province.

MEASURE (IN PERCENT)				
REPUBLIC/ PROVINCE	RURAL TOTAL	AGED TOTAL	AGED % IN RURAL TOTAL	% OF AGED IN RURAL AREAS
Bosnia-Hercegovina	17.3	6.1	11.3	30.8
Montenegro	13.5	8.3	13.4	21.3
Croatia	15.2	11.5	20.4	25.9
Macedonia	21.7	6.7	10.9	33.3
Slovenia	9.4	11.6	17.1	14.2
Serbia (Proper)	27.6	10.0	18.7	49.4
Kosovo	24.6	4.6	6.6	34.7
Vojvodina	19.9	11.3	18.9	32.2

Source: Savezni Zavod za Statistiku. *Statisticki Godisnjak Jugoslavije 1989.* (Belgrade: Savezni zavod za statistiku), 1989, pp. 452-456.

number of firms and institutions supplement this basic pension, thereby permitting retirees to live more comfortably. In Serbia, for example, a pensioner is guaranteed an income according to a formula which is based on the average family income in the commune computed in the previous month.[3] In those circumstances when the pensioner's firm cannot pay, the republic makes a direct contribution and utilizes those statutory provisions which require working children of the elderly to provide assistance. Retired peasants receive remuneration depending upon the market price of the commodities they would have produced, if able.

Approximately half of the aged population is covered under the Serbian social security system, and only a small fraction of those who receive benefits derive a significant share of their pension from the social assistance (i.e., public welfare) provisions. On average, in Yugoslavia in 1988, 66.3 percent of pension income was derived from savings or the personal income of the pension holder; 28 percent was derived from the work organization, and only 5 percent from the federation or republic (i.e., social assistance) (Posrkaca 1989).

Again, there is dramatic variation among the republics in their level of support and in their legal requirements and accounting procedures (Table 5). In Montenegro, for example, 14.7 percent of all pension income is derived from the republics or federation, reflecting its weak economic and industrial structure. Sixty-two percent of pension income in Serbia is contributed by the work unit, while only a negligible 1 percent is contributed by the work unit in Macedonia and Slovenia.

The pension and compensation system in Yugoslavia is rapidly approaching a crisis point. The contributing base of active workers has increased by only 8 percent during the 1984-88 period, and the worker base may have shrunk dramatically with the 1990 depression in the Yugoslav economy. Nevertheless, total pension holders increased 27 percent during the 1984-88 period, which suggests that the pension system is under increasing strain (Posrkaca 1989). In some republics, such as Slovenia, the ratio of pension recipients to participants in the social security fund approaches two pension holders per five contributors (Table 6). The high pensioner/worker ratio can have a significant negative impact on future productivity, economic growth, and social peace.

As the current economic depression deepens in Yugoslavia, the financial base of the pension funds becomes seriously endangered. The work unit and state pension contributions are paid out of current revenues; and as these revenues decline, there will be mounting pressure to avoid responsibility and to erode the level of pension benefits. In the 1984-88 period, the typical Yugoslav firm increased its pension burden from 15.7 percent of total firm revenue in 1984 to 19.3 percent of total firm revenue in 1988. The five year increase in pension payments was 43 percent in Bosnia, which had 17.4

TABLE 6. Total number of pension holders by republic and province, 1984 and 1988.

REPUBLIC/ PROVINCE	YEAR				
	1984		1988		AVERAGE ANNUAL GROWTH RATE
	TOTAL	PER INSURED	TOTAL	PER 1000 INSURED	
Yugoslavia (Total)	1,944,195	280	2,336,044	294	4.7
Bosnia-Hercegovina	272,126	242	340,970	273	5.8
Montenegro	54,321	308	64,769	309	4.5
Croatia	501,704	310	559,850	318	2.8
Macedonia	109,301	205	143,418	241	7.0
Slovenia	270,381	307	355,923	388	7.1
Serbia (Proper)	472,025	272	565,704	275	4.6
Kosovo	47,341	220	57,652	238	5.0
Vojvodina	216,986	325	247,758	361	4.4

Source: Dragan Posrkaca, "Penzijsko i invalidsko osiguranje," *Jugoslovenski Pregled,* (July-August 1989), p. 306.

and relative size of the retired population threatens the social security system with overload and collapse. Third, efforts to maintain or enhance the quality of life for the retired members of the Yugoslav community would come at the expense of future productivity gains and would endanger further Yugoslavia's fragile federation. Finally, the economic crisis of the 1980s has led to the deterioration in the income and living standards of the elderly. The future suggests a worsening situation for the aged in Yugoslavia.

THE POLICY PROCESS

As a decentralized federal nation, Yugoslavia has not initiated and adopted a national policy for the elderly. As is the case in virtually all Yugoslav social policy arenas, policy-making responsibility has been devolved to the republics and provinces. Thus, the level and type of services provided may vary greatly, depending upon the republic in which the elderly citizen resides. In no republic, however, does the level of services approach that of Western Europe or the other members of the Organization for Economic Cooperation and Development (OECD).

Within Yugoslavia, the level of services provided to the elderly vary by the wealth of one's republic and by one's proximity to the major urban centers. Thus, the level of service in Slovenia tends to be the highest in the federation, while the Macedonian and Montenegrin service delivery system for the aged is almost nonexistent.

Responsibility for articulating the needs of the elderly is held by the Gerontological Society. Each such society is republic specific and is funded from republic sources. As can be expected, there is little coordination among the societies, and few commonalities in their approaches and concerns. One result is that national level data on service needs or the evaluation of service delivery simply do not exist.

Each republic government approaches the issues related to the aged in its own way. Most republics, in fact, have no comprehensive policy regarding the elderly, and most republics have decentralized the elderly's policy concerns among the housing, health, and social welfare sectors. Serbia, for example, did not adopt its first republic policy on the aged until 1986; and prior to that time, any services which were provided were supposedly covered by the broad-based social interest agencies (e.g., adult education, housing, health, etc.) (Nedeljkovic 1981). Not surprisingly, little or no funds were made available to implement the 1986 Serbian comprehensive policy for the elderly.

The policy neglect of the aged and failure to establish a comprehensive scheme were indicative of the Yugoslav approach toward special populations overall. Each one has suffered similarly, and the republic governments intervened only episodically following the public emergence of major scandals.

A primary problem associated with the implementation of broad-based social policy for the elderly was the competitive public choice model (i.e., self-management) that was applied to social service delivery systems by the republics and provinces after 1974 (Figure 1). Each social policy, such as elementary education or mental health, was organized on the basis of "self-managed interests of the community." These, in turn, were arranged hierarchically to parallel the government structure within the republic or province. Governing boards were established at the local, regional, and republic levels. The republic level self-management interests of the community imposed standards, audited units that were lower in the hierarchy, and lobbied the republic governments to increase the obligatory minimum contributions required from the enterprises. Regional associations coordinated the delivery of services within the region's boundaries, attempting to achieve some economies of scale. Finally, the communal (i.e., local) interests of the community had the primary responsibility to provide service, to contract with local employers for specialized services, and to solicit funds from the local enterprises.

As far as the interests of the elderly population were concerned, the Self-Managed Interest of the Community (SIZ) structure contained some serious flaws. First, interest communities were established for housing, health, education, higher education, science, and social welfare to parallel the state ministries and the state bureaucracies. SIZs were not established, however, for special populations such as the elderly, children, or the handicapped. This meant that the needs of the elderly were fragmented over an entire spectrum of social policy agencies and, often, one local SIZ had no idea what another local SIZ was doing.

A second flaw in the system was the competitive nature of the process. The needs of the elderly had to compete at the local level with the needs of every other group in society. Since the elderly, unlike the youth and education communities, lacked an organizational focus to articulate their interests and to pressure the commu-

FIGURE 1. Structure of the self-managed interests of the community (SIZ) in Yugoslavia.

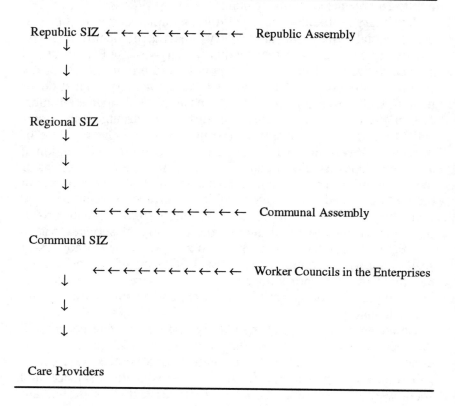

nal assembly, this population regularly stood at a competitive disadvantage. Compounding the problem was that the elderly were disproportionately located in the economically disadvantaged communes which had fewer resources to distribute and fewer profitable firms to tap for new programs and essential projects.

The third flaw was the lack of coordination among the interests of the community. The housing health and education interests perceived one another as competitors and potential antagonists, and they rarely cooperated. The enterprises which were solicited for funds and support also felt overwhelmed and abused by the process. Thus, as the economy worsened, the enterprises responded by cutting their contributions across the board, particularly for those social interests that were more marginal to the enterprise (e.g., the elderly). By 1989, the system had become so overloaded, and the firms so overburdened, that a collapse was imminent. Self-management of social services, in short, did not work in the Yugoslav context.

MEETING THE NEEDS OF THE ELDERLY– AN EVALUATION

Each republic and province in Yugoslavia has authorized the creation of a number of locally-based institutions to assist the elderly with some of their basic needs. These institutions include senior citizen centers, nursing care facilities, senior citizen residential homes, meals-on-wheels plans, and homemaker services for the elderly. None of these services, however, are mandated; and with the exception of old-age pensions and medical care, there are no entitlements for the elderly.

As a result of the voluntary nature of the service delivery program, very few of the above-mentioned services are provided by the commune. In fact, it has been estimated that in Serbia less than 2 percent of the elderly have access to any one of these services, even though an estimated 39 percent of the elderly are in need of one or more such programs (Manojlovic 1989; Manojlovic 1981). Nursing homes, residential care, meals-on-wheels, etc., appear to be limited solely to some of the major urban centers; and even in these centers, Yugoslav researchers note that there are extraordinarily long waiting lists for the services, and republics such as Macedonia and Montenegro provide almost no institutional care for the elderly outside the hospital system.

For practical purposes, the republics and communes provide few services to only a tiny proportion of the elderly in need. The elderly tend to take care of one another, rather than rely on publicly supported institutions. Those who are chronically ill are sent to the overcrowded hospitals, or if they are in better health they may be sent to the spas and mineral water springs for treatment. Throughout Yugoslavia, there are also insufficient numbers of senior citizen centers which provide a place for socialization and few specialized centers. In fact, particularly in the southern republics, the senior citizen centers are often little more than subsidized cafes for elderly men to socialize with each other in the bazaar or farmer's market.

Adequate housing is an acute need among many of the elderly Yugoslavs. In an all-Yugoslav study conducted in 1973, 44 percent of the elderly were found to live in unsatisfactory housing conditions. Nine percent reported no kitchen facilities, 40 percent lacked a bathroom, 30 percent had no toilet, 27 percent lacked sewage, and 23 percent had no water (Zivkovic 1973). In 1980, 20 percent of the elderly polled described their housing accommodations as miserable or worse (Manojlovic 1981, 23).

The need for assistance with cooking and simple household tasks by the aged is also substantial. In a Serbian survey, 21 percent of the elderly reported great difficulties in shopping for food, and 12 percent were not able to undertake even simple household tasks, such as preparing tea or coffee (Manojlovic 1981, 25).

Most of the elderly in Yugoslavia have had to rely upon one another or on their families for support and assistance. However, as the Yugoslav nation urbanizes and the elderly remain in rural areas distant from their children, the possibilities for family support diminish. Research from the Institute for Social Policy in Yugoslavia, for example, revealed that 43 percent of the elderly respondents did not see their children even once in the course of a year, and only about a fifth of the elderly reported that their children provide them with significant monetary or material assistance. Nearly two-thirds of the elderly population acknowledge persistent loneliness or social neglect (Institut za Socijalnu Politiku 1980).

Laws in republics, such as Serbia, mandate that children provide material assistance to their elderly parents. Nevertheless, there has been little enforcement of these laws, and most elderly are unlikely or are unwilling to use legal mechanisms to force compliance by their children. Although the elderly believe that their children should provide some assistance to them, the location of their children in distant cities reduces the effectiveness of social pressures to enhance intergenerational obligation. Finally, the extremely acute housing crisis throughout Yugoslavia has made it very difficult or impossible for the elderly to move in with their children's families. There is simply, in most cases, no space available.

The extended family tradition has withered even in traditional rural areas. A comprehensive survey of the elderly in 1984 in Stari Pazov, a rural, traditional commune in Vojvodina, showed that over 40 percent of the aged with grown children received no assistance from their children, and less than 20 percent received assistance beyond the occasional family visit (Sokolovic 1985). It is not surprising, therefore, that only 18 percent of the elderly polled agreed that their children are providing them with all the help that they need (Manojlovic 1981, 35). Finally, only 17 percent believe that their life as a retired person did not entail a considerable loss of status and respect (Manojlovic 1981, 34).

Health care is a major concern for the elderly in Yugoslavia, and it is a social policy area where considerable improvement is imperative. Preventive care is particularly lacking. In Serbia, for example, only 14 percent of the communes regularly provide vaccinations for the elderly, and 59 percent of the communes never provide vaccination services (Manojlovic 1988, 68). Only 6 percent of the communal health facilities have personnel who are trained to provide gerontological medicine, 19 percent of communes have no ambulatory facilities, and 90 percent have no home health care provisions (Manojlovic 1988, 68). Even when medical services are available, they are often delivered poorly. Seventy-nine percent of the Serbian elderly complained about long waits at medical facilities; 63 percent complained about neglect; and 31 percent complained about rudeness or the lack of common courtesies (Manojlovic 1988, 70).

Services for the Yugoslav elderly who live in rural areas are considerably poorer than those provided in the cities. The level of poverty among this population is acute. Rural elderly can never really retire, and approximately one-third of this population has no younger relatives or children upon which to rely. Access to medical care is difficult, and housing conditions tend to be much more primitive than in the city (Manojlovic 1983). In mountainous rural areas, entire villages have become populated solely by the elderly, and the republic or commune is unable to provide even a minimal level of care (Sinadinovski 1984). The reality is that many of the elderly who are stronger and healthier take care of those who are weaker and infirm.

Overall, we must conclude that the social welfare system for the elderly in Yugoslavia is overwhelmed by the economic and demographic crises it faces, and that it has not yet met the basic needs of its population. Neither social services, housing, nor medical services are adequate. Finally, there are serious gaps in the distribution of services, with the rural and economically depressed area residents suffering disproportionately.

FROM SOCIAL WELFARE STATISM TO SOCIAL WELFARE PLURALISM

Under the Marxist-Leninist model, the state assumed responsibility for a cradle-to-grave welfare system, and the state used this important benefit as a primary externality to assure compliance of the population with the political system. This welfare system bonded individuals and entire generations to the continuance of the system, and the comprehensiveness of such a welfare model rendered the cost of noncompliance to the individual much too high for most to bear. Thus, throughout Eastern Europe and the Soviet Union, the state monopoly over educational, employment, housing, and retirement resources served the interests of the authorities, increased the dependence of the population on the system, and provided a strong sense of stability for the regime.

The state also severely limited the participation of the individual, as well as the market and other nongovernmental institutions, in the social welfare delivery system. The accumulation of private assets and investment capital was sharply restricted through collectivization of land, closure of investment mechanisms, and nationalization of capital. Church or voluntary social welfare institutions were closed or merged into the state-run organizations. Small businesses were heavily taxed, personal income limits were strictly controlled, and inheritance taxes and other statutory limitations effectively eliminated the transfer of assets and working capital to younger cohorts. In short, the capacity for individuals to prepare for their old age was severely limited and sharply curtailed.

For the regime, welfare statism entailed significant risks, as well as important political benefits. The regime, for example, was expected to deliver on its promises to provide for the common good and social welfare, or lose its legitimacy to rule; but in Yugoslavia, as well as the remainder of Eastern Europe, the state was forced by a deteriorating economy to renege on these pledges. For the elderly, there was no security; for the youth, there was no future; for the worker, there were few, if any, profits to be distributed; and for the family, there was no long-term support or stability. Most grating of all, however, was that the elite lived much better than the non-elites and enjoyed more stable and more secure benefits. Overall, the elderly had given their lives to a regime, but failed to reap any of the rewards.

The Yugoslav government was not able to escape its responsibility to its elderly through devolution or decentralization. Medical care was of poor quality or poorly distributed. Income support for pensioners was insufficient. Housing conditions for the aged were deplorable, and social services and recreational outlets for the aged were a rarity. For the majority of the Yugoslav elderly, retirement had become a grim matter of survival, and with the collapse of the currency and the inflation of the 1980s, the final blow occurred. Throughout Yugoslavia, the aged felt betrayed, and this betrayal was perceived by nearly every household in the nation. Despite the glowing words of the leaders, socialist self-management did not perform as predicted; those who had given the most to the system for the longest time experienced this failure most acutely.

It should not be implied that the protests associated with the collapse of the Yugoslav regimes were led or orchestrated by the elderly. Nevertheless, unlike other periods of civil unrest, this generatio–the war-time generation–chose not to defend the regime, and did not grant it further legitimacy. The erosion of support from the generation that had led the revolution during the war was very significant to the rapid, but unbloody, dissolution of the communist regimes in the Yugoslav federation.

Today, there is a sense of fatalism throughout Yugoslavia. The system of pensions, social services, and income support is running on its own inertia, and there is no comprehensive or even piecemeal program of reform. The economy is in desperate shape. The government's decision to undergo economic shock therapy and become a market economy has fostered a domino effect leading to plant closures and layoffs. Yugoslavia has an acute shortage of investment capital and an accompanying increase in the demand for social welfare payments. Productivity has fallen dramatically and demand for locally produced products has evaporated. The enterprises, in short, can no longer afford to maintain their pension payments.

The Yugoslav political climate has changed dramatically as well. Multiparty elections and parliamentary democracy have raised expectations as the nationalist-populist leaders promise security, stability, prosperity, and economic growth overnight. They have used tensions among the republics to transfer attention from the economic collapse to symbolic issues of nationalist pride. Politically, the public choice self-management model has died, but its institutions carry on for lack of a replacement.

Within Yugoslavia, there are no social bases upon which the Yugoslav welfare model can be resuscitated. Enterprises have no funds to contribute and are fighting for their own survival. The overwhelming majority of pensioners or soon-to-be pensioners have negligible personal savings as a result of a forty-year legacy of state dependency. In brief, the situation is critical.

Only one avenue is open to Yugoslav society and politics at this time; namely, a rapid transition from welfare statism to welfare pluralism. At its core, welfare pluralism demands the diffusion of responsibility for social welfare programs, such as care for the elderly. The concept is based upon the diffusion of responsibility away from the state monopoly to a shared responsibility of the state, individual, market, and voluntary associations.

Under the type of social pluralism that is being experimented with in Yugoslavia, the state shifts its role from the primary vendor of social welfare policy to a coordinator and regulator of the system. The source of pension payments becomes net profit rather than the gross income of the firm. In place of the seizure of individual investment capital, as occurred in the past, the state protects and encourages individual assumption of responsibility for old-age support, where possible. In place of state monopoly and state responsibility, responsibility under social pluralism is shared. Finally, the government recognizes the true market contribution of the rural sector and applies a greater percentage of its resources to enhance the security of the elderly in those regions.

Slovenia has begun to experiment with social welfare pluralism in Yugoslavia with mixed results. This republic has found that the elderly prefer to have some control over their security and not to surrender all control to the state. The republic also has found that the voluntary sector is often more efficient in the delivery of services, but this benefit is balanced by a strong need to regulate the process to prevent exploitation and misuse of the elderly's savings. Finally, the Slovenian republic has found that the introduction of a free marketplace for the sale of agricultural land has permitted many of the poor rural elderly to accumulate the assets necessary to support themselves through sale of their property, and no longer be a burden on the state.

In summary, social welfare statism has collapsed in Yugoslavia, and it is collapsing throughout Eastern Europe. These formally socialist states can no longer support their welfare systems. There is a strong political demand for the state to withdraw from such direct and obtrusive intervention. The only alternatives now are a free and generally unregulated market as in the U.S., or the form of cooperative social welfare pluralism found in much of Western Europe. The first choice is unacceptable in the context of East European politics and society. The second choice, while not ideal, does buy time for the new regimes and can accommodate itself well to the goals and aspirations of these nations for democratic pluralism and prosperity.

POSTSCRIPT

Since this chapter was written, the Yugoslavia we have known for the past seventy years has disappeared to be succeeded by five separate and antagonistic entities. The dissolution, however, was preceded by the break up of the social welfare system and the collapse of the government's capacity to honor the social contract and to provide even the minimum standard of support for its pensioners.

During the 1980s, socialist Yugoslavia's inability to support those who had given the most to the preservation of the system and had sacrificed their personal welfare to construct the socialist self-managed state, sent a message that reverberated throughout all strata of society. In the 1990s when the Communist parties, the federal institutions and the Republics began to compete for support among the electorate, the elderly turned their backs on the regime; and, in many cases, they encouraged their sons and daughters to abandon the system that had betrayed them. Yugoslavia's tragedy demonstrates that when a regime loses its moral respect and legitimacy and ignores its social responsibility and generational covenant, it may soon lose its own mandate to rule.

NOTES

1. The Gini Index of Inequality for Yugoslavia is less than the figures in the United States and in other Western nations. This is primarily a result of the fact that Yugoslavia does not have a class of very wealthy individuals to skew the measure. From a public policy perspective, however, income disparities among the political units in Yugoslavia (i.e., republics and provinces) are greater than income disparities among the states in the United States.

2. Elderly is defined as age sixty and over in confirmity with Yugoslav statistics and pension policies.

3. This was particularly significant in 1989 when inflation exceeded 100 percent per month. Pensioners, during this time, encountered a severe income crunch. The pension was 40 percent of the average family income for a single retiree, 60 percent for a two member household; 75 percent for a three member household; 90 percent for a four member household; and 100 percent for five or more members in the household.

4. The high rate of Montenegrin pension payments is explained by the facts that Montenegro is a small and poor republic in which a disproportionate number of citizens participated in the National Liberation war and received federal pension payments as veterans or as retired military officers.

REFERENCES

Bilten za Pitanja Zdravstenog, Invalidskog i Penzijskog Osiguranja. 1989, March-April.

Institut za Socijalnu Politiku. 1980. "Analiticko-dokumentacione osnove Srednjorocnog plana razvoja SR Srbije za period 1981 do 1985 godine-socijalna zastita." Belgrade: Institut za socijalnu politiku.

Breznik, Dusan. 1977. "Demographic process of aging with special reference to the situation in Yugoslavia." First Gerontological Congress of Yugoslavia. Belgrade.

Manojlovic, Petar. 1981. *Starenje i Starost.* Belgrade. Institut za Socijalnu Politiku.

Manojlovic, Petar. 1983. "Socijalna sigurnost poljoprivrednika i sistem njihovog socijalnog obezbedenja u starosti." *Gerontoloski Zbornik '82*, edited by Vitomir Stojakovic. Belgrade: gerontolosko Drustvo SR Srbije, 7-11.

Manojlovic, Petar. 1988. "Humanizacija uslova i postupka u ostvarivanju zdravstvene zastite penzionera i drugih starih osoba." *Gerontoloski Zbornik '87*, edited by Vitomir Stojakovic. Belgrade: Gerontolosko Drustvo SR Srbije.

Manojlovic, Petar. 1989. "Mesto i uloga dnevnih centara i klubova za pensionere i druge starije ljude u sistemu drustvene brige o humanizaciji zivotnih uslova u starosti." *Gerontoloski Zbornik 88* edited by Vitomir Stojakovic, Belgrade" Gerontolosko Drustvo SR Srbije, 10.

Markovic, Mihajlo. 1985. "Donet zkon o penzijskom i invalidskom osiguranju zemljoradnika." *Opstina,* December, 49-56.

Nedeljkovic, Ives Rastimir. 1981. "Cvorista i praznine u mrezama drustvenih delatnosti namenjenih starosti." *Gerontoloski Zbornik 1981* edited by Vitomir Stojakovic. Belgrade: Gerontolosko Drustvo SR Srbije, 19-26.

Posrkaca, Dragan. 1989. "Invalidsko osiguranje 1984-1988." Jugoslovenski Pregled, July-August, 306-312.

Savezni Zavod za Statistiku. 1989. *Statisticki Godisnjak SFRJ,* Belgrade: Savezni Zavod za Statistiku.

Sinadinovski, Jakim. 1984. "Drustveno-ekonomski polozaj seoskih starackih domacinstava i njihove proizvodne mogucnosti u SR Makedoniji." *Zbornik '84*, edited by Vitomir Stojakovic. Belgrade: Gerontolosko Drustvo SR Srbije, 58-73.

Socialist Federal Republic of Yugoslavia, Federal Committee for Labor, Health and Social Welfare. 1987. *National Report for the World Assembly on Aging.* June, Belgrade.

Sokolovic, Mirjana. 1985. "Socijalni polozaj i potrebe starih lica na teritoriji opstine Stara Pazova. *Gerontoloski Zbornik '85,* edited by Vitomir Stojakovic. Belgrade: Gerontolosko Drustvo SR Srbije.

Stojakovic, Vitomir. 1990. Internal Records of the Republicki Zavod za Socijalnu Zastitu, May, S.R. Serbia.

Zenenovic, Mira. 1986. "Socijalna (ne)sigurnost penzionera." *Socijalni Rad,* February, 23-29.

Zivkovic, Miroslav. 1973. "Starost u Jugoslaviji." *Gerontolosko-Socioloska Studija,* Belgrade.

Index

Abuse of elderly
  in Britain, 147
  in China, 261
  in United States, 45,48
Alzheimer's disease
  in Germany, 213
  in Israel, 113-115
  in United States, 26,42
Ambulatory care in Germany, 216-219
Arab population in Israel, 108,109, 112
  day care centers for, 119

Barefoot doctors of China, 274-275
Bedridden elderly
  in China, 279,280
  in Germany, 212
  in Japan, 247,248,250,254-257
Board and Care Homes in United States, 47-48
Bosnia-Hercegovina
  number of pension holders in, 301
  pension and worker's compensation income in, 299
  percent of aged population in, 295
  and rural population, 297
  personal income per worker in, 291
  population actively engaged in economy of, 292
Britain, 18-19,23,129-157
  abuse of elderly in, 147
  case management approach in, 154

changing role of state in, 136-152
consumerism in, limitations of, 151-152
Conventry Project in, 153-154
day care centers in, 137,138
disabilities of elderly in, 130-131, 146
familism ideology in, 19,133,150
family caregivers in, 14,19,132-136
  needs of, 150
  as primary providers of care, 136,137
  supportive services for, 154-155
  traditional roles of, 156
future supply of informal care in, 132-136
health care and medical services in, 6,136
home and community-based services in, 12,139-156
  compared to Japan, 258-259
  Griffiths Report on, 148,149, 150,151
  number of clients in, 138
  recent innovations in, 152-156
  role of state in, 136,137
  White Paper on, 148,151
housing options in, 138,140,141
  choices of residents concerning, 145-147,151
institutional care in, 9,136
marketization of services in, 19, 144,147,150
mental hospitals in, 11
mixed economy of care in, 145-148,150

in Japan, 249-254
  compared to Britain, 258-259
  compared to Sweden, 257-258
  preventive programs in, 249
in Sweden. *See* Sweden, home and
    community-based services in
in United States, 11,16,35-39,
    46-47
  cost of, 36,38
  public funding of, 30,36
  workers in, 46-47
Home Help program
  in Britain, 153-154
  in Finland, 95-96
  in France, 193-194,195,205,208
    cost of, 199
  in Germany, 216,217
  in Japan, 250,251,257
    compared to Sweden, 257-258
  in Sweden, 63,65-66,67-70
    caregivers in, 75
    client satisfaction with, 72
    compared to Japan, 257-258
    cost of, 61
    services provided by, 64,75
Housing, 5,6
  in Britain, 138,140,141,145-147
    choices of residents concerning,
      145-147,151
  in Canada, 167
  in Finland, 93-94
  in France, 195-196,198
    conditions of, 198,200
  in Germany, 21,214
  in Israel, 124,125
  in Sweden, 60,61,71
  in United States, 47-49
    for low-income elderly, 47-48
    for middle and upper income
      elderly, 48-49
  in Yugoslavia, 306

Immigrants
  in Britain, 134
  in Israel, 18,103-104,105

aging of, 106
disabilities and mental health
  problems of, 112
employment of, 110-111
future needs of, 125-126
from Soviet Union, 109-110
Income of elderly
  in France, 191-192
  in Germany, 214
  from pension systems. *See*
    Pension systems
  in Sweden, 60
  in United States, and housing
    options, 47-49
Independent lifestyle of elderly
  in Britain, 131-132
  in France, and dependency, 196-
    198,201-203
  in Sweden, 60,62-64,68
  in United States, 27,45,50
Individualism, in United States, 2,28
Industrial areas in Japan, population
  of elderly in, 236-237
Institutional care, 8-11
  in Britain, 9,136
  in Canada, 9-10,12,167-168
    criteria for, 167
  in China, 10,273,274,279-280
  in Finland, 8,91-95
  in France, 10,194,195,208
    cost of, compared to cost of
      home care, 199-203
    dependency of population in,
      197,201-203
  in Germany, 10,21,219-221
    characteristics of elderly in, 216
    quality of, 226
  in Israel, 9,104,122-124
    cultural traditions against, 104
    future trends in, 125
    population at risk for, 107
  in Japan, 10,252
  in nursing homes. *See* Nursing
    homes
  in Sweden, 8-9, 78-81